MW00743729

Chinese
Herbal
Medicine
MADE EASY

Thomas Richard Joiner is a nationally certified acupuncturist and herbalist (NCCA) and a graduate of the Institute of Traditional Chinese Medicine/First World Acupuncture in New York City. He conducted advanced studies in acupuncture and herbology at the Academy of Chinese Culture and Health Sciences in Oakland and the Institute of Chinese Herbology in Berkeley. He was a personal student of Mantak Chia at Taoist Esoteric Yoga from 1980 to 1983. During that time he studied Taoist Philosophy and Internal Martial Arts, including Microcosmic Orbit Meditation, Iron Shirt Chi Kung, and Taoist Sexology (seminal ovarian Kung Fu).

Joiner has over twenty years of martial arts experience and is a Yondan fourth-degree black belt and a certified instructor in Chinese Goju martial arts and Tien Tao Chi Kung. He has been a member of the Chinese National Chi Kung Institute for over ten years and was inducted into the Martial Arts Hall of Fame in 1994. He is currently a member of the West Oakland Mental Health Advisory Board and is the founding president of a Chinese herbal mail order company, Treasures From the Sea of Chi. He also conducts lectures and workshop programs in Oakland on the use of Chinese herbs.

He has also written *The Warrior as Healer,* a book focusing on the historic use of Chinese herbs in healing injuries, increasing vitality, and focusing meditation in the martial arts.

Ordering

Trade bookstores in the U.S. and Canada, please contact:

Publishers Group West
1700 Fourth Street, Berkeley CA 94710
Phone: (800) 788-3123   Fax: (510) 528-3444

Hunter House books are available at bulk discounts for textbook course adoptions; to qualifying community, health care, and government organizations; and for special promotions and fund-raising. For details please contact:

Special Sales Department
Hunter House Inc., PO Box 2914, Alameda CA 94501-0914
Phone: (510) 865-5282   Fax: (510) 865-4295
E-mail: ordering@hunterhouse.com

Individuals can order our books from most bookstores or
by calling toll-free:

(800) 266-5592

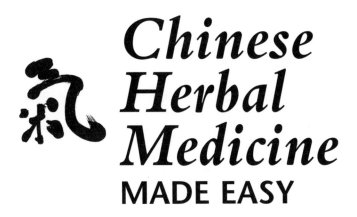

Chinese Herbal Medicine

MADE EASY

Natural and Effective Remedies for Common Illnesses

Thomas Richard Joiner

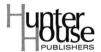

Hunter House
PUBLISHERS

Hunter House Inc., Publishers
PO Box 2914
Alameda CA 94501-0914

Library of Congress Cataloging-in-Publication Data
Joiner, Thomas Richard, 1943–
Chinese herbal medicine made easy : natural and effective remedies for common illnesses / by Thomas Richard Joiner.—1st ed.
p. cm.
Includes bibliographical references and index.
ISBN 0-89793-276-5 — ISBN 0-89793-275-7 (paper)
1. Herbs—Therapeutic use—Encyclopedias. 2. Medicine, Chinese—Encyclopedias. I. Title.
RM666.H33 J647 2000
615'.321'095103—dc21
99-058835

Project Credits
Cover Design, Book Design and Production: *osprey*design
Developmental Editor: Lydia Bird
Line and Copy Editor: Kelley Blewster
Proofreader: John David Marion
Indexer: Judy Joiner
Graphics Coordinator: Ariel Parker
Acquisitions Editor: Jeanne Brondino
Associate Editor: Alexandra Mummery
Editorial and Production Assistant: Melissa Millar
Publicity Manager: Sarah Frederick
Marketing Assistant: Earlita Chenault
Customer Service Manager: Christina Sverdrup
Order Fulfillment: Joel Irons
Administration: Theresa Nelson
Publisher: Kiran S. Rana

Printed and Bound by Publishers Press, Salt Lake City, Utah

Manufactured in the United States of America
9 8 7 6 5 4 3 2 1   First Edition   00 01 02 03 04

Contents 中草藥

Chapter Three: Illnesses and Their Treatments **35**

中
草
藥

The Pinyin System, which is the most common method for transliterating Chinese into the Latin alphabet, has been used for all of the individual herbs and formulas mentioned in this book.

Important Note

The information in this book reflects current therapeutic knowledge. The self-treatment recommendations and information are appropriate in most cases; however, they are not a substitute for medical diagnosis. For specific information concerning your personal medical condition, consult a physician. Anyone using information offered in Chinese Herbal Medicine Made Easy does so at his or her own risk. The author and publisher cannot be held responsible for the results of self-treatment attempted on the basis of anything read in this book.

The names of organizations, products, or alternative therapies appearing in this book are given for informational purposes only. Their inclusion does not imply endorsement, nor does the omission of any organization, product, or alternative therapy indicate disapproval.

Acknowledgments

Y ou could say that I began writing this book in the spring of 1979, when the spiritual seed that my grandfather had planted in me during my childhood and nurtured until his passing finally came to fruition. As I recall, it was in early April, on a day that began much like any other day, that I experienced what can only be described as a spiritual awakening. The soul-stirring event that took place that fateful morning through the grace of God put an end to the moral degeneration that had brought me to the brink of spiritual bankruptcy. In the aftermath of that religious experience, two significant events occurred. Not only would they have an impact on my mental and physical health, they would ultimately change the course of my life. The first was an introduction to traditional Chinese medicine. The second was my decision to make a number of lifestyle changes, including (1) a turn to vegetarianism, motivated by a newfound reverence for life that would no longer allow me to kill animals for food; (2) learning to subordinate the sexual urge, which led to more regulated and less impulsive sexual activity; and (3) a spiritual reaffirmation that inspired me to adopt prayer and meditation as a daily practice.

It is now the spring of 2000. As this book takes final form, I'd like to express my gratitude for the quality of life I have experienced, due in part to a twenty-year odyssey that began with an introduction to traditional Chinese medicine, conceivably China's greatest contribution to the world community. Indeed a blessing, that introduction was made possible by the following people who, because of their generosity and dedication, have earned my admiration and respect: Urayoana Trinidad, Jackie Haught, Elaine Nurse, Tertentch Hetep, the class of 1987 at the Institute of Traditional Chinese Medicine in New York City (First World Acupuncture Advisory Association—FWAAA), and Lai Fu Chai, Professor of Herbology at the Academy of Chinese Culture and Health Sciences, Oakland, California. My deepest appreciation to "My Little Sweetie," Judy Joiner, whose love, support, and tireless effort made this project possible; my spiritual mother, Carmen Quinones, whose guidance and advice has been instrumental in my spiritual growth; my grandparents, Daddy Bennie and Grandma Lessie, the family patriarchs whose struggle made survival possible for all of us that followed; Ma "T"; and Uncle Bennie. Last, but certainly not least, this book is dedicated to my mom, Ruby Blanchard.

Introduction

I believe that all plants possess curative powers. Even though a great deal of the healing ability of plants remains undiscovered, I am convinced that God has provided us with the means to cure every human affliction through the use of botanical medicines.

Plant medicines are the original medicine of mankind, and their use for treating disease can be traced all the way back to a time when the primary health-care providers were shamans, sages, and medicine men. Physical evidence obtained from burial sites of many ancient cultures (Egyptian, African, Chinese, Aztec, and others) suggests that throughout human history plant medicines have played an important role in the treatment of disease. This role, I might add, is not limited to humans. Documented evidence compiled from field studies has shown that, much like their human counterparts, injured or sick animals will instinctively search for particular botanical substances in an attempt to heal injuries and effect a cure.

Not until the twentieth century—with the increase in the number of trained physicians and the rapid development of the pharmaceutical industry—was the use of herbal remedies that had been passed down by word of mouth from elders to their offspring replaced by Western allopathic medicine as the primary source of medical treatment.

Another contributing factor to the decline of herbal remedies is the lack of scientific research into their effectiveness, which the Western medical establishment often cites as its principal reason for discrediting alternative medicine in general and herbology in particular. To that, I can only reply that centuries of use by members of indigenous populations has validated the effectiveness of herbal systems as diverse as Ayurvedic, African, Western, and Chinese. Perhaps the best known and most documented is the highly regarded five-thousand-year-old Chinese herbal system.

In recent years, Western allopathic medicine has come under increased criticism, mainly because of its excessive use of chemical drug therapy and the invasive life-threatening nature of surgery. Many concerned consumers, seeking an alternative to chemical drugs and their often dangerous side effects, are looking to Chinese herbal medicine as a way to safely manage their health.

This increased level of public interest has recently given rise to a new movement. Primarily spearheaded by American-trained Chinese acupuncturists/herbalists, an attempt is currently underway to explain in terms everyone can understand how to use Chinese herbs for treating common illnesses. Hopefully, this book will be among those that eliminate the confusion that has made using Chinese herbs so difficult.

In the past, anyone curious about using Chinese herbs was usually frustrated by deterrents that seemed to fall into three main categories: cultural differences, complicated medical language, and a tendency to make this five-thousand-year-old herbal system appear mysterious and unnecessarily complex. It was a desire to overcome cultural differences, to avoid complicated medical language, and to demystify this practical healing art that provided the inspiration for my writing *Chinese Herbal Medicine Made Easy.*

Herbs are often referred to as "the people's medicine." Their popularity is due in part to their affordability compared to prescription drugs and the fact that they can be administered with minimal training and experience. While treatment by a professional herbalist is certainly required in complicated cases, centuries of use by the Chinese people have proven that self-treatment can be performed successfully—when simple instructions are given and complicated medical language is avoided.

Since becoming a Chinese herbalist over a decade ago, I have worked to develop a private practice whose focus centers on treating illness as well as encouraging the regular use of Chinese herbs for promoting a healthier lifestyle. I take great personal pride in the fact that through my conscious effort to use simple, understandable language, many of my patients have gained insights into some of the underlying principles of traditional Chinese medicine and have acquired the ability to use Chinese herbs for maintaining their health.

In my continued effort to keep the language in this book uncomplicated, I have drawn upon some advice my grandmother gave me many years ago. Although she encouraged education, she cautioned me against succumbing to the intellectual disease that impairs the ability of the educated to use common sense and plain talk, a malady she referred to as "analysis paralysis." I will consider this book a success only if it is considered by the reader to be both informative and comprehensible.

How This Book Is Organized

To facilitate use, I have divided *Chinese Herbal Medicine Made Easy* into three chapters. The first chapter contains a brief historical overview, followed by an explanation of principles and diagnostic methods of Chinese medicine. In the second chapter, I discuss some ingredients frequently used in Chinese herbal formulas and provide detailed instructions on how to make an herbal decoction (tea) and medicinal wine. I also explain what patent formulas are and discuss tonics used for life extension and general health maintenance. The third chapter—which makes up the bulk of the book—is devoted entirely to listing common illnesses in alphabetical order; a brief discussion about the illness and its symptoms is followed by the herbal formula or formulas used to treat it.

Also included are a glossary of terms commonly used in Chinese medicine but perhaps unfamiliar to the layperson. There is also a general index, which includes medical terms, disorders, and symptoms; indexes for raw and patent formulas; a cross-reference of the

Chinese, English, and Latin names of ingredients found in the raw herbal formulas; resources for purchasing Chinese herbs; and a bibliography.

How to Use This Book

In all cases of illness, diagnosis by a skilled physician is highly recommended. If any doubt exists about the first diagnosis, a second opinion should be sought. Once the nature of the illness has been determined, only then does a responsible health-care practitioner encourage the patient to make a decision about the type and manner of treatment.

If the decision is made to use herbal remedies, this information should be shared with the primary physician. Some will take a positive attitude, others will prefer to wait and see, and some may be less than encouraging. In any event, it should not be forgotten that making choices concerning the type of medical care used for treating your body is a basic human right! It should also be remembered that although herbal medicine is an effective remedy for a host of illnesses, it should by no means be considered a panacea. Herbal medicine can and should be used safely and effectively, and as the reader knows, prudence is recommended when taking any form of medicine.

My suggestions to ensure the greatest likelihood of success with this book are

- Comply with the recommended dosage.
- Use the formula whose "description" most closely corresponds with your symptoms.
- If relief is not experienced after a reasonable period of time (approximately four to ten days), reconsider self-treatment and seek the advice of a professional traditional Chinese doctor or Western medical doctor with whom you're comfortable.

Ten Rules for Good Health

I also encourage following the ten "rules" for good health:

- Remember that an ounce of prevention is worth a pound of cure. If you have any doubts about your health, seek professional help.
- Adopt a balanced diet: eat more grains, fresh vegetables, and

fruit; consume less fat and sugar and fewer products containing artificial additives.

- Drink copious amounts of filtered, distilled, or boiled water daily—a minimum of eight glasses.
- Engage regularly in a gentle form of exercise.
- Be moderate in all that you do: diet, alcohol, exercise, rest, sex, sleep, work, and play.
- Avoid the vices of casual sex, drugs, gambling, and alcohol.
- Practice personal hygiene, including carefully cleaning all foods.
- Worry less; laugh more.
- Work with—not against—nature.
- Abide by the golden rule, which reminds us to "do unto others as you would have them do unto you," and keep in mind the five virtues of Confucius: wisdom, justice, charity, honesty, and propriety.

Needless to say, it is doubtful that the use of herbs by the Chinese people, which dates back five millennia, would have endured for so many centuries if herbs' effectiveness had not been well proven. In spite of this system's five-thousand-year history, there still exists a reluctance on the part of the Western medical establishment to acknowledge its legitimacy. I have no doubt that the unwilling acceptance of Chinese herbal medicine is to a large extent motivated by a concern for profit. I sincerely hope that the antagonism that has persisted between so-called alternative therapies and conventional Western medicine will soon be reconciled and that a "New World Medicine" will emerge—one that is based on mutual respect, that incorporates all proven therapies, and that truly serves the needs of all people, rich and poor alike

Finally, I would like to conclude by affirming my belief that all healing comes from God. I consider it a supreme privilege to be chosen as an instrument for his work, always knowing that the final decision concerning our health and ultimate destiny is his alone.

Thomas Richard Joiner
Oakland, California

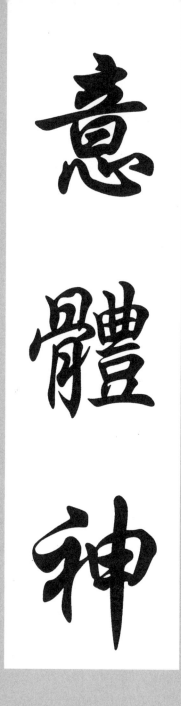

意

體

神

Body, Mind, and Spirit

I 中草藥

Basics of Chinese Medicine

lthough the following pages contain some of Chinese medicine's most important principles, they should not be considered a continuum of Chinese medical theory. My intention is to offer a brief, understandable explanation of Chinese medicine's historical origins, along with an overview of its diagnostic methods. A detailed account of the highly technical workings of the science and art of Chinese medicine is beyond the scope of this book and probably not particularly interesting to the average reader. In spite of its brevity, I believe this overview will provide some useful insights for anyone using this book, as well as for those who have a more general interest in traditional Chinese medicine.

An Ancient Philosophy

The concepts that became the foundation for traditional Chinese medicine can be traced back to the earliest stages of human history—before there was industry, technology, or organized political systems—when mankind primarily interacted with its environment, lived according to the laws of nature, and held a fundamental belief in God. Different cultures certainly embraced different concepts of God and the universe, but certain essential principles were consistently observed among the various primeval groups, and there existed a shared belief that only through adherence to these principles could humans exist in harmony with nature. Opposing these elemental forces was considered taboo. Doing so was thought at the very least to cause illness and, more likely, death. The fundamental idea of living in harmony with nature and the environment is the basis for China's religious and philosophical concepts, as well as the theoretical foundation for the five-thousand-year-old traditional Chinese medical system.

This is particularly significant when you consider the fact that in all cultures the medicine practiced is merely a reflection of the beliefs of the people. Religion, philosophy, and nature play a much more important role in Chinese medicine than they do in the modern high-tech medicine practiced here in the West. In fact, one of the defining features setting Chinese medicine apart from its Western counterpart is the attention given in Chinese medicine to nature and environmental factors when it comes to diagnosing and treating disease.

Principles of Chinese Medicine

Yin and Yang

There is no question that our understanding of all aspects of Asian culture and traditional Chinese medicine in particular is advanced when there is clarification of the theory of opposites, known as yin and yang. Even though the majority of us are familiar with the Asian concept of duality, a certain amount of ambiguity still exists. Unfortunately, because of complications created by language and culture, a simple descriptive definition has not always been readily available. I believe that the key to comprehending the principle governing the mutually interdependent forces of yin and yang rests with our ability to understand that, according to this ancient philosophy, the ideal or perfect state of everything that exists in nature, including health, can only be achieved when there are equal amounts of these two primal elements.

This theory of harmony between opposite yet complementary forces is exemplified in traditional Chinese medicine's belief that when one of these elements is in excess of the other, illness occurs. And, conversely, only when there exists balance between or equal portions of both yin and yang can we experience optimal health. It is also helpful to understand that in traditional Chinese medicine, the body's two primary substances—blood (yin) and Chi (yang)—are also represented by these two rudimental forces. (See Blood and Chi, below, for a discussion of the roles played by these substances in maintaining optimal health.)

Taoism

During China's long history three major religions or schools of thought have borne the most profound influence on all aspects of Chinese culture: Buddhism, Confucianism, and Taoism.

Of the three, Buddhism most closely conforms to the Western definition of religion. Generally speaking, Buddhist teaching centers around meditation and the pursuit of the eight-fold path, which is similar to the Ten Commandments of the Judeo-Christian tradition. Confucianism, which is based on the teaching and writing of the philosopher Confucius, relies more on ethics that emphasize the proper way for people to behave in society. At the center of its teaching are guidelines which, if upheld, lead to a just and harmonious society as well as a stable government. Taoism, by contrast, which is deeply rooted in China's folk traditions, is a complex system of philosophical thought, mysticism, and ancient health practices.

Among these Taoist health practices is a body of knowledge concerning the use of herbs for promoting health that was developed from experiments conducted in an effort to discover herbal formulas capable of producing immortality (see Blood and Chi, below, for more about these experiments). Life extension, which lies at the heart of Taoist philosophy, is accomplished through conforming to the laws of nature, practicing health-promoting exercises and diet, and the use of herbal decoctions. Many of these principles and health practices form the basis for traditional Chinese medicine.

External Causes of Illness: Perverse Energies

Traditional Chinese medicine teaches that perverse atmospheric conditions—*perverse energies*—are often the primary cause of, or at least contributing factors in, a long list of common illnesses. Perverse energies include

Wind, the primary transport system for hundreds of airborne viruses associated with a great number of respiratory diseases;

Cold, which causes the body's fluids to congeal, impeding the circulation of fluid to the joints and blood through the body;

Heat, which causes pronounced sweating and dehydration;

Dampness, associated with inflammatory muscle and joint disease such as rheumatism and arthritis;

Dryness, which attacks the body's fluids and is associated with, among other things, increased thirst and constipation.

This simple explanation demonstrates Chinese medicine's theory concerning humans' physiological responses to their environment and the relationship of those responses to health and disease. The Chinese believe that perverse energies occur most often when normal environmental conditions are excessive. Examples are extreme cold spells in winter and unseasonable conditions such as a warm spell in winter or the period of transition from one season to another.

Of course, it is impossible to avoid exposure to environmental elements. Therefore, Chinese medicine emphasizes a preventive rather than a curative approach by offering strategies for protecting the body from perverse energies. Mainly, these preventive strategies are carried out in two ways: via the diet and through the use of botanical, mineral, and zoological substances (Chinese herbs). Combined, these two factors afford one of the most powerful tools available for increasing the body's natural defenses. Used on a regular basis, herbs become an extension of nutrition that assists in providing protection against pernicious external influences. This practice has proven to be effective for general health maintenance as well as for promoting life extension.

More specifically, certain recommendations involve the use of particular herbal formulas for strengthening individual internal

organs. This health regimen is based on the presumption that certain climatic conditions known to be more prevalent during a particular season often demonstrate an adverse effect on a specific organ. The table below lists examples of the relationship between atmospheric conditions, corresponding seasons, and the internal organs affected by them:

Climatic Condition	Season	Internal Organ
Wind	Spring	Liver
Cold	Winter	Kidneys
Heat	Summer	Heart
Dampness	Late Summer	Spleen
Dryness	Autumn	Lungs

Internal Causes of Illness: Emotions

In addition to the cause-and-effect relationship between perverse climatic conditions and disease, another important concept is Chinese medicine's belief that emotions (namely, anger, fear, grief, joy, and anxiety) also influence one's health. Unlike Western medicine, which has too often in the past labeled as psychosomatic those illnesses related to emotional matters, Chinese medicine holds that when certain emotions are experienced in excess, they will affect particular organs. Specifically, anger is associated with the liver, fear with the kidneys, grief with the lungs, joy with the heart, and anxiety with the spleen. While the explicit connection between emotions and the vital organs is not always obvious to the layperson, examples such as the affect of grief and weeping on the lungs or how anxiety can affect the spleen or stomach (by causing digestive problems in general or a nervous or upset stomach in particular) are more apparent.

Not only are matters of temperament an important source of diagnostic information, Chinese medicine assigns even greater importance to them by stating that the combined effects of *external* climatic elements and *internal* emotional factors are major precipitating factors in all forms of disease.

In fact, the scrutiny afforded by traditional Chinese medicine to psychological and climatological factors is rivaled only by the attention given to what are considered the two primary substances in human physiology: the blood and the Chi.

Blood and Chi

Nourishing and strengthening the blood and the Chi (the vital energy that flows through the body) is considered by Chinese medicine to be the key to health and longevity. Modern practitioners of traditional Chinese medicine still follow the same basic guidelines for doing so set down by ancient physicians. The early herbal experiments that later became the basis for Chinese medicine's life-extension principles date all the way back to imperial China. They, for the most part, resulted from attempts to satisfy royal demands for an elixir —one that would serve as a cure-all but would also guarantee eternal life. These experiments, which involved the use of precious metals (such as gold) as well as botanical and zoological substances, were conducted by highly motivated Taoist sages and herbalists who knew that failure to produce such a potion could result in their death!

In spite of the experimenters' obvious failure to develop a medicine that would insure immortality, they did discover herbal formulas that invigorate and strengthen the body while minimizing many of the health problems associated with aging. Perhaps more than any other culture, China is well known for its large population of senior citizens, a fact that is by some accounts largely attributable to the use of herbal formulas discovered centuries ago.

Why, you may ask, is nourishing the blood and the Chi so important? Perhaps a brief description of their individual functions will provide the answer.

Every organ in the body depends upon blood for nourishment. Using herbs to enrich the blood can be compared to using high-octane fuel to improve an automobile's performance. Enriched blood improves overall bodily performance by improving the functioning of all of the organs, which promotes maximum organ efficiency, better health, and longevity. Likewise, by nourishing the Chi, energy levels are increased—providing greater vitality, strength, and endurance.

Lifestyle Choices

In addition to emphasizing the importance of the quality of blood and Chi, Chinese medicine also recommends moderation in life activities. This means practicing temperance in eating, drinking, and sexual activity, combined with proportionate amounts of work, exercise, and rest. By practicing self-control and using herbal formulas, we can correct the imbalances that occur as a result of overindulgence in dietary and sexual matters and underindulgence in exercise and rest.

Interestingly, while there is some agreement between Western and Chinese medicine on the basic principles of diet and health, the two systems hold completely divergent opinions regarding sexual overindulgence and its negative effects on overall health and long life. Western medicine makes little or no mention of the consequences of sexual excess, whereas Chinese medicine teaches that it causes more harm than is commonly realized. According to Chinese medical theory, sexual or reproductive functioning corresponds with the kidneys, and sexual excess can contribute to kidney emptiness. This *deficiency* or *weakening of the kidneys* is characterized by health problems that range from urinary bladder dysfunction (incontinence) to impotence (in men). These conditions, commonly seen in the elderly, are treatable.

Treatment of kidney weakness consists of herbal therapy and internal exercises that strengthen the kidneys and invigorate the urogenital system. Normally, during the course of such treatment, the traditional Chinese physician will prescribe temporary abstinence from sexual activity in conjunction with taking herbal formulas and performing internal exercises to correct the imbalance that has been created as a result of too much sex. The length of treatment usually depends on the age of the patient and the extent of the abuse. An effective cure is always accompanied by a suggestion of sexual temperance.

The importance of daily exercise, followed by inactivity or relaxation, is also emphasized. Unfortunately, many people, especially the elderly, lack sufficient energy for such a regimen. In those cases, herbal formulas are recommended to strengthen the body and increase overall energy levels, making exercise possible.

Restful sleep should occur naturally as a result of daily activity. Meditation and Chi Kung (breathing exercises) are highly recommended as a means of improving the quality of sleep by eliminating the tendency toward excessive mental activity.

Diet

In spite of many differences in theory and application that distinguish one form of medicine from another, they all share certain basic concepts considered essential for maintaining good health; the importance of good nutrition and its relationship to health is one of them.

I have always found it interesting that some people who are introduced to Chinese medicine/herbology tend to become preoccupied with elements that seem "strange" or "weird." Typical things that engage such people's curiosity are the medical use of precious minerals like jade, pearls, and gold or the medical use of animal parts like deer antler and tiger bone in some of the more exotic prescriptions. Regrettably, this fascination with the unusual aspects of traditional Chinese medicine often overshadows the tradition's basic commonsense advice with regard to things like the importance of diet for maintaining good health.

The dietary recommendations put forth by traditional Chinese medicine are based on Taoist dietary principles. While some of them may be familiar, others that are more of a departure from Western dietary concepts may not be. I can assure you that these minor differences in no way undermine the general consensus concerning the important role played by diet in maintaining health.

The first recommendation is to eat fresh, raw fruit regularly. Contrary to Western medical belief that the skin of the fruit should be eaten because it is full of vitamins, Taoists insist that all fruit should be peeled and the skin discarded and that the seeds, which contain the primordial essence of the fruit, should be chewed and eaten.

The second recommendation is to eat whole foods in a form as close to their natural state as possible, including whole grains, fresh fruit, and vegetables. Believing that vitamin pills can make up for vital nutrients in foods is a mistake!

The third recommendation is to combine foods wisely, taking into consideration the acid and alkaline balance of the food. This means ingesting equal portions of each food item—not too much of one or the other.

Examples of acid and alkaline foods are:

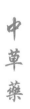

Acid Foods	*Alkaline Foods*
onion	banana
orange	spinach
cabbage	bread
coffee	carrot
pepper	broccoli

sugar	potato
tomato	eggplant
alcoholic beverage	rice

The fourth recommendation is not to eat when you are extremely tired. Fatigue creates sluggish and inefficient digestion of the fuel (food), which clogs down the digestive system.

The fifth recommendation is not to drink liquids with your meal. Liquids dilute saliva and thus undermine the effectiveness of the enzymes that are an important part of digestion.

The sixth recommendation is not to eat immediately following sexual intercourse. Immediately following and during sex, all systems are subordinate to sensory receptors.

The seventh and final recommendation is not to consume food or drink that is too hot or too cold. A tepid or neutral temperature is recommended for anything taken into the digestive system.

Strict adherence to these dietary guidelines and the use of herbal therapy (when needed) will correct imbalances that often begin as mild digestive disturbances and if left unattended often escalate. Such complications then risk becoming contributing factors in more serious diseases of the digestive system, such as gastritis, pancreatitis, gallstones, intestinal abscess, colitis, acid reflux, ulcers, and kidney stones.

Diagnostic Methods

An integral part of traditional Chinese medicine's diagnostic process is the asking of questions by the physician, a procedure similar to what may occur in the office of a Western physician. The gathering and analysis of this information, however, differs significantly between the two traditions. In Western medicine, diagnosis is usually limited to taking vital signs (blood pressure, listening to heart and lungs, temperature), followed by treatment based on symptomatic complaints. By contrast, Chinese medicine is based on holism, the fundamental theory that isolated symptoms are secondary to treating the whole person. Therefore, the diagnostic process is considerably more comprehensive.

Visual Observation

First, the Chinese physician will complete a visual examination of the patient, which involves observing the patient's facial expression, muscle tone, posture, energy levels, and overall general appearance.

Interview

In addition to considering prevailing seasonal and climatic conditions, the physician will query the patient about any emotional trauma that may have occurred as a result of a recent life experience. Discussions may include questions about medical history, the patient's living and working environment, and general lifestyle, including sexual habits.

Palpation

Palpation, or examination by touch, takes two forms. The first form, common to both Chinese and Western medicine, involves palpating local areas on the body that may be painful or swollen to determine the degree of sensitivity. This can provide information about whether the problem is superficial or deeper, possibly involving one of the internal organs. The other form of palpation, which requires an extraordinary amount of skill and sensitivity, is unique to Chinese medicine and is known as "reading the pulses."

Although there are several places on the body where the pulse can be taken, in traditional Chinese medicine the principal site used for diagnosis is the radial pulse on the wrist. The information gained from this subtle art provides insights into the condition of each of the vital organs (heart, lungs, kidneys, liver, and spleen) and therefore refines the data obtained by palpating the body. Reading the pulses requires that the physician pay strict attention to the pulse's *pace,* or the number of beats per minute; *strength,* or how strong or weak it is; and overall *quality,* or the smoothness and regularity of the rhythm.

Next, the tongue is analyzed (this is technically part of the visual diagnosis). Although the information supplied by this technique is to some extent nonspecific, it does have analytical value. The doctor will ask the patient to stick out the tongue, then he or she will study its color, which may or may not indicate the presence of a febrile, or feverish, disease. The tongue's thickness or thinness will be considered for relevant information about fluid retention, followed by observation of the "fur," or tongue coating, which can provide clues to the condition of the patient's digestive system.

A Treatment Plan

Finally, after reviewing and analyzing all of the information, the Chinese physician is able to make a determination about the nature and cause of the disease. A treatment plan is designed that incorporates the appropriate therapies, usually including one or a combination of the following: acupuncture, herbal medicine, moxabustion, cupping, five star plum blossom, and tui na massage.

Acupuncture is a therapy that uses needles inserted into specific acupuncture points to affect the flow of vital energy. Herbal medicine involves the use of botanical, mineral, and zoological substances for curing disease. Moxabustion is a form of heat therapy that uses the herb mugwort applied to specific areas of the body to treat illness. Cupping is a technique that involves the use of suction cups made of bamboo or glass. Five star plum blossom (also known as dermal needles) uses five needles bound together (and resembling a plum blossom) to stimulate yang energy by tapping areas of the body. Tui na massage is Chinese therapeutic massage.

While all of these traditional Chinese therapies are useful and complementary to one another, the two main ones are acupuncture and herbal medicine. Of the two, by far the therapy most often used is traditional Chinese herbal medicine, which not coincidentally is the subject of this work.

2

Herbs and
Their Preparation

All of the herbal formulas in this book are presented in two basic forms: either in raw form, which requires that the herbs be decocted (made into tea) or cured in an alcohol solution (made into a medicinal wine), or in patent formulas, which are commercially prepared packaged herbs in pill form, tablets, salves, syrup, herbal oils, and ointments.

Each form (raw or patent) offers its own distinct advantages. For example, if your primary concern is convenience, the prepackaged patent formulas would be the form of choice. It should be pointed out, however, that decocting raw herbs or preparing them as medicinal wine produces a potion that is more potent and that usually provides a quicker cure than the patent formula.

Another consideration is tolerance for the taste of the medicine. Decocted raw herbal formulas are normally taken "as is" and are in some cases considered to have an unpleasant taste. Medicinal wine, on the other hand, is usually sweetened with honey or crystallized rock sugar, which can make the taste rather pleasant. With herbs in pill form (patent formulas), taste is not likely to be an issue.

The best way to make a choice is to use the form most appropriate to the urgency of the situation, taking into consideration the amount of time required for cooking and curing the herbs.

From my perspective, the form you choose is secondary to encouraging you to use Chinese herbs in any form discussed in this book. That way, you can experience their benefits, enabling you to establish your own opinions concerning the various forms' effectiveness.

Important Ingredients in Chinese Herbal Formulas

The term "herbal medicine," contrary to popular belief, is not limited to botanical substances. It refers to any ingredient that has medicinal value. Although 85 percent of the ingredients used in Chinese herbology are of plant origin—roots, bark, leaves, seeds, and flowers—15 percent are animal by-products and minerals.

While some of the animal products (such as deer and antelope horn) are harvested without injuring the animal, others such as tiger bone have largely contributed to widespread killing and subsequently to the endangerment of the species. As a result, many Western countries have made it illegal to trade in substances made from the body parts of endangered species. In spite of the ongoing controversy, the ingredients in question continue to be sold "under the counter" in many Chinese herb shops.

This raises both ethical and legal issues that must be considered when using certain ingredients that are part of the Chinese herbal system. For anyone like myself who is sensitive to the issue of animal cruelty, it should be mentioned that there are botanical ingredients that can be substituted for zoological ones. In the final analysis, however, the decision about their use should in my opinion be left entirely up to the individual. (*Note:* Just because a formula has the word "tiger" in its name doesn't mean that it contains tiger parts. Some manufacturers of patent formulas will include the word "tiger" in the names of their products because the animal signifies power and strength to the Chinese people.)

I would like to introduce some of the major ingredients used in Chinese herbology. Heading the list is the herb that by some estimates is the most precious known to man—ginseng.

Ginseng

Botanical name: Radix panax ginseng
Part of the plant used: Root

Ginseng's growing reputation has aroused the curiosity of many people, who have tried it in at least one of its many forms (teas, tinctures, pills). Unfortunately, misinformation concerning proper dosage and the length of time it should be taken and, perhaps most importantly, inexperience in choosing high-quality ginseng (due to lack of experience) have resulted in widespread improper use of this legendary herb. Consequently, most users have not truly experienced ginseng's powerful tonifying (strengthening and invigorating) effects and wrongfully assume that its reputation is unfounded.

Let me assure you that ginseng's power should not be underestimated! It is for good reason considered the greatest Chinese tonic herb. Of all the herbal plant medicines, ginseng is unquestionably the most powerful for effectively increasing the body's vital energy (Chi).

In order to experience the extraordinary tonifying capabilities of ginseng, three important points must be considered:

- The quality of the root
- The dosage or amount taken
- The length of time it is taken

Since ginseng's introduction to the Western world by Jesuit priests in the late seventeenth century, the high price of this herb has created a great temptation for unscrupulous merchants to adulterate it with other substances and misrepresent its quality to uninformed consumers. Regrettably, these deceptive practices continue; therefore, I advise restricting use to the raw ginseng root, avoiding teas, pills, capsules, and tinctures.

The exorbitant price of ginseng, which can range from $25 to $1,000 or more per pound, can somewhat be justified by the stringent methods required to cultivate and grow it. Cultivation from seed to maturity normally requires seven years! Due to supply and demand, many roots are harvested prematurely. It is unfortunately these poor-quality three- to four-year-old roots that proliferate in the ginseng market.

The quality of ginseng is determined by (1) its age (the older herb is more potent), (2) where it is grown, and (3) whether it is grown wild or is cultivated. The highest-quality ginseng is grown wild in Manchuria and is known as heaven's grade. Seven years or older, it is both rare and extremely expensive.

Second only to Manchurian is North Korean (red) ginseng, also known as heaven's grade. It is seven years or older, it is grown wild, and although supplies are limited, it is available—albeit for a price that may be beyond the average person's budget. Lesser grades of Korean ginseng that are younger (three to six years old) are cultivated and grown in South Korea. They are readily available and are more afford-able for the average consumer. I should mention that the exportation of ginseng is controlled by the governments of both North and South Korea; therefore, all Korean ginseng bears a government seal, which is helpful in determining its authenticity.

Last but not least is Chinese ginseng. The highest quality is known as Yi Sun ginseng; it is grown wild and is normally harvested at six to seven years old. The second Chinese ginseng worth consideration is called Shiu Chu ginseng; it is of a somewhat lesser quality but still considered excellent. Shiu Chu ginseng is cultivated (rather than grown wild), is three to six years old, and is relatively expensive. Third, there is Kirin (red) ginseng, which is of an average quality but is also more commonly available. It is cultivated, is normally four to six years old, and is more affordable for the average consumer.

It cannot be overstated that the supply of wild ginseng (Korean, Manchurian, and Chinese) is extremely limited, so unless you are certain about the integrity of the source from which it is purchased, buyer beware!

Ginseng, like all tonics, should be used over an extended period of time for its effects to be fully realized. It is not unusual to encounter Chinese people who have used ginseng continuously for many years.

Variations in quality can make it difficult to determine effective dosage; therefore, each person needs to experiment to discover the dosage that works best for him or her. Generally, one can avoid confusion by using the traditional Chinese dosage. If it is used in a formula with other herbs, take the dosage recommended for that formula; if it is taken alone, one to two grams a day should suffice.

The length of time needed to experience the effects of ginseng varies, but after approximately thirty to sixty days the effects should be obvious. It is interesting to note, however, that people with moderate diets often experience ginseng's effects sooner than people who indulge in rich, highly spiced diets that include a lot of meat.

Although ginseng is considered a "safe" ingredient, persons suffering from high blood pressure are advised to substitute American ginseng for the Asian varieties mentioned.

Huang Qi

Botanical name: Radix astragali membranacai
Part of the plant used: Root

Often used to support ginseng in Chinese herbal formulas, Huang Qi is famous in its own right for strengthening the immune system and combating fatigue and lack of appetite. Its use in Chinese herbology can be traced back nearly five millennia. Included in a list of what are considered superior herbs, Huang Qi is mentioned in the ancient classical text *Shen Nong Ben Cao Jing,* by Shen Nong, the founder of Chinese herbology. This work first appeared around 200 B.C.

In recent years Huang Qi has been the focus of scientific research conducted in China and abroad. The result has been a number of reports published about its use as an immune-system enhancer for patients who suffer from immune deficiency disorders, as well as patients undergoing radiation or chemotherapy treatment. Further experiments have indicated a positive result in lowering blood pressure and treating pulmonary disease.

Dang Gui

Botanical name: Radix angelicae sinesis
Part of the plant used: Root

Since ancient times Dang Gui has been held in high esteem, and it is often a chief ingredient in blood formulas. Although valuable to both sexes, it is especially important for women. Shen Nong, the founder of Chinese herbology, writes in his classical text *Shen Nong Ben Cao Jing* that in addition to being effective for a full range of gynecological complaints, Dang Gui is a superior herb that should be included in all formulas designed to promote the circulation of blood. Its ability to influence viscosity by thinning blood that is too thick or nourishing blood that is too thin makes it an invaluable ingredient in blood formulas in either a supporting role or as a main ingredient.

Few Chinese herbs have been as extensively studied by modern scientists as Dang Gui. Modern medicine's interest in this herb is a direct result of reports made by Chinese clinicians who have used it for treating conditions caused by poor peripheral circulation, such as thrombosis and vasculitis. Dang Gui has also recently attracted the attention of a few Western gynecologists, who prescribe it primarily for managing symptoms associated with premenstrual syndrome and menopause.

Although Dang Gui is considered a "safe" ingredient, there are contraindications that should be mentioned. Patients suffering from diarrhea are normally not prescribed Dang Gui because of its mild laxative effect, and it is also contraindicated during pregnancy, except when administered by a qualified herbal practitioner.

Ju Hua (Chrysanthemum Flowers)

Botanical name: Flos chrysanthemi morifolii
Part of the plant used: Flower

Ju Hua comes in two varieties: yellow and white. The yellow flower is generally prescribed for treating colds with accompanying fever, dizziness, sore throat, and bloodshot eyes. Interestingly, in addition to the typical method of preparation (decoction or herbal tea), Ju Hua is sometimes used to treat colds by stuffing pillows with chrysanthemum flowers. Still, the most popular method of preparation is the highly touted restorative beverage known as chrysanthemum wine.

Ju Hua was first mentioned in the classical text *Shen Nong Ben Cao Jing*. Today, Ju Hua in the form of white flowers (also known as Gan Ju Hua or Bai Ju Hua) can often be found in formulas used for treating high blood pressure and arteriosclerosis. Its use for the treatment of hypertension is based on its ability to stabilize the central nervous system and dilate blood vessels, thus increasing blood flow.

Gan Cao (Licorice)

Botanical name: Radix glycyrrhizae uralensis

Part of the plant used: Root

Gan Cao is without a doubt one of the most commonly used Chinese herbs. In China it is used not only medicinally, but also for sweetening food and as a coloring agent in manufactured food products. In recent studies involving both animals and humans, Gan Cao has proven effective for treating stomach and duodenal ulcers. It has been used for many centuries and is mentioned in practically every Chinese herbal text ever written. Shen Nong, the founder of Chinese herbology, credited Gan Cao with being in the superior class of herbs.

Seldom a main ingredient, Gan Cao's role in most Chinese formulas is a secondary one. It is often used to improve the flavor of bitter or otherwise unpleasant-tasting herbs, as well as to mitigate or harmonize toxicity.

Gan Cao is considered a demulcent (soothing agent) for the lungs and throat and is widely used in the United States in cough syrups and cough drops. Although by and large a safe herb, its use in large doses and over a long period of time is contraindicated. Gan Cao should never be combined or used with the following herbs as their combined use will cause negative side effects: Gan Sui (Euphorbiae kansui), Da Ji (Euphorbiae seu knoxiae), Yuan Hua (Flos daphnes genkwa), Hai Zao (Herba sargassii).

He Shou Wu

Botanical name: Radix polygoni multiflori
Part of the plant used: Root

In the United States this herb is often called Fo-ti, rumored to be so nicknamed in the 1970s by a Western marketer of Chinese herbs. So that this renaming will not create unnecessary confusion, if you attempt to purchase the herb, be aware that among Chinese herbalists and operators of herb shops it is known as He Shou Wu or simply Shou Wu.

Known and used in Chinese herbology for thousands of years, He Shou Wu is also famous in Japan, where it is called Kashuu.

He Shou Wu is revered for its ability to promote longevity, nourish the vital energy (Chi), and increase fertility. It is often used as a main ingredient in formulas prescribed for premature graying of hair, angina pectoris, deficiency of Chi (fatigue), and impotence.

He Shou Wu is one of the most widely used herbs in Chinese

herbology, and experiments have shown that in addition to the healing abilities listed above, it also effectively reduces the formation of plaque and fatty deposits in the arteries. For that reason it is undergoing extensive clinical study for the treatment of high cholesterol.

Sheng Jiang (Ginger Root)

Botanical name: Radix zingiberis officinalis recens
Part of the plant used: Root

Sheng Jiang is used in approximately 50 percent of all Chinese herbal formulas. Truly a universal herb, it is valued throughout the world for both its medicinal worth and its use as a culinary ingredient.

Ginger's hot, spicy flavor makes it valuable for warming the lungs, expelling cold, and eliminating phlegm. It also helps abate nausea and will settle an upset stomach. Studies have shown that Sheng Jiang is effective for inhibiting vomiting as well as providing analgesic and anti-inflammatory benefits. Its reputation as a stomachic that can also benefit gastric ulcers has been confirmed by recent laboratory tests.

Sheng Jiang's most important function, however, and the reason for its frequent use in Chinese herbal formulas, is its ability to mitigate the potentially toxic effects of other ingredients. Its mention in *Shen Nong Ben Cao Jing,* the ancient herbal classic, is clearly a testimonial to Sheng Jiang's importance.

Raw Herbal Formulas: Methods of Preparation

Below I provide detailed instructions for preparing a decoction (tea) and medicinal wine. Although herbs can be prepared in other ways—oils, liniments, pills, capsules, etc.—the two methods described herein are considered the most functional and are by far the most popular methods for preparing Chinese herbs for consumption.

Decoction

Even though tea drinking is a daily rite in many parts of the world, such as the Middle East, Japan, North Africa, and India, tea seems mostly to be associated with China and the Chinese people.

Undoubtedly, this is influenced by the fact that tea is one of China's most important agricultural commodities, but it could also be attributed to the esteem and ceremonial reverence tea is afforded in Chinese culture. Unlike other cultures that consider tea to be just one choice of many beverages, in China it is the primary beverage. There, it is not only considered a refreshment but is believed to be therapeutic and life-sustaining.

According to Chinese history, tea-drinking was first introduced around 2737 B.C. by Emperor Shen Nong, who is also credited with being the founder of Chinese herbal medicine. Author of the classic *Shen Nong Ben Cao Jing* (also called *Divine Husbandman's Classic of Materia Medica)*, perhaps the earliest text on Chinese herbal medicine, Shen Nong is often referred to in classical Chinese literature as one of the "immortals," that is, a legendary figure in Chinese history.

Given China's long history of tea-drinking as well as the culture's use of herbs for treating disease, no wonder the technique of decoction (which is essentially the same as brewing tea) is by far the most popular method for preparing and consuming herbs. Decoction is especially effective for acute disorders, because the herbal tea is quickly assimilated into the bloodstream and the healing effects are felt more rapidly.

Although preparation is quite simple, several important points should be remembered:

- Never cook a decoction in an aluminum pot. Use porcelain, Pyrex, enamel, or glass.
- When preparing a decoction, first bring the water to a rolling boil and then add the herbs; this is necessary to extract the therapeutic properties.
- Always simmer the decoction over a low flame.
- Never store the decoction in a plastic container.

Exact instructions for preparing a decoction are as follows:

- Bring the required quantity of room-temperature water to boil in a large pot.
- Add the herbs, stir, and return to a boil;
- Lower the heat to simmer and cover the pot.
- Simmer over a low flame for thirty minutes.

- Remove pot from heat with the lid on, and allow the cooked tea to cool in the pot for another thirty minutes.
- Strain off the herbs and discard them.
- Place the strained herbal tea into a glass container for storage.

To make enough decoction for one day, add one to two ounces of fresh herbs to twenty-four fluid ounces (three cups) of boiling water. Brew the tea as instructed above. After the cooking process, the water will be reduced to approximately sixteen ounces of fluid. Drink one-half cup (four fluid ounces) at room temperature three times daily, in the morning, afternoon, and evening.

To prepare larger quantities, simply double, triple, or quadruple the amounts of water and herbs and prepare the decoction as above. Herbal decoctions can be stored in the refrigerator for about ten to fourteen days.

Taoists believe that neither hot nor cold is a desirable temperature for substances to be ingested; a tepid or neutral temperature is recommended. After preparing an herbal decoction, allow the tea to come to room temperature before drinking it.

Medicinal Wine

The ancient practice of aging herbs in alcohol is the simplest and, by some accounts, the oldest method known for making medicinal preparations. The Yao Jiu or medicinal wine is made by leaving the herbs in an alcohol solution and allowing the herbal properties to be extracted or drawn out by the alcohol. The spirit (or wine) itself is considered to possess nourishing, blood-invigorating properties that enhance the therapeutic effects of the herbs prepared with it.

Alcohol ranks second only to water as the most frequently used solvent in herbal preparation. Although other solvents such as milk, vinegar, and infant's urine are occasionally used, to the layman they remain mostly unheard of.

When Yao Jiu preparations are intended for internal consumption, sweet rice wine, vodka, or fine brandy is the spirit of choice. For external preparations such as liniments, ethanol or rectified turpentine is used.

Making a medicinal wine is quite simple. The most important consideration after the quality of the ingredients (herbs and alcohol)

is the environment. The best conditions for properly aging or curing the wine are those most similar to the dark, cool, dry, and neutral conditions found in commercial wine cellars.

A medicinal wine is made by adding 1.5 to 2.5 ounces of fresh herbs to a fifth or liter of alcohol. If vodka is used, honey can be added to improve the taste. For internal consumption, the alcohol used should be no more than 80 proof.

Exact instructions for preparing a medicinal wine are as follows:

Uncap the bottle of alcohol and pour off enough to make room for the herbs. Add the herbs and recap the bottle. Store it in a cool, dry place for a minimum of sixty to ninety days. Gently shake the bottle once a week during this time.

When the aging process is completed, leave the herbs in the bottle until all of the wine has been consumed. The longer the medicinal wine is aged, the more potent it will become. It is not uncommon to age a medicinal wine for a year or more.

Once the Yao Jiu has aged properly, the standard dose is one ounce of wine at room temperature three times daily, in the morning, afternoon, and evening. You can dilute the medicinal wine in four ounces of tepid water or drink it straight up.

Tonics: What They Are and How to Use Them

To quote the famous Chinese physician Sun Shu Mao (581–682 A.D.), whose life spanned 101 years, "Anyone under forty should use herbs occasionally to naturally regulate and strengthen the body; anyone over fifty should use tonics daily to nourish the blood, strengthen the body and promote longevity." Tonics, often called the elixir of life, invigorate and strengthen the body. They can be used for maintaining health in the absence of illness, as well as for restoring strength and energy after surgery, childbirth, or chronic illness. Many of the tonic formulas used in modern Chinese medicine were developed centuries ago during the imperial dynasties and have enjoyed continued use by the Chinese people for the past five thousand years.

While they are simple to use, several things should be pointed out about using herbal tonics:

- Most important, just as with losing weight, bodybuilding, or any other process to improve physical condition, tonics require uninterrupted use over a period of time for their beneficial effects to be fully realized. Needless to say, taking tonics for a couple of days or a week is in no way harmful, but nor is that enough time to be very helpful.
- Second, herbal tonics should be taken after meals.
- Finally, herbal tonics should never be taken when you are in the early stages of a cold, because they will drive the cold deeper into the body!

Although tonics can be decocted into tea, traditionally the preferred method of preparation for tonic formulas is medicinal wine, mainly because it is the nature of tonics to stimulate, an action reinforced by alcohol. The standard dosage is one ounce of medicinal wine at room temperature three times daily, in the morning, afternoon, and evening. You can dilute the medicinal wine in four ounces of tepid water, or drink it straight up.

What follows are nine time-proven tonic formulas that increase energy (Chi) and strength, extend endurance, alleviate anemia, improve circulation, and invigorate the vital organs:

Ba Zhen Tang (Eight Treasure Decoction)

Original Source: *Zheng Ti Lei Yao* (according to *Chinese Herbal Medicine Formulas and Strategies*)

Ingredients:

Quantity (Grams)	Chinese Herbs	English Translation
9	Ren Shen	Ginseng Root
12	Bai Zhu	Atractylodes Rhizome
15	Fu Ling	Tuckahoe Root
6	Zhi Gan Cao	Honey-Cooked Licorice Root
18	Shu Di Huang	Chinese Foxglove Root, Wine-Cooked
15	Bai Shao	White Peony Root
15	Dang Gui	Tangkuei
9	Chuan Xiong	Szechuan Lovage Root
3 pieces★	Sheng Jiang	Fresh Ginger Root
2 pieces	Da Zao	Jujube Fruit

*each the size of a quarter (twenty-five-cent piece)

Description: Ba Zhen Tang is composed of ten ingredients highly valued for their ability to increase the Chi (six herbs) and nourish the blood (four herbs). This formula increases energy level, nourishes and improves circulation of the blood, and reduces shortness of breath, lightheadedness, and vertigo.

Analysis: Ren Shen increases energy levels, Shu Di Huang enriches the blood, and Bai Zhu and Fu Ling strengthen the spleen and resolve dampness. Bai Shao and Dang Gui assist in enriching the blood, and Chuan Xiong circulates it. Da Zao and Sheng Jiang benefit the stomach and spleen while aiding digestion and absorption of nutrients. Zhi Gan Cao harmonizes all the herbs in the formula and improves the taste of the decoction.

Dosage and Method of Preparation: Make a decoction or a medicinal wine. For a decoction, drink four ounces of Ba Zhen Tang tea at room temperature three times daily, or drink six ounces twice daily. For a medicinal wine, drink one ounce of medicinal wine at room temperature three times daily.

Shi Quan Da Bu Tang (All Inclusive Great Tonifying Decoction)

Original Source: *Tai Ping Hui Min He Ji Ju Fang* (according to *Chinese Herbal Medicine Formulas and Strategies*)

Ingredients:

Quantity (Grams)	Chinese Herbs	English Translation
9	Ren Shen	Ginseng Root
12	Bai Zhu	Atractylodes Rhizome
15	Fu Ling	Tuckahoe Root
6	Zhi Gan Cao	Honey-Cooked Licorice Root
18	Shu Di Huang	Chinese Foxglove Root, Wine-Cooked
15	Bai Shao	White Peony Root
15	Dang Gui	Tangkuei
9	Chuan Xiong	Szechuan Lovage Root
9	Rou Gui	Saigon Cinnamon Inner Bark
18	Huang Qi	Milk-Vetch Root

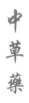
中草藥

Description: The first eight ingredients in this formula are the same as those in Ba Zhen Tang (Eight Treasure Decoction); the last two are what make it different. You should use the formula whose indications most accurately address your particular symptoms. This formula increases energy levels, nourishes and circulates the blood, improves the appetite, eliminates coughing caused by physical exertion, and strengthens the lower extremities.

Analysis: Ren Shen strengthens the entire body by increasing Chi levels. Bai Zhu and Fu Ling strengthen the spleen and resolve dampness. Shu Di Huang, Bai Shao, and Dang Gui, when combined, powerfully enrich the blood, and Chuan Xiong improves its circulation. Rou Gui benefits the kidneys, and Huang Qi increases Chi, strengthens the immune system, and benefits the lungs. Zhi Gan Cao harmonizes the herbs and improves the taste.

Dosage and Method of Preparation: Make a decoction or medicinal wine. For a decoction, drink four ounces of Shi Quan Da Bu Tang tea at room temperature three times daily, or drink six ounces twice daily. For a medicinal wine, drink one ounce of medicinal wine at room temperature three times daily.

Tze Pao Sanpien Extract (Priceless Treasure Three Whip Extract); also known as Zhi Bao San Bian Jing Wan

Description: What might be considered a "super tonic," Tze Pao Sanpien Extract is a broad-spectrum nutritive tonic that should be taken for extended periods (six months minimum; one to two years preferred) to experience its full effects. This patent medicine contains forty-two different ingredients that strengthen the entire body, improve the mind and spirit, strengthen the lower back, empower sexual function, counter fatigue, eliminate spontaneous sweating, improve poor memory, relieve insomnia and chronic asthma, and improve the immune system and weak extremities.

Dosage: It usually comes in a box containing ten vials (10cc each), in a 32-ounce bottle of liquid, or in pill form—all with complete instructions on dosage.

Wan Nian Chun Zi Pu Ziang (Thousand Year Spring Nourishing Syrup); also known as Wan Nian Jun Zi Bu Jiang

Description: This general tonic benefits the lungs, liver, spleen, pancreas, and kidneys. It is recommended for health maintenance and cases where there is general weakness and chronic illness, including asthma and arthritis. It is nourishing and addresses problems associated with malnutrition and is considered an excellent tonic for aging persons.

Dosage: This patent medicine comes in bottles of 100cc, with complete instructions on dosage.

Yang Rong Wan (Support Luxuriant Growth Pills); also known as Yang Ying Wan, or Ginseng Tonic Pills

Description: Yang Rong Wan nourishes the blood while it supports the kidneys. This patent formula is used for maintaining and promoting health when there is general weakness as a result of chronic illness. This is a good multipurpose tonic whose use will promote longevity.

Dosage: This patent medicine comes in bottles of two hundred pills, with complete instructions on dosage.

Ching Chun Bao (Recovery of Youth Tablets); also known as Shuang Bao Su Kou, Qing Chun Bao Fu Ye, or Antiaging Tablets

Description: This tonic formula dates back to Ming Cheng Zu, the third emperor of the Ming Dynasty (1368–1644 A.D.). This patent medicine strengthens the brain, enhances memory, alleviates insomnia, increases vigor, resists fatigue, preserves and strengthens sexual function, enhances immunity, improves heart function, delays development of coronary heart disease by reducing blood fat, and aids in the prevention of vascular sclerosis.

Dosage: This patent formula comes in bottles of eighty pills, with complete instructions on dosage.

Quan Lu Wan (Complete Deer Pills); also known as Alrodeer Pills

Description: Quan Lu Wan is primarily made from various parts of the spotted deer. It tonifies and invigorates the Chi, increases energy, nurtures the blood, and strengthens the lungs, spleen, kidney, and heart. This patent medicine is an excellent tonic for nourishing the Chi and the blood and is recommended for general weakness, for the aging, and for those recovering from surgery, trauma, or difficult childbirth.

Dosage: This patent medicine comes in bottles of one hundred pills, with complete instructions on dosage.

Jen Shen Lu Jing Wan Condensed (Ginseng Deer Horn Pill); also known as Ren Shen Lu Rong Wan

Description: This patent formula containing ginseng and deer antler strengthens the kidneys, improves digestion, and nourishes the blood. It is an excellent rehabilitation tonic following surgery, illness, or childbirth and improves memory and appetite, corrects anemia, strengthens weak legs and back, abates mental restlessness and insomnia, heart palpitations, and poor memory.

Dosage: This patent medicine comes in bottles of one hundred pills, with complete instructions on dosage.

Ren Shen Shou Wu Jing (Ginseng Polygona Root Extract)

Description: This patent medicine is an excellent general tonic for both men and women. It benefits the liver and nourishes the blood; it corrects symptoms of insomnia, dizziness, poor memory, poor appetite, fatigue, aching joints, and diminished sex drive.

Dosage: This comes as an alcohol liquid extract in bottles of 50cc, with complete instructions on dosage.

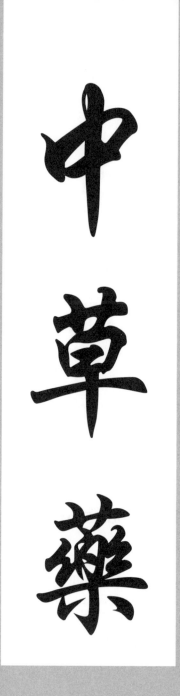

中草藥

Chinese Herbal Medicine

3

Illnesses and
Their Treatments

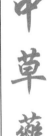

This chapter discusses common illnesses and conditions from the Chinese medical perspective as well as the more familiar Western medical approach. Symptoms and basic etiology will be considered, followed by a list of herbal formulas that can be used for treating the particular illness.

Success in using these formulas will depend on a number of considerations. An accurate diagnosis by a medical professional and strict compliance with the recommended dosage are imperative. Because illness does not always exhibit exactly the same symptoms in each individual case, care should be taken in choosing the formulas whose description most closely correspond with your particular symptoms. Finally, prudence should be exercised when using any form of medicine; if relief is not experienced within a reasonable length of time (four to ten days), attempts at self-treatment should be abandoned and a professional Chinese or Western doctor should be consulted.

Acid Reflux (see also Indigestion)

One of the many colorful terms used in traditional Chinese medicine is the term that describes acid reflux. Referred to as "rebellious Chi," acid reflux occurs when acid or fluid in the stomach travels upward into the throat—instead of along its normal downward course through the digestive system—causing a burning sensation associated with heartburn. Left untreated, acid reflux can lead to esophagitis (inflammation of the esophagus).

In some instances acid reflux can be corrected simply by avoiding spicy and highly acidic foods and beverages such as citrus, tomatoes, peppers, onions, coffee, tea, and sodas. Repeated episodes may indicate a hiatal hernia, in which case it may be advisable to seek professional help. The following formulas can be used to treat the symptoms of acid reflux:

Wu Zhu Yu Tang (Evodia Decoction)

Original Source: *Shang Han Lun* (according to *Chinese Herbal Medicine Formulas and Strategies*)

Ingredients:

Quantity (Grams)	Chinese Herbs	English Translation
12	Wu Zhu Yu	Evodia Fruit
18	Sheng Jiang	Fresh Ginger Root
9	Ren Shen	Ginseng Root
4 pieces	Da Zao	Jujube Fruit

Description: This is an excellent raw herb formula for excessive stomach acid. It relieves acid regurgitation, dry heaves, and the spitting up of clear fluids and controls the desire to vomit immediately after eating.

Analysis: The chief ingredients, Wu Zhu Yu and Sheng Jiang, both calm the stomach and relieve vomiting. Ren Shen strengthens the spleen, and Da Zao supports the action of Ren Shen.

Dosage and Method of Preparation: Make a decoction. Drink four ounces of Wu Zhu Yu Tang tea at room temperature three times daily, or drink six ounces twice daily, as needed.

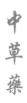

Ping Wei San (Calm the Stomach Decoction)

Original Source: *Tai Ping Hui Min He Ji Ju Fang* (according to *Chinese Herbal Medicine Formulas and Strategies*)

Ingredients:

Quantity (Grams)	Chinese Herbs	English Translation
15	Cang Zhu	Atractylodes Cangzhu
12	Huo Po	Magnolia Bark
12	Chen Pi	Ripe Tangerine Peel
6	Zhi Gan Cao	Honey-Cooked Licorice Root
9	Sheng Jiang Fresh	Ginger Root
4 pieces	Da Zao	Jujube Fruit

Description: This formula relieves acid reflux, bloated stomach, nausea, and excessive belching.

Analysis: The chief herb, Cang Zhu, is one of the most important herbs in Chinese herbology for strengthening the spleen. Da Zao benefits the stomach, Huo Po works synergistically with the chief herb, Chen Pi and Sheng Jiang calm the stomach and relieve vomiting, and Zhi Gao Cao harmonizes the actions of the other herbs and improves the taste of the formula.

Dosage and Method of Preparation: Make a decoction. Drink four ounces of Ping Wei San tea at room temperature three times daily, or drink six ounces twice daily, as needed.

Wei Te Ling "204" (Stomach Especially Effective Remedy)

Description: This patent medicine is effective for acid reflux because of the calcium mineral salts (from the cuttlefish bone) that neutralize excessive stomach acids. It is also useful for acute gastritis, abdominal bloating, excessive belching, and gas.

Dosage: Wei Te Ling "204" comes in bottles of 120 pills, with complete instructions on dosage.

Lui Jun Zi Tablets (Six Gentlemen Tablets)

Description: Excellent for poor digestion, acid regurgitation, nausea, and heartburn.

Dosage: This patent medicine comes in bottles of ninety-six tablets, with complete instructions on dosage.

Wei Yao (Gastropathy Capsules); also known as 707 Gastropathy Capsules

Description: This patent formula reduces excess stomach acid, stops stomach or related chest pain caused by heartburn, and reduces belching and regurgitation of stomach acid.

Dosage: It comes in bottles of forty-two capsules, with complete instructions on dosage.

Acne

Although there is general agreement between traditional Chinese and Western medicine on the cause of acne—which is in most cases a result of clogged hair follicles or sebaceous glands producing excessive amounts of oil—when treating acne, Chinese herbalists usually place greater emphasis than Western practitioners on the patient's overall health and diet and the condition of the blood and bowels. Much like their Western counterparts, Chinese herbalists might also recommend the elimination of certain foods such as meat, poultry, shellfish, eggs, dairy products, oily or fatty foods, refined sugar, chocolate, cocoa, soda, tea, coffee, tomatoes, and avocados. They might also suspect certain drugs as a possible cause (for example, barbiturates, isoniazid, rifampin, bromides, and iodides). On rare occasions acne can be caused by exposure to hydrocarbons (a class of aliphatic, cyclic, or aromatic compounds containing only hydrogen and carbon, including methane, benzene, and others).

In addition to adhering to the above-mentioned changes in diet, acne sufferers should drink large quantities of water and pay strict attention to sanitary habits. Regular elimination of the body's waste from the bowel and purifying the blood through the use of medicinal herbs have been shown to do more for improving the complexion than drugstore cosmetic preparations that clog the pores and often destroy natural protective oils. The following patent formulas are excellent remedies for acne:

Cai Feng Zhen Zhu An Chuang Wan (Margarite Acne Pills); also known as Colorful Phoenix Precious Pearl Hide Skin Boil Pills

Description: This patent formula dispels toxins from the blood, relieves itching, and eliminates pus-filled bumps, rashes, and hives.

Dosage: It comes in bottles of thirty-six pills, with complete instructions on dosage.

Chuan Shan Jia Qu Shi Qing Du Wan (Armadillo Counter Poison Pill); also known as Anteater Scale Remove Damp or Clear Toxin Pills

Description: This patent acne medicine relieves itching and reduces inflammation, sores, carbuncles, dermatitis, acne sores, and hives.

Dosage: It comes in bottles of forty-eight pills, with complete instructions on dosage.

Acquired Immune Deficiency Syndrome (AIDS)

Acquired immune deficiency syndrome, better known as AIDS, is a deficiency of the immune system caused by infection with the HIV virus. There is no cure for AIDS. Regrettably, once AIDS is diagnosed, the condition is considered fatal, but, interestingly, AIDS is not present in all individuals infected with the HIV virus. The percentage of those infected whose condition progresses to AIDS varies widely in different countries and in different risk groups. The main risk groups in the West are homosexual or bisexual men and people who inject themselves with drugs. Also at risk are heterosexuals who have sex with infected partners, children of infected women, and people who have received transfusions with tainted or infected blood. Prior to the early 1980s hemophiliacs were members of the high-risk group as a result of receiving infected blood; however, better screening of blood and treatment of blood products has practically eliminated any possibility of infection as a result of blood transfusion.

In its most severe form, HIV infection lowers the immune system, which makes the individual susceptible to a variety of infections and cancers, including Kaposi's sarcoma—a rare, slow-developing form of skin cancer—and lymphoid tumors. Infections commonly seen in HIV-infected patients are herpes simplex, shingles, tuberculosis, a rare form of pneumonia called pneumocystis carinii, and candidiasis, better known as thrush.

Some individuals who first become infected with the HIV virus may exhibit no symptoms, while others experience a short-term illness resembling infectious mononucleosis. Preliminary examination often reveals abnormalities such as high fever, sore throat, and enlarged lymph glands. As the disease progresses, a wide range of symptoms develop, including weight loss, diarrhea, fever, infections, and neurological disorders that can include dementia. The features of full-blown AIDS include cancers such as Kaposi's sarcoma, lymphomas of the brain, chronic herpes simplex, and a full range of uncontested infections due to immune deficiency.

Since there is no cure for AIDS, and until a cure or vaccine is found, the importance of prevention cannot be overemphasized. The major form of transmission is sexual contact, specifically between penis and anus, penis and vagina, or penis and mouth. The virus can also be passed in the blood via transfusions, via needles shared by drug addicts, and from a pregnant women to her unborn fetus.

Risk of contraction can be reduced by practicing "safe sex." Safe-sex techniques include reducing the number of sex partners. Ideally, sex should be restricted to partners whose sexual histories are known. The use of condoms during anal, vaginal, and oral sex is strongly recommended. Hugging, dry kissing, and mutual masturbation are all considered safe.

Both Western and traditional Chinese medicine can only offer supportive treatment for complications and symptoms associated with AIDS. Many reports have suggested that the most effective approach to treatment involves the use of both forms of medicine. Chinese herbal formulas can be useful as part of a continuing effort to improve the quality of life of HIV- and AIDS-infected persons by managing the symptoms of the disease until either a curative treatment or a vaccination is found.

Huang Bing Shan has written an excellent book on this disease called *AIDS and Its Treatment by Traditional Chinese Medicine*. It claims to have witnessed clinical success treating AIDS with the herbal formulas that follow.

These formulas treat the following symptoms of AIDS: abdominal distention, acid regurgitation, belching, cough and wheezing, chronic diarrhea, cold limbs, diarrhea, dizziness, dry cough with little or no phlegm, dry mouth and throat, emaciation, fatigue, fever, foul-smelling bowel movements, fullness in the chest, hiccups, inability to drink water, insomnia, Kaposi's sarcoma, labored breathing, large or small tubercles, loss of appetite, loss of sleep, low back pain, night sweats, pain, pale complexion, palpitations, poor appetite, red-flushed face, thirst (constant), tidal fever, tinnitus, ulcerating that will not heal, ulceration of the lips, tongue, and mouth, vomiting, weakness in the lower back and knees. In addition, two patent formulas are included that will resolve lumps all over the body, stop pain, and increase white-blood-cell counts in cancer patients undergoing chemo or radiation therapy. For information on additional herbal formulas used to treat these diseases or other symptoms of AIDS, refer to the appropriate entry in this chapter.

Sha Shen Mai Men Dong Tang Jia Jian (Glehnia and Ophiopogonis Decoction)

Original Source: *Wen Bing Tiao Bian* (according to *Chinese Herbal Medicine Formulas and Strategies*)

Ingredients:

Quantity (Grams)	Chinese Herbs	English Translation
9	Sha Shen	Root of Silvertop Beech Tree (Glehnia)
9	Mai Men Dong	Lush Winter Wheat Tuber
6	Yu Zhu	Rhizome of Solomon's Seal
4.5	Sang Ye	White Mulberry Leaf
6	Chuan Bei Mu	Fritillaria Bulb
4.5	Tian Hua Fen	Heavenly Flower Root
9	Shu Di Huang	Chinese Foxglove Root, Wine-Cooked
6	Mu Dan Pi	Tree Peony Root, Bark of
6	Ze Xie	Water Plantain Rhizome
3	Gan Cao	Licorice

Description: This herbal formula is used to treat the symptoms of AIDS, including cough and wheezing, dry cough with little or no phlegm, labored breathing, night sweats, emaciation, and insomnia.

Analysis: Sha Shen, Mai Men Dong, Yu Zhu, and Tian Hua Fen all moisten the lungs and stop thirst, Shu Di Huang benefits the kidneys and strengthens the blood, and Chuan Bei Mu transforms phlegm and stops coughing. Mu Dan Pi, Sang Ye, and Ze Xie disperse lung and kidney heat, and Gao Cao harmonizes the actions of the other herbs and improves the taste of the decoction.

Dosage and Method of Preparation: Prepare a decoction. Drink four ounces of Sha Shen Mai Men Dong Tang Jia Jian three times daily, as needed.

Dang Gui Liu Huang Tang (Tangkuei and Six Yellow Decoction)

Original Source: *Lan Shi Mi Cang* (according to *Chinese Herbal Medicine Formulas and Strategies*)

Ingredients:

Quantity (Grams)	Chinese Herbs	English Translation
9	Dang Gui	Tangkuei
15	Sheng Di Huang	Chinese Foxglove Root, Raw
15	Shu Di Huang	Chinese Foxglove Root, Wine-Cooked
6	Huang Lian	Golden Thread Root
12	Huang Qin	Baical Skullcap Root
6	Huang Bai Amur	Cork Tree Bark
9	Mu Li	Oyster Shell
9	Fu Xiao Mai	Wheat Grain
9	Huang Qi	Milk-Vetch Root

Description: This herbal formula is used to treat the symptoms of AIDS, including night sweats, tidal fever, tinnitus, insomnia, and red-flushed face and cheeks.

Analysis: Dang Gui, Shu Di Huang, and Sheng Di Huang all nourish the fluids (moisten or lubricate the intestines) as well as enrich the blood. Sheng Di Huang also cools the blood, and Shu Di Huang benefits the kidneys. Huang Qin, Huang Lian, and Huang Bai Amur clear heat; Huang Qi strengthens immunity and eliminates

中
草
藥

excessive sweating. Mu Li calms the spirit, and Fu Xiao Mai benefits the stomach. The combination of these herbs is based on the theory that by clearing heat and strengthening the blood and Chi, pores and intestines will constrict, thereby reducing excess sweating.

Dosage and Method of Preparation: Make a decoction. Drink four ounces of Dang Gui Liu Huang Tang tea three times daily, as needed.

Huo Xiang Zheng Qi San Jia Jian (Agastache Decoction to Rectify the Qi)

Original Source: *Tai Ping Hui Min He Ji Ju Fang* (according to *Chinese Herbal Medicine Formulas and Strategies*)

Ingredients:

Quantity (Grams)	Chinese Herbs	English Translation
12	Huo Xiang	Patchouli
9	Fu Ling	Tuckahoe Root
6	Ze Xie	Water Plantain Rhizome
12	Bai Zhu	Atractylodes Rhizome
6	Shen Qu	Medicated Leaven
9	Shan Zha	Hawthorne Fruit
6	Mu Xiang	Costus Root
9	Sha Ren	Grains of Paradise Fruit/ Seeds★
6	Huo Po	Magnolia Bark
6	Chen Pi	Ripe Tangerine Peel
9	Ban Xia	Half Summer
9	Da Fu Pi	Betel Husk
3 pieces	Da Zao	Jujube Fruit
3	Gan Cao	Licorice

★ the fruit or seeds must be smashed.

Description: This herbal formula is used for symptoms of AIDS, including diarrhea, abdominal distention, vomiting, loss of appetite, fatigue, fever, and pain.

Note: Use this formula with caution if you are suffering from a cold.

Analysis: Huo Xiang settles the stomach and promotes spleen activity; Ban Xia calms the stomach and stops vomiting; Huo Po and Da Fu Pi improve digestion and transform dampness; Fu Ling and Bai

Zhu strengthen the spleen; Chen Pi regulates the energy in the spleen and stomach while it dries dampness; Sha Ren and Mu Xiang assist in carrying out these functions and also stop pain; Shen Qu and Shan Zha aid digestion by eliminating sluggishness and dispersing food; Ze Xie resolves toxicity (or sour stomach); and Da Zao and Gan Cao settle the stomach and transform dampness.

Dosage and Method of Preparation: Prepare a decoction. Drink four ounces of Huo Xiang Zheng Qi San Jia Jian tea three times daily, as needed.

Fu Zi Li Zhong Tang Jia Wei (Prepared Aconite Decoction to Regulate the Middle)

Original Source: *Tai Ping Hui Min He Ji Ju Fang* (according to *Chinese Herbal Medicine Formulas and Strategies*)

Ingredients:

Quantity (Grams)	Chinese Herbs	English Translation
90	Fu Zi	Accessory Root of Szechuan Aconite
90	Dang Shen	Relative Root
90	Bai Zhu	Atractylodes Rhizome
90	Fu Ling	Tuckahoe Root
90	Huang Qi	Milk-Vetch Root
90	Bu Gu Zhi	Scuffy Pea Fruit
90	Wu Wei Zi	Schizandra Fruit
90	He Zi	Myrobalan Fruit
90	Gan Jiang	Dried Ginger Root
90	Rou Dou Kou	Nutmeg Seeds
30	Gan Cao	Licorice

Description: This herbal formula is used to treat the symptoms of AIDS, including diarrhea, chronic diarrhea, abdominal pain, pale appearance, cold limbs, and low back pain.

Analysis: Fu Zi warms and increases kidney energy; Dang Shen strengthens the spleen; Gan Jiang regulates the stomach and increases digestion; Bai Zhu strengthens the spleen and dries dampness; Bu Gu Zhi benefits the kidneys; Rou Dou Kou warms the spleen and disperses cold; Huang Qi increases overall energy and treats prolapse; Fu Ling suppresses dampness and strengthens the spleen; Wu Wei Zi and He Zi combined assist in astringing and stopping diarrhea; and Gan Cao harmonizes the other herbs in the formula and improves the taste of the decoction.

Dosage and Method of Preparation: Have the herbs ground into a fine powder and mixed together. Store in a glass jar. Mix three grams of the powdered herbal formula with honey to form a pill. Take the pill with warm water on an empty stomach, as needed.

Xiao Yao San Jia Jian (Rambling Decoction)

Original Source: *Tai Ping Hui Min He Ji Ju Fang* (according to *Chinese Herbal Medicine Formulas and Strategies*)

Ingredients:

Quantity (Grams)	Chinese Herbs	English Translation
9	Dang Gui	Tangkuei
9	Fu Ling	Tuckahoe Root
9	Bai Shao	White Peony Root
9	Bai Zhu	Atractylodes Rhizome
9	Chai Hu	Bupleurum Hare's Ear Root
9	Dang Shen	Relative Root
6	Mu Xiang	Costus Root
6	Gan Cao	Licorice

Description: This herbal formula is used for symptoms of AIDS, including loss of appetite, belching, hiccups, and fullness in the chest.

Analysis: Chai Hu benefits the liver; Bai Shao and Dang Gui strengthen the blood; Bai Zhu and Fu Ling resolve dampness and strengthen the spleen; Dang Shen improves energy (Chi); Mu Xiang benefits the liver and spleen; and Gan Cao harmonizes the other herbs in the formula and improves the taste.

Dosage and Method of Preparation: Prepare a decoction. Drink four ounces of Xiao Yao San Jia Jian tea three times daily, as needed.

Li Zhong Tang Jia Wei (Regulate the Middle Decoction)

Original Source: *Shang Han Lun* (according to *Chinese Herbal Medicine Formulas and Strategies*)

Ingredients:

Quantity (Grams)	Chinese Herbs	English Translation
9	Ren Shen	Ginseng
9	Bai Zhu	Atractylodes Rhizome
9	Gan Jiang	Dried Ginger Root
9	Ban Xia	Half Summer
9	Chen Pi	Ripe Tangerine Peel
9	Ding Xiang	Clove Flowerbud
9	Wu Zhu Yu	Evodia Fruit
3	Zhi Gan Cao	Honey-Cooked Licorice Root

Description: This herbal formula is used for the symptoms of AIDS, including vomiting, frequent vomiting accompanied by diarrhea, pale complexion, fatigue, and cold limbs.

Analysis: Ren Shen strengthens the body by increasing energy while it aids digestion; Gan Jiang harmonizes or settles the stomach and stops vomiting; Bai Zhu dries dampness and strengthens the spleen; Ban Xia settles the stomach and reduces nausea and vomiting; Chen Pi settles the stomach and strengthens the spleen; Ding Xiang warms the stomach and spleen as it disperses cold and assists in stopping vomiting; Zhi Gan Cao harmonizes the other herbs in the formula and improves the taste of the decoction; and Wu Zhu Yu stops vomiting, relieves diarrhea, and reduces pain.

Dosage and Method of Preparation: Prepare a decoction. Drink four ounces of Li Zhong Tang Jia Wei tea three times daily, as needed.

Bao He Wan Jia Jian (Preserve Harmony Decoction)

Original Source: *Dan Xi Xin Fa* (according to *Chinese Herbal Medicine Formulas and Strategies*)

Ingredients:

Quantity (Grams)	Chinese Herbs	English Translation
9	Bai Zhu	Atractylodes Rhizome
9	Fu Ling	Tuckahoe Root
9	Shen Qu	Medicated Leaves
15	Shan Zha	Hawthorne Fruit
9	Ban Xia	Half Summer
9	Chen Pi	Ripe Tangerine Peel

中
草
藥

9	Lai Fu Zi	Radish Seed
6	Lian Qiao	Forsythia Fruit
9	Ji Nei Jin	Chicken Gizzard Lining
9	Mai Ya	Barley Sprout

Description: This herbal formula is used for symptoms of AIDS, including loss of appetite, pale appearance, acid regurgitation, abdominal distention, and foul-smelling bowel movements.

Analysis: Bai Zhu and Fu Ling dry dampness and strengthen the spleen, and Shan Zha and Shen Qu combined improve sluggish digestion, disperse food, and benefit the spleen. Ban Xia and Chen Pi strengthen the spleen and settle the stomach, and Lai Fu Zi assists in the previous actions. Lian Qiao disperses heat, while Mai Ya and Ji Nei Jin combine to disperse food and calm the stomach as well as improve the appetite.

Dosage and Method of Preparation: Make a decoction. Drink four ounces of Bao He Wan Jia Jian tea three times daily, as needed.

Sheng Ma Xiao Du Yin (Cimicifugae Evil Toxins Decoction)

Source: *AIDS and Its Treatment by Traditional Chinese Medicine*
Ingredients:

Quantity (Grams)	Chinese Herbs	English Translation
6	Sheng Ma	Black Cohosh Rhizome (Cimicifugae)
9	Huang Qi	Milk-Vetch Root
6	Chai Hu	Burpleurum Hare's Ear Root
6	Dang Gui	Tangkuei
9	Jin Yin Hua	Honeysuckle Flower
9	Lian Qiao	Forsythia Fruit
3	Zhi Zi	Gardenia Fruit
6	Chi Shao	Red Peony Root
6	Ji Xue Teng	Millettia Root and Vine
9	Mu Dan Pi	Tree Peony Root, Bark of
6	Yi Yi Ren	Seeds of Job's Tears
6	Nan Xing	Jack in the Pulpit Rhizome

Description: This herbal formula is used to treat symptoms of AIDS, including Kaposi's sarcoma, large or small tubercles, ulcerating that will not heal, fatigue, and poor appetite.

Analysis: Huang Qi improves energy, eliminates toxins, and generates new flesh, while Sheng Ma and Chai Hu assist Dang Gui and Ji Xue Teng to enrich and cool the blood. Zhi Zi and Mu Dan Pi assist in cooling the blood while removing toxins. Jin Yin Hua and Lian Qiao reduce fever and resolve toxins (infection), Chi Shao improves circulation of blood and clears heat and infection, and Nan Xing and Yi Yi Ren assist in clearing infection as well as strengthen the spleen, thus improving appetite.

Dosage and Method of Preparation: Make a decoction. Drink four ounces of Sheng Ma Xiao Du Yin three times daily, as needed.

Liang Ge San Jia Jian (Cool the Diaphragm Decoction)

Original Source: *Tai Ping Hui Min He Ji Ju Fang* (according to *Chinese Herbal Medicine Formulas and Strategies*)

Ingredients:

Quantity (Grams)	Chinese Herbs	English Translation
9	Huang Qin	Baical Skullcap Root
9	Huang Lian	Golden Thread Root
6	Zhi Zi	Gardenia Fruit
9	Sheng Di Huang	Chinese Foxglove Root, Raw
9	Mai Men Dong	Lush Winter Wheat Tuber
6	Dan Zhu Ye	Bland Bamboo Leaves
3	Gan Cao	Licorice
6	Bo He★	Peppermint

★See special instructions for preparation on the next page.

Description: This herbal formula is used to treat symptoms of AIDS, including thrush; ulceration of the lips, tongue, and mouth accompanied by a white curd-like substance in the oral cavity; excessive thirst; and fever.

Analysis: Huang Qin, Dan Zhu Ye, Huang Lian, and Zhi Zi combine to clear heat, eliminate infection (toxins), and reduce fever. Dan

中
草
藥

Zhu Ye also clears heat and generates fluids, reducing dryness and thirst. Bo He solidifies the energies of the other herbs. Sheng Di Huang and Mai Men Dong cool the blood and generate fluids, eliminating thirst. Gan Cao harmonizes the other herbs in the formula and improves the taste of the decoction.

Dosage and Method of Preparation: Make a decoction. Do not add Bo He to the decoction until the last five minutes of cooking time. Overcooking Bo He will cause it to lose its effectiveness. Drink four ounces of Liang Ge San Jia Jian tea three times daily, as needed.

Chen Pi Zhu Ru Tang Jia Wei (Tangerine Peel and Bamboo Shavings Decoction)

Original Source: *Jin Gui Yao Lue* (according to *Chinese Herbal Medicine Formulas and Strategies*)

Ingredients:

Quantity (Grams)	Chinese Herbs	English Translation
30	Ren Shen	Ginseng
30	Chen Pi	Ripe Tangerine Peel
30	Zhu Ru	Bamboo Shavings
30	Mai Men Dong	Lush Winter Wheat Tuber
30	Tian Hua Fen	Heavenly Flower Root
30	Zhi Mu	Anemarrhena Root
5 pieces	Da Zao	Jujube Fruit
3	Sheng Jiang	Fresh Ginger Root

Description: This herbal formula is used to treat symptoms of AIDS, including vomiting, severe vomiting with difficulty eating, and dry mouth and throat accompanied by an inability to drink water.

Analysis: Chen Pi harmonizes the stomach and stops vomiting. Zhu Ru clears the stomach and also stops vomiting. They are combined with Ren Shen, which benefits energy levels and generates fluids to stop thirst. Sheng Jiang settles the stomach and assists in stopping vomiting. Zhi Mu and Tian Hua Fen act together to reduce fever and replenish fluids, counteracting dehydration. Mai Men Dong benefits the stomach and generates fluids as well. Da Zao settles the stomach and harmonizes the other herbs in the formula.

Dosage and Method of Preparation: Grind the ingredients into a powder and make a decoction. Drink four ounces of Chen Pi Zhu Ru Tang Jia Wei tea three times daily, as needed.

Huang Lian E Jiao Tang Jia Wei (Coptis and Ass-Hide Gelatin Decoction)

Original Source: *Shang Han Lun* (according to *Chinese Herbal Medicine Formulas and Strategies*)

Ingredients:

Quantity (Grams)	Chinese Herbs	English Translation
12	Huang Lian	Golden Thread Root (Coptis)
9	E Jiao★	Donkey-Skin Glue (Ass-Hide)
6	Huang Qin	Baical Skullcap Root
6	Bai Shao Yao	White Peony Root
9	Shu Di Huang	Chinese Foxglove Root, Wine-Cooked
9	Bai Zi Ren	Arborvitae Seeds
9	Suan Zao Ren	Sour Jujube Seeds

★See special preparation instructions below.

Description: This herbal formula is used to treat the symptoms of AIDS, including insomnia, palpitations, and loss of sleep, accompanied by dizziness, tinnitus, tidal fever, night sweats, and weakness in the lower back and knees.

Analysis: Huang Lian reduces fever and clears infection, E Jiao nourishes the blood, and Huang Qin assists in relieving infection. Bai Shao Yao nourishes the blood, while Suan Zao Ren and Bai Zi Ren provide a sedative effect that helps to correct insomnia. Shu Di Huang cools the blood and nourishes the kidneys.

Dosage and Method of Preparation: Make a decoction. E Jiao should not be cooked with the formula. After finishing the cooking process, strain off herbs, then add E Jiao. Stir well and allow the herb to dissolve. It will not be necessary to re-strain the decoction. Drink four ounces of Huang Lian E Jiao Tang Jia Wei tea three times daily, as needed.

Xi Huang Wan (West Gallstone Pills)

Description: This patent formula is used to fight the symptoms of AIDS, including reducing swollen lymph nodes, stopping pain, and resolving lumps and nodules all over the body.

Caution: This formula is prohibited for use during pregnancy.

Dosage: This patent medicine comes in boxes containing eight vials, with complete instructions on dosage.

Ji Xue Teng Qin Gao Pian (Millettia Reticulata Liquid Extract Tablets); also known as Caulis Millentiae Tablets

Description: This patent formula is used to treat the symptoms of AIDS, specifically lowered white-blood-cell counts. The formula is said to increase the white-blood-cell count in cancer patients who have undergone chemotherapy or radiation therapy.

Dosage: This patent formula comes in bottles of one hundred tablets, with complete instructions on dosage.

Addiction to Alcohol

Both Western allopathic and traditional Chinese medicine view alcohol dependence as an illness characterized by habitual, compulsive, long-term consumption of alcohol and the development of withdrawal symptoms when drinking is suddenly stopped. Generally referred to as alcoholism, the development of alcohol dependence can be divided into four main stages:

(1) Tolerance increases, whereby the person is able to drink more and more alcohol before experiencing ill effects.

(2) The drinker experiences memory lapses relating to events that occurred during the drinking episode.

(3) The drinker experiences loss or lack of control over alcohol and can no longer be certain of the ability to discontinue drinking whenever he or she wants to.

(4) The drinker undergoes prolonged binges of intoxication, suffering observable mental and physical complications.

The following formulas are excellent for treating the liver disease that is the usual result of long-term alcohol abuse. However, due to the complicated psychological dynamics accompanying alcoholism, the type of therapy provided by twelve-step programs such as Alcoholics Anonymous is strongly recommend.

Important Note: Detoxification from alcohol, which can include delirium tremors, requires supervised medical treatment.

Da Huang Zhe Chong Tang (Rhubarb and Eupolyphaga Tea)

Original Source: *Jin Gui Yao Lue* (according to *Chinese Herbal Medicine Formulas and Strategies*)

Ingredients:

Quantity (Grams)	Chinese Herbs	English Translation
30	Da Huang	Rhubarb Root
3	Tu Bie Chong	Wingless Cockroach
6	Tao Ren	Peach Kernel
3	Gan Qi	Dried Lacca Sinica
6	Qi Cao	Dried Larva of Scarab
6	Shui Zhi	Leech
6	Meng Chong	Horse Flies
6	Huang Qin	Baical Skullcap Root
6	Xing Ren	Almond Kernel
30	Sheng Di Huang	Chinese Foxglove Root, Raw
12	Bai Shao	White Peony Root
9	Gan Cao	Licorice Root
9	Chai Hu	Bupleurum Hare's Ear Root

Description: An excellent raw herb formula for those suffering from alcoholism, this formula brings relief from the following symptoms: emaciation, abdominal bloating, loss of appetite, dry scaly skin, dark discolored eyes, fever, and aches.

Analysis: Huang Qin clears heat; Da Huang cools the blood; Tu Bei Chong, Shui Zhi, Meng Chong, Tao Ren, Gan Qi, and Qi Cao all clear stagnation and improve circulation. Sheng Di Huang and Bai Shao nourish the blood, Chai Hu benefits the liver, Xing Ren nourishes the fluids, and Gan Cao harmonizes the formula.

Dosage and Method of Preparation: Make a decoction. Drink four ounces of Da Huang Zhe Chong Tang tea at room temperature three times daily, or drink six ounces twice daily. This formula can be taken over an extended period.

Shu Gan Li Pi Tang (Spread the Liver and Regulate the Spleen Decoction)

Original Source: *Yi Fang Xin Jie* (according to *Chinese Herbal Medicine Formulas and Strategies*)

Ingredients:

Quantity (Grams)	Chinese Herbs	English Translation
12	Chai Hu	Bupleurum Hare's Ear Root
12	Bai Zhu	Atractylodes Rhizome
9	Xiang Fu	Nut Grass Rhizome
15	Dang Shen	Relative Root
9	Ze Xie	Water Plantain Rhizome
12	He Shou Wu	Polygonum Shouwu Root
12	Dan Shen	Salvia Root
3	San Qi (powdered)	Pseudo Ginseng Root

Description: Excellent raw herb formula used to strengthen the liver and spleen. Patients addicted to alcohol will find this formula helpful to combat symptoms including irritability, insomnia, fatigue, reduced appetite, diarrhea, and pain in the chest. This formula is commonly used for chronic hepatitis as well as the early stages of cirrhosis.

Analysis: Chai Hu and Xiang Fu both benefit the liver, Bai Zhu benefits the spleen and improves the appetite, and Dang Shen improves the function of the spleen and stomach. Ze Xie benefits the kidneys, He Shou Wu benefits both the kidneys and liver as well as nourishes the blood, Dan Shen circulates the blood, and San Qi reduces swelling and pain.

Dosage and Method of Preparation: Make a decoction. Drink four ounces of Shu Gan Li Pi Tang tea at room temperature three times daily, or drink six ounces twice daily.

Addiction to Drugs

Similar to the epidemic of drug use that now confronts Western society, one of the major problems facing postrevolutionary China was the widespread addiction to opium among the Chinese population. One of the first orders of business of the revolutionary Communist government was to establish programs whose aims were drug rehabilitation and political reform. Nearly half a century later the same techniques that were used for treating opium addiction (using auricular/ear acupuncture and Chinese herbal therapy) are currently being studied as possible prototypes for drug-treatment programs in several Western countries, including the United States.

In spite of the differences in the chemical makeup of the drugs in question (for example, opium versus crack cocaine), all drug addiction takes on two forms: psychological and physical dependence. A person is psychologically dependent if he or she experiences cravings or emotional distress when the drug is withdrawn and is physically dependent when the body has adapted to the presence of the drug, causing physical symptoms of withdrawal when the drug is not taken.

Psychological symptoms include irritability, confusion, and emotional instability. Physical symptoms include yawning, sneezing, running nose, watering eyes, sweating, diarrhea, vomiting, trembling, cramps, and, rarely, seizures and coma.

Detoxing from drugs, which is always difficult, is seldom life-threatening. However, due to the extreme discomfort experienced when a person attempts to stop abusing drugs, medical supervision is recommended. The herbal formulas listed below have proven useful for reducing withdrawal symptoms, strengthening the body, and restoring energy levels lowered as a result of excessive drug use. Due to the complicated psychological dynamics accompanying drug abuse, the therapy provided by twelve-step programs like Narcotics Anonymous is strongly recommended.

Green Tiger Liver Harmony

Description: This patent formula reduces the symptoms of drug withdrawal, such as irritability, headaches, dizziness, insomnia.

Dosage: It is available in packages of 10 tablets, bottles of 75 tablets, or boxes of 150 to 300 tablets, and in bottles of 1/4 ounce to 1 ounce concentrated liquid extract, all with complete instructions on dosage.

Chai Hu Mu Li Long Gu Tang (Ease Plus)

Description: This patent medicine relieves drug-withdrawal symptoms including tremors, muscular spasms, insomnia, irritability, nervousness, chills, and sweating.

Dosage: It comes in bottles of thirty or ninety pills, with complete instructions on dosage.

Additionally, the following herbal tonics are very useful for strengthening the body and restoring energy levels lowered by excessive drug use.

Ba Zhen Tang (Eight Treasure Decoction)

Original Source: *Zheng Ti Lei Yao* (according to *Chinese Herbal Medicine Formulas and Strategies*)

Ingredients:

Quantity (Grams)	Chinese Herbs	English Translation
9	Ren Shen	Ginseng Root
12	Bai Zhu	Atractylodes Rhizome
15	Fu Ling	Tuckahoe Root
6	Zhi Gan Cao	Honey-Cooked Licorice Root
18	Shu Di Huang	Chinese Foxglove Root, Wine-Cooked
15	Bai Shao	White Peony Root
15	Dang Gui	Tangkuei
9	Chuan Xiong	Szechuan Lovage Root
3 pieces★	Sheng Jiang	Fresh Ginger Root
2 pieces	Da Zao	Jujube Fruit

★Each the size of a quarter (twenty-five-cent piece).

Description: Ba Zhen Tang is composed of ten ingredients highly valued for their ability to increase the Chi (six herbs) and nourish the blood (four herbs). This formula increases energy

中草藥

level, nourishes and improves circulation of the blood, and reduces shortness of breath, lightheadedness, and vertigo.

Analysis: Ren Shen increases energy levels, Shu Di Huang enriches the blood, and Bai Zhu and Fu Ling strengthen the spleen and resolve dampness. Bai Shao and Dang Gui assist in enriching the blood, and Chuan Xiong circulates it. Da Zao and Sheng Jiang benefit the stomach and spleen while aiding digestion and absorption of nutrients. Zhi Gan Cao harmonizes all the herbs in the formula and improves the taste of the decoction.

Dosage and Method of Preparation: Make a decoction or a medicinal wine. For a decoction, drink four ounces of Ba Zhen Tang tea at room temperature three times daily, or drink six ounces twice daily. For a medicinal wine, drink one ounce of medicinal wine at room temperature three times daily.

Tze Pao Sanpien Extract (Priceless Treasure Three Whip Extract); also known as Zhi Bao San Bian Jing Wan

Description: What might be considered a "super tonic," Tze Pao Sanpien Extract is a broad-spectrum nutritive tonic that should be taken for extended periods (six months minimum; one to two years preferred) to experience its full effects. This patent medicine contains forty-two different ingredients that strengthen the entire body, improve the mind and spirit, strengthen the lower back, empower sexual function, counter fatigue, eliminate spontaneous sweating, improve poor memory, relieve insomnia and chronic asthma, and improve the immune system and weak extremities.

Dosage: It usually comes in a box containing ten vials (10cc each), in a 32-ounce bottle of liquid, or in pill form—all with complete instructions on dosage.

Addiction to Nicotine

Nicotine, a drug in tobacco that acts as a stimulant and is responsible for tobacco addiction, is absorbed into the bloodstream by either chewing or smoking tobacco. Although Chinese medicine's use of auricular (ear) acupuncture and herbal therapy for treating addiction is normally associated with withdrawal from what are classified as class A drugs (crack cocaine, heroin, and methamphetamine), these techniques are also used for treating nicotine dependence. Arguably, it is the tar in tobacco smoke and not the nicotine that damages lung tissue and causes diseases like lung cancer, throat cancer, emphysema, and cardiovascular disease. Undeniably, however, it is the nicotine that creates the dependence leading to long-term habitual use.

Withdrawal symptoms from tobacco use/nicotine addiction (which include headache, drowsiness, fatigue, difficulty concentrating, and depression) are weaker than with other addictive drugs. But the length of time needed for treatment is usually the same. The following herbal formulas can be used in addition to acupuncture treatment or alone for withdrawal from tobacco use/nicotine addiction.

Green Tiger Liver Harmony

Description: This formula calms restlessness, relieves headache and insomnia, and is useful for withdrawal from tobacco, nicotine, and other drugs.

Dosage: It comes in packages of 10 tablets, bottles of 75 tablets, or boxes of 150 to 300 tablets, with complete instructions on dosage.

233 Detox

Description: This patent formula calms restlessness, reduces fever, and pacifies the lungs; it is useful for drug withdrawal of various kinds.

Dosage: It comes in bottles of twenty-four tablets, with complete instructions on dosage.

Aging—see Tonics (in chapter 2)

AIDS—see Acquired Immune Deficiency Syndrome

Alcoholism—see Addiction to Alcohol

Allergies

Hypersensitivity to environmental substances has created a branch of Western medicine devoted entirely to identifying and treating its many causes, whereas traditional Chinese medicine does not even recognize the words "allergy" or "allergen." What Chinese medicine does recognize is the fact that the body will react unfavorably to certain environmental conditions. Its approach to treatment, however (since it is based on an entirely different concept of humans' relationship to nature), does not include the use of high doses of antibiotics and antihistamines routinely prescribed by Western allergists. Normally when a Chinese herbalist is presented with the typical allergy symptoms of running eyes, stuffy nose, sneezing, and the like, he or she will recommend a two-part treatment consisting of herbal blood cleansers to remove allergens and toxic waste from the bloodstream and emollients to soothe sensitive mucus membranes in the mouth, nose, and throat. Often it is also necessary to harmonize the center (the stomach) to offset the nausea brought on by postnasal drip, which occurs when infected sinus material is inadvertently swallowed or drains into the stomach.

Hypersensitive reactions (allergies) can be caused by exposure to chemicals or reaction to flowers, grasses, tree pollen, animal dander (tiny particles of animal skin and hair), house dust, dust mites, yeast, certain drugs and foods, and bee or wasp venom. Of the food allergies, the most common are caused by milk, eggs, shellfish, dried fruits, nuts, and certain food dyes or coloring.

The symptoms created by hypersensitive reactions are upset stomach, running or stuffy nose, running or itchy eyes, rash or hives, fever, sneezing, coughing, headache, dizziness or lightheadedness, and sinus and ear infection. The following patent formulas can be used to relieve the symptoms associated with allergies:

Bi Yan Pian (Nose Inflammation Pills)

Description: This formula provides relief from sneezing, itchy eyes, facial congestion, sinus congestion, rhinitis, sinusitis, and hay fever.

Dosage: It comes in a bottle of one hundred tablets, with complete instructions on dosage.

Bi Tong Tablet (Nose Open Tablet); also known as Tablet Bi-Tong

Description: This patent medicine provides relief from rhinitis, sinusitis, hay fever, nasal congestion, watery eyes, and facial congestion.

Dosage: It comes in bottles of one hundred tablets, with complete instructions on dosage.

Yao Zhi Gui Ling Gao (Herbal Tortoise Jelly)

Description: This patent formula provides relief from allergic skin reactions, hives, rashes, furuncles (surface-level skin boils), carbuncles (boils under the skin level), infected skin lesions, and abscesses.

Dosage: It comes in three hundred-gram bottles of syrup, with complete instructions on dosage.

Lien Chiao Pai Tu Pien (Forsythia Defeat Toxin Tablet); also known as Lian Qiao Bai Du Pian

Description: This patent medicine is indicated for acute infections and inflammation, including abscess, carbuncles with pus, and itching skin with rash and redness.

Caution: This formula is prohibited for use during pregnancy.

Dosage: It comes in boxes containing twelve vials with eight tablets per vial, with complete instructions on dosage.

Hsiao Yao Wan (Bupleurum Sedative Pills); also known as Xiao Yao Wan

Description: This patent medicine provides relief from allergies including the symptoms of abdominal bloating, hiccups, headache, belching, hypoglycemia, and dizziness.

Dosage: It comes in bottles of two hundred pills, with complete instructions on dosage.

Alzheimer's Disease

Alzheimer's is a progressive condition in which nerve cells in the brain degenerate. Its exact cause is unknown, but theories range from chronic infection to toxic poisoning by heavy metals (e.g., aluminum). There has also been speculation about the possibility of a genetic factor, since 15 percent of Alzheimer's sufferers have a family history of the disease.

Incidence of Alzheimer's disease, which is rare before age sixty, steadily increases with age. Approximately 30 percent of people over the age of eighty-five are affected. The features of the disease vary among individuals, but there are three distinct stages. In the first stage the sufferer becomes increasingly forgetful. Problems with memory can cause the person to feel anxious and depressed. Forgetfulness gradually progresses to the second stage, when the sufferer begins to experience severe memory loss, particularly short-term memory loss. Victims often become disoriented and experience progressive loss of the ability to concentrate. This causes increased anxiety, unpredictable mood changes, and altered personality. In the third stage, sufferers experience severe disorientation and confusion, which can be accompanied by hallucinations and paranoid delusions. Soon signs of nervous-system disease begin to emerge (such as involuntary reflexes and incontinence). While some patients become unpleasant and sometimes violent, others become docile and somewhat helpless. Neglect of personal hygiene and purposeless wandering are very common. Eventually the patient becomes bedridden, and the immobility, which creates bedsores, along with feeding problems and a high incidence of pneumonia makes life expectancy very short.

Neither Western nor traditional Chinese medicine offer specific remedies for Alzheimer's disease. Instead, treatment is directed at managing symptoms by, for example, providing nutrient supplementation through the use of herbal tonics and using antibiotic herbal formulas for treating the urinary tract infection that may result from urinary incontinence. The effort of the care provider should be applied to addressing and treating individual symptoms as they occur, making the patient's circumstances as comfortable as possible for the duration of his or her life.

For more information on herbal formulas that can be used to treat the symptoms of Alzheimer's disease, refer to the entries in this chapter for specific symptoms.

Amenorrhea

Although Chinese herbal therapy has proven to be very effective for treating amenorrhea (cessation of the menstrual period), the process of initiating menstruation has been shown to be somewhat slower when herbs are used exclusively. Therefore, acupuncture is highly recommended to "jump-start" the menstrual period, followed by herbal therapy to regulate it.

Of the two kinds of amenorrhea—primary and secondary— primary amenorrhea (which is delayed puberty or a failure to begin menstruating by age sixteen) is the more complicated. The delay of the onset of puberty may be natural, it may result from endocrine disorders, or in rare cases it can be caused by Turner's syndrome (a disorder in which one female chromosome is missing).

The most common cause of secondary amenorrhea is pregnancy. Other than that, periods may temporarily cease after a women has stopped taking birth control pills (this usually lasts for no more than six to eight weeks, although it has been known to last as long as a year). Other possible causes are emotional stress, depression, anemia, anorexia nervosa, excessive physical training, and use of drugs. Disorders of the ovaries such as polycystic ovary or a tumor such as those found in ovarian cancer are other possible causes (see also Ovarian Cyst). Amenorrhea occurs permanently after menopause or after a hysterectomy (surgical removal of the uterus). The following herbal formulas will relieve amenorrhea.

Gui Zhi Fu Ling Tang (Cinnamon Twig and Poria Tea)

Original Source: *Jin Gui Yao Lue* (according to *Chinese Herbal Medicine Formulas and Strategies*)

Ingredients:

Quantity (Grams)	Chinese Herbs	English Translation
12	Gui Zhi	Saigon Cinnamon Twig

12	Fu Ling	Tuckahoe Root
15	Chi Shao Yao	Red Peony Root
12	Mu Dan Pi	Tree Peony Root, Bark of
12	Tao Ren	Peach Kernel

Description: This is an excellent formula for treatment of amenorrhea. It relieves abdominal cramps, mild uterine bleeding of purple or dark blood during pregnancy, and amenorrhea with abdominal distention and pain.

Analysis: The chief herbs, Gui Zhi and Fu Ling, when combined, unblock blood vessels, promote circulation, and benefit the heart and spleen. Chi Shao Yao eliminates blood clots and promotes circulation; Mu Dan Pi and Tao Ren cool the blood, reduce abdominal masses, and assist in circulating the blood.

Dosage and Method of Preparation: Make a decoction. Drink four ounces of Gui Zhi Fu Ling Tang tea at room temperature three times daily, or drink six ounces twice daily.

Wu Ji Bai Feng Wan (Black Chicken White Phoenix Pills/Condensed); also known as Wu Chi Pai Feng Wan, or Wu Ji Bai Feng Wan Nong Suo

Description: This patent medicine is for amenorrhea, infertility, menstrual cramps, and deficient blood (anemia).

Dosage: It comes in bottles of 120 pills, with complete instructions on dosage.

Note: The next two patent formulas can be used alone; however, a more powerful effect will result from combining Bu Xue Tiao Jing Pian and Dang Gui Pian.

Bu Xue Tiao Jing Pian (Nourish Blood Adjust Period Pills); also known as Bu Tiao Tablets

Description: This patent medicine is for anemia, amenorrhea, fatigue, and bloating.

Dosage: It comes in bottles of one hundred pills, with complete instructions on dosage.

Dang Gui Pian (Angelica Dang Gui Tablets); also known as Angelicae Tablets

Description: This patent medicine is for amenorrhea, fatigue, weakness, and anemia.

Dosage: It comes in bottles of one hundred pills, with complete instructions on dosage.

Anemia

Deficient blood, or blood that is defective or lacking nutrient quality, is the Chinese medical term for what Western medicine commonly refers to as anemia. It occurs when the hemoglobin (a component of red blood cells that carries oxygen from the lungs to the tissues) is below normal, or when there is hemorrhaging or loss of blood.

There are three basic forms of anemia; by far the most common form is iron-deficiency anemia, which results from a lack of iron, an essential component of hemoglobin. The second type of anemia is aplastic anemia, which is often seen in patients undergoing treatments using radiation or anticancer drugs, or in people who have had long-term exposure to benzene (a chemical found in gasoline) or insecticides. And finally there is megaloblastic anemia, more commonly called pernicious anemia, which is caused by a vitamin B12 deficiency.

Both pernicious and iron-deficiency anemia can be corrected through diet, vitamin supplements (iron and B12), and the use of herbs—which is the preferred method because of herbs' ability to correct the vitamin and mineral deficiency as well as improve circulation, remove plaque from the blood vessels (veins and arteries), and counteract the fatigue characteristic of this condition. It should be noted that anemia usually affects more women than men because of the blood loss experienced during the menstrual period.

When aplastic anemia is a result of radiation or anticancer drugs, transfusions are given to correct the anemia. In persistent cases, bone-marrow transplantation may be necessary. Recovery usually occurs in mild forms of the disease; however, in severe cases without a bone-marrow transplant, aplastic anemia can be fatal.

The following formulas are excellent for treating pernicious and iron-deficiency anemia:

Dang Gui Bu Xue Tang (Dang Gui Decoction to Tonify the Blood)

Original Source: *Nei Wai Shang Bian Huo Lun* (according to *Chinese Herbal Medicine Formulas and Strategies*)

Ingredients:

Quantity (Grams)	Chinese Herbs	English Translation
30	Huang Qi	Milk–Vetch Root
6	Dang Gui	Tangkuei

Description: This decoction is used for treating anemia with fatigue, sallow complexion, and headaches.

Analysis: The large dose of Huang Qi in this formula is used to strengthen the spleen and lungs, thereby reinforcing the source of blood. Dang Gui is chosen as an assistant because it also strengthens as well as invigorates or circulates the blood.

Dosage and Method of Preparation: Make a decoction. Drink four ounces of Dang Gui Bu Xue Tang tea at room temperature three times daily, or drink six ounces twice daily.

Si Wu Tang (Four Substance Decoction)

Original Source: *Tai Ping Hui Min He Ji Ju Tang* (according to *Chinese Herbal Medicine Formulas and Strategies*)

Ingredients:

Quantity (Grams)	Chinese Herbs	English Translation
21	Shu Di Huang	Chinese Foxglove Root, Wine–Cooked
15	Bai Shao	White Peony Root
12	Dang Gui	Tangkuei
6	Chuan Xiong	Szechuan Lovage Root

Description: This is an excellent herbal formula for treating anemia with resulting fatigue, sallow complexion, and headaches.

Analysis: This classical formula consists of what are considered four superior ingredients: Shu Di Huang strongly nourishes the blood while benefiting the liver and kidneys; this action is assisted by Bai Shao, Dang Gui, and Chuan Xiong. When used together, they strengthen (or enrich) the blood, improve circulation, and moisten the intestines.

Dosage and Method of Preparation: Make a decoction. Drink four ounces of Si Wu Tang tea at room temperature three times daily, or six ounces twice daily.

Dang Gui Pian (Angelica Dang Gui Tablets); also known as Angelicae Tablets

Description: This formula nourishes the blood. Use Dang Gui Pian for chronic anemia (pernicious and iron deficiency) following traumatic injury, surgery, or childbirth.

Dosage: It comes in bottles of one hundred pills, with complete instructions on dosage.

Dang Gui Gin Gao (Angelica Dang Gui Syrup); also known as Tankwe Gin for Tea

Description: Use for anemia to eliminate fatigue and improve blood quality following surgery or illness.

Dosage: This patent medicine comes in bottles of 100 or 200cc, with complete instructions on dosage.

Angina

In both traditional Chinese and Western medicine the heart is considered the chief organ, and in typical Chinese fashion it is illustriously referred to as "emperor of the body." In addition to controlling all of the other organs, the heart also controls the circulation of blood. Without effective blood circulation the body becomes cold, which makes it understandable why traditional Chinese medicine also refers to the heart as the fire organ.

Defects of the heart are various and include aneurysm, coronary thrombosis (blockage of one or more coronary arteries), and heart-valve disease. The most common heart problem is angina pectoris, which is a term used to describe pain in the chest, arms, or jaw due to lack of oxygen to the heart muscle. Normally, angina is most severe during exercise or periods of stress.

Angina's primary cause is inadequate blood supply, usually due to coronary heart disease, in which the coronary arteries are narrowed by arteriosclerosis (fatty deposits on the walls of the arteries). Other causes include coronary artery spasm, in which the blood vessels narrow suddenly for a short period of time with no permanent obstructions, and arrhythmia (abnormal heart rhythm). In addition to the pain of angina, other symptoms can include nausea, dizziness, sweating, and difficulty breathing.

The Chinese herbal formulas recommended for angina are useful for eliminating pain by reducing the plaque that has built up in the arteries. However, if any of the angina symptoms described above are experienced, do not attempt self-diagnosis—the risks are too great. I recommend seeing a qualified heart specialist, who will determine the cause of the symptoms. Then consideration can be given to using the following herbal formulas.

Huo Lou Xiao Ling Dan (Fantastically Effective Formula to Invigorate the Collaterals)

Original Source: *Yi Xue Zhong Zhong Can Xi Lu* (according to *Chinese Herbal Medicine Formulas and Strategies*)

Ingredients:

Quantity (Grams)	Chinese Herbs	English Translation
15	Dang Gui	Tangkuei
15	Dan Shen	Salvia Root
15	Ru Xiang	Frankincense Resin
15	Mo Yao	Resin of Myrrh

Description: This formula relieves pain in the chest, back, or neck caused by angina.

Analysis: The chief ingredient, Dang Gui, enriches the blood, and when combined with Dan Shen, improves circulation and cools the blood. Ru Xiang and Mo Yao improve circulation and relieve pain.

Dosage and Method of Preparation: Make a decoction. Drink four ounces of Ho Lou Xiao Ling Dan tea at room temperature three times daily, or drink six ounces twice daily.

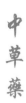

Mao Dong Ching (Ilex Root); also known as Mao Dang Qing

Description: It is used for blood stagnation, numbness in the arms, and poor blood circulation and is useful for prevention of heart disease including arteriosclerosis, stroke, and embolism.

Dosage: This patent medicine comes in bottles of thirty capsules, with complete instructions on dosage.

Kuan Hsin Su Ho Wan (Cardiovascular Styrax Pills); also known as Guan Xin Su He Wan, or Guan Xin Su Ho Capsules

Description: This formula relieves angina, numbness in the arms, and heart disease. It is also useful for the prevention of myocardial infarction (heart attack) as well as for treatment afterward.

Caution: This formula is prohibited for use during pregnancy.

Dosage: It comes in bottles of thirty pills, with complete instructions on dosage.

Anorexia and Bulimia

Bulimia is an illness characterized by overeating usually followed by self-induced vomiting in an effort to expel food as quickly as possible. In some cases large doses of laxatives are used in addition to or instead of vomiting. Cycles of binge eating followed by purging may occur once a day or several times a day. Severe bulimia can lead to dehydration and loss of potassium, causing symptoms such as lethargy and muscle cramping.

The majority of bulimics are females between ages fifteen and thirty. Distressed about their compulsive behavior, sufferers of bulimia may be depressed and/or suicidal. Quite often bulimia is a variant of another psychiatric disorder, anorexia nervosa, in which dieting is carried to an extreme. Sufferers of both illnesses share a morbid fear of becoming obese.

Anorexia and bulimia are treated similarly. Treatment consists of supervised regulation of eating habits, psychotherapy for resolving the emotional problems at the root of both illnesses, and herbal tonics to support the nutritional effort and increase energy levels.

Voluntary abstention from eating, such as that seen in anorexia nervosa, is practically unheard of in China, which most likely can be attributed to the widespread hunger and starvation that was a part of Chinese history prior to the Communist revolution. Sufferers of anorexia—a disease primarily seen in affluent Western cultures—exhibit the same symptoms (malnutrition and emaciation) normally seen in underdeveloped countries, where there is a shortage of food due to natural disasters, poverty, or overpopulation.

Various opinions exist concerning the precise causes of anorexia. Some theorize that anorexics typically are highly conforming people anxious to please to the point of being obsessive. Others suggest that anorexia is a true phobia of gaining weight, which leads to a fear of eating. Still others insist that it is merely a symptom rather than a separate disease, citing depression, personality disorders, or even schizophrenia as the real cause.

The use of herbal tonics to support the nutritional effort, restore strength, and increase energy levels is highly recommended for treating both anorexia and bulimia. The following herbal tonics can be used to combat the effects of anorexia.

Shi Quan Da Bu Tang (All Inclusive Great Tonifying Decoction)

Original Source: *Tai Ping Hui Min He Ji Ju Fang* (according to *Chinese Herbal Medicine Formulas and Strategies*)

Ingredients:

Quantity (Grams)	Chinese Herbs	English Translation
9	Ren Shen	Ginseng Root
12	Bai Zhu	Atractylodes Rhizome
15	Fu Ling	Tuckahoe Root
6	Zhi Gan Cao	Honey-Cooked Licorice Root
18	Shu Di Huang	Chinese Foxglove Root, Wine-Cooked
15	Bai Shao	White Peony Root
15	Dang Gui	Tangkuei
9	Chuan Xiong	Szechuan Lovage Root
9	Rou Gui	Saigon Cinnamon Inner Bark
18	Huang Qi	Milk-Vetch Root

中
草
藥

Description: The first eight ingredients in this formula are the same as those in Ba Zhen Tang (Eight Treasure Decoction); the last two are what make it different. You should use the formula whose indications most accurately address your particular symptoms. This formula increases energy levels, nourishes and circulates the blood, improves the appetite, eliminates coughing caused by physical exertion, and strengthens the lower extremities.

Analysis: Ren Shen strengthens the entire body by increasing Chi levels. Bai Zhu and Fu Ling strengthen the spleen and resolve dampness. Shu Di Huang, Bai Shao, and Dang Gui, when combined, powerfully enrich the blood, and Chuan Xiong improves its circulation. Rou Gui benefits the kidneys, and Huang Qi increases Chi, strengthens the immune system, and benefits the lungs. Zhi Gan Cao harmonizes the herbs and improves the taste.

Dosage and Method of Preparation: Make a decoction or medicinal wine. For a decoction, drink four ounces of Shi Quan Da Bu Tang tea at room temperature three times daily, or drink six ounces twice daily. For a medicinal wine, drink one ounce of medicinal wine at room temperature three times daily.

Wan Nian Chun Zi Pu Ziang (Thousand Year Spring Nourishing Syrup); also known as Wan Nian Jun Zi Bu Jiang

Description: This general tonic benefits the lungs, liver, spleen, pancreas, and kidneys. It is recommended for health maintenance and cases where there is general weakness and chronic illness, including asthma and arthritis. It is nourishing and addresses problems associated with malnutrition and is considered an excellent tonic for aging persons.

Dosage: This patent medicine comes in bottles of 100cc, with complete instructions on dosage.

Tze Pao Sanpien Extract (Priceless Treasure Three Whip Extract); also known as Zhi Bao San Bian Jing Wan

Description: What might be considered a "super tonic," Tze Pao Sanpien Extract is a broad-spectrum nutritive tonic that should be taken for extended periods (six months minimum; one to two years preferred) to experience its full effects. This patent medicine contains forty-two different ingredients that strengthen the entire body, improve the mind and spirit, strengthen the lower back, empower sexual function, counter fatigue, eliminate spontaneous sweating, improve poor memory, relieve insomnia and chronic asthma, and improve the immune system and weak extremities.

Dosage: It usually comes in a box containing ten vials (10cc each), in a 32-ounce bottle of liquid, or in pill form—all with complete instructions on dosage.

Anxiety

Although Chinese medicine believes that emotional disturbances are for the most part psychosomatic, it recognizes that emotional distress can have physical causes that range from cerebral disorders, to headaches caused by inadequate blood supply to the brain, to hormonal and chemical imbalances (including excess levels of adrenaline). Treating these symptoms is integral to treating the accompanying emotional disorders. Although there is no equivalent to Western psychiatry in Chinese medicine, the use of acupuncture and herbal therapy to calm the spirit are effective for treating minor emotional disorders such as nervousness, agitation, and anxiety.

Anxiety can be either mild or severe. In mild cases it may simply cause feelings of being ill at ease, while in more severe cases it can create feelings of intense fear. A certain amount of anxiety or nervousness is normal; only when it inhibits thoughts and disrupts daily activity is it considered a disorder.

Anxiety is often a symptom of another psychological disorder, such as hypochondria (an abnormal concern about health with the false belief of suffering from illness), depression, or psychosexual disorders. Symptoms of anxiety include palpitations, hyperventilation, dryness of the mouth, tension headaches, restlessness, or an inability to relax, tremors of the hands, nausea, difficulty swallowing, sweating, and blushing.

Traditional Chinese medicine offers several herbal formulas that are useful for anxiety. Their primary functions are to abate restlessness, calm the spirit, and tranquilize the mind.

Tian Wang Bu Xin Wan (Heavenly Spirit Benefit Heart Pill); also known as Tien Wang Pu Hsin Tan, Emperor's Tea, or Tien Wang Bu Xin Wan

Description: This patent formula calms the spirit. It is useful for restlessness, anxiety, palpitations, and insomnia.

Dosage: It comes in bottles of two hundred pills, with complete instructions on dosage.

Bai Tzu Yang Hsin Wan (Biota Seed Support Heart Pill)

Description: This patent formula calms the spirit; it is useful for treating insomnia, anxiety, and mental restlessness, and accompanying dryness of the mouth or lips.

Dosage: It comes in bottles of two hundred pills, with complete instructions on dosage.

Deng Xin Wan (Stabilize Heart Pill); also known as Ding Xin Wan

Description: This patent medicine calms the spirit. Use it to treat restlessness, anxiety, insomnia, palpitations, and poor memory.

Dosage: It comes in bottles of one hundred pills, with complete instructions on dosage.

Appetite, Loss of

Loss of the desire for food is usually temporary and is most often caused by minor illness, fever, emotional disorders, anorexia nervosa, and cold or flu. Persistent or long-term loss of appetite can be symptomatic of a more serious psychological or physical disorder and should be investigated by a physician. Abuse of amphetamine drugs, depression or anxiety, stroke, brain tumors, intestinal disorders, stomach tumors, gastric ulcers, and liver disorders such as hepatitis are all possible causes.

For a person who is generally healthy, appetite usually returns to normal once any underlying cause is diagnosed and treated. The following Chinese herbal formulas can be used to stimulate the appetite.

Xiao Yao San Jia Jian (Rambling Decoction)

Original Source: *Tai Ping Hui Min He Ji Ju Fang* (according to *Chinese Herbal Medicine Formulas and Strategies*)

Ingredients:

Quantity (Grams)	Chinese Herbs	English Translation
9	Dang Gui	Tangkuei
9	Fu Ling	Tuckahoe Root
9	Bai Shao	White Peony Root
9	Bai Zhu	Atractylodes Rhizome
9	Chai Hu	Bupleurum Hare's Ear Root
9	Dan Shen	Salvia Root
6	Mu Xiang	Costus Root
6	Gan Cao	Licorice

Description: This herbal formula is used to resolve loss of appetite.

Analysis: Fu Ling and Bai Zhu benefit the spleen and improve appetite; Chai Hu benefits the liver; Bai Shao, Dan Shen, and Dang Gui all benefit the blood; Mu Xiang benefits the spleen and stomach; and Gan Cao harmonizes all the herbs in this formula and improves the taste.

Dosage and Method of Preparation: Make a decoction. Drink four ounces of Xiao Yao San Jia Jian tea three times daily, as needed.

Bao He Wan Jia Jian (Preserve Harmony Decoction)

Original Source: *Dan Xi Xin Fa* (according to *Chinese Herbal Medicine Formulas and Strategies*)

Ingredients:

Quantity (Grams)	Chinese Herbs	English Translation
9	Bai Zhu	Atractylodes Rhizome
9	Fu Ling	Tuckahoe Root
9	Shen Qu	Medicated Leaven
15	Shan Zha	Hawthorne Fruit
9	Ban Xia	Half Summer
9	Chen Pi	Ripe Tangerine Peel
9	Lai Fu Zi	Radish Seed
6	Lian Qiao	Fruit

| 9 | Ji Nei Jin | Chicken Gizzard Lining |
| 9 | Mai Ya | Barley Sprout |

Description: This herbal formula is used for loss of appetite.

Analysis: Bai Zhu and Fu Ling strengthen the spleen and improve appetite; Shan Zha disperses stagnation of food and benefits digestion, assisted by Shen Qu. Ban Xia and Chen Pi benefit the spleen and calm the stomach, Lai Fu Zi assists in calming the stomach, Lian Qiao clears heat and reduces nodules, and Ji Nei Jin and Mai Ya support the action of the spleen, as well as improving digestion and settling the stomach.

Dosage and Method of Preparation: Make a decoction. Drink four ounces of Bao He Wan Jia Jian tea three times daily, as needed.

Arteriosclerosis

Arteriosclerosis, popularly known as hardening of the arteries, is a condition in which the arteries lose elasticity due to calcium deposits within their lining (Monckeberg's arteriosclerosis) or due to muscle and elastic fibers being replaced by fibrous tissue (medial arteriosclerosis). Both types are characterized by a thickening of the arteries' walls and a narrowing of their channels, which causes hypertension. The impaired circulation of blood through arteries, always a cause for concern, triggers even greater concern when it affects the coronary artery, which supplies blood to the heart.

Although arteriosclerosis mainly affects older people, it can affect anyone regardless of age who is indifferent to his or her health, particularly with regard to diet and exercise. To improve circulation and maintain elasticity of the arteries, traditional Chinese medicine recommends herbal therapy, walking, massage, and participation in Tai Chi Chuan, one of the gentler styles of the martial arts. Additionally, a low-fat diet is recommended to inhibit the formation of cholesterol, whose deposits narrow the channels of the arteries. Consumption of red meat, dairy products, salt, refined sugar, and alcohol should be avoided. Obesity and smoking are also known to exacerbate arteriosclerosis.

Traditional Chinese medicine recommends a single-herb formula as well as some patent formulas to treat arteriosclerosis.

Shan Zha Tang (Hawthorne Berry Tea)

Ingredient:

Quantity (Grams)	Chinese Herb	English Translation
15	Shan Zha	Hawthorne Fruit

Description: Shan Zha tea when consumed several times daily reduces fatty lipids in the blood, lowers cholesterol, and softens the arteries. This formula should be used over a long period of time, preferably two to three years.

Analysis: Shan Zha improves digestion, improves circulation of blood, removes lipids from the arterial walls, and benefits hypertension and coronary heart disease.

Dosage and Method of Preparation: In a tea cup, prepare an infusion by adding eight ounces of boiling water to approximately two tablespoons of Shan Zha; cover the cup and steep for ten to fifteen minutes. Strain off the herb and drink the tea. This formula should be prepared and consumed several times daily for extended periods of time (two to three years recommended).

Du Zhong Pian (Cortex Eucommiae Tablets); also known as Compound Cortex Eucommiae Tablets, and Fu Fang Du Zhong Pian

Description: This formula lowers high blood pressure, decreases cholesterol, reduces hardening of the arteries and blood vessels.

Dosage: It comes in bottles of one hundred tablets, with complete instructions on dosage.

Jing Ya Ping Pian (Hypertension Repressing Tablets); also known as Jiang Ya Ping Pian

Description: This formula is useful for lowering blood pressure and cholesterol levels and for prevention of hardening of the arteries.

Dosage: It comes in boxes of twelve bottles, twelve tablets per bottle, with complete instructions on dosage.

An Sheng Pu Shin Wan (Peaceful Shen Tonify Heart Pill); also known as An Shen Bu Xin Wan

Description: This patent formula relieves obstructions in the blood vessels and is useful for reducing arteriosclerotic plaque that causes hardening of the arteries. It is known for its soothing, tranquilizing effects.

Dosage: It comes in bottles of three hundred pills, with complete instructions on dosage.

Bao Jian Mei Jian Fei Cha (Bojenmi Chinese Tea)

Description: This tea reduces fatty deposits that have accumulated on the walls of the blood vessels, arterial plaque, and high blood pressure.

Dosage: It comes in cans of one hundred grams or as tea bags, with complete instructions on dosage.

Arthritis

Those who suffer from arthritis are well aware that certain climatic conditions are the greatest contributors to the pain and suffering that characterize this disease. These climatic conditions coincide with the name that traditional Chinese medicine has given arthritis, which is wind damp disease or bi-syndrome. Arthritis or wind damp disease is the inflammation of a joint characterized by pain, swelling, stiffness, and redness.

Arthritis may involve one or many joints and can vary in severity from mild aching and stiffness to severe pain. In severe cases arthritis can cause deformity of the joint. Osteoarthritis, also known as degenerative arthritis, is the most common type and is a result of wear and tear on the joints.

Rheumatoid arthritis, the most severe type of inflammatory joint disease, is an autoimmune deficiency disorder in which the body's immune system acts against and damages the joints and surrounding soft tissues, causing many joints—most commonly those in the hands, feet, and arms—to become painful, stiff, and deformed.

Still's disease, or juvenile rheumatoid arthritis, is most common in children under age four. It usually clears up after a few years, but even then it may stunt growth and leave the child with permanent deformities.

Seronegative arthritis is a group of disorders that causes symptoms and signs of arthritis in a number of joints. Although blood-test results for rheumatoid arthritis are negative with this disease, the two share many of the same symptoms. It can be associated with skin disorders such as psoriasis, inflammatory intestinal disorders such as Crohn's disease, or autoimmune deficiency disorders.

Infective arthritis (also known as septic or pyogenic arthritis) is a joint disease caused by the invasion of bacteria into the joint from a nearby infected wound or as a result of an infection in the bloodstream. The affected joint usually becomes hot, swollen, and painful. Infective arthritis may also occur as a complication of an infection elsewhere in the body, such as chicken pox, German measles, mumps, rheumatic fever, or gonorrhea. It may also be a complication of nonspecific inflammation of the urethra (the canal that discharges urine, which extends from the bladder to the body's exterior), in which case it is referred to as Reiter's syndrome.

Ankylosing spondylitis is arthritis of the spine, wherein the joints linking the vertebrae become inflamed and the vertebrae fuse. This type of arthritis may spread to other joints, most often to the hips. Gout is associated with another form of arthritis in which uric acid (one of the body's waste products) accumulates in the joints in the form of crystals, causing inflammation and usually affecting one joint at a time.

The following herbal formulas can be successfully used to combat the symptoms associated with arthritis.

Gui Zhi Shao Yao Zhi Mu Tong (Cinnamon Twig, Peony and Anemarrhena Decoction)

Original Source: *Jin Gui Yao Lue* (according to *Chinese Herbal Medicine Formulas and Strategies*)

Ingredients:

Quantity (Grams)	Chinese Herbs	English Translation
12	Gui Zhi	Saigon Cinnamon Twig
6	Ma Huang	Yellow Hemp
6	Fu Zi	Accessory Root Szechuan Aconite
6	Zhi Mu	Anemarrhena Root
9	Bai Shao Yao	White Peony Root
15	Bai Zhu	Atractylodes Rhizome
12	Fang Feng	Guard Against the Wind Root

中草藥

| 15 | Sheng Jiang | Fresh Ginger Root |
| 6 | Gan Cao | Licorice Root |

Description: This formula can be used for painful, swollen joints that are warm to the touch, especially the legs, knees, and ankles, with stiffness and reduced range of motion. It is also useful for rheumatoid arthritis, connective-tissue disorders, and gout.

Analysis: The chief herb, Gui Zhi, unblocks the channels (the meridians) and improves circulation. It is assisted by Ma Huang and Fu Zi, which both strengthen this effect while also relieving pain. Zhi Mu and Bai Shao Yao clear heat and prevent dryness (thus preventing lack of lubrication). Bai Zhu assists by removing dampness and, with the aid of Fang Feng, strengthens the formula's function of expelling wind and dampness. Sheng Jiang stimulates movement and strengthens the action of the other herbs in the formula. Gan Cao harmonizes their action (allowing them to work together without upsetting the stomach) and improves the taste of the formula.

Dosage and Method of Preparation: Make a decoction. Drink four ounces of Gui Zhi Shao Yao Zhi Mu Tong tea at room temperature three times daily, or drink six ounces twice daily.

Juan Bi Tang (Remove Painful Obstruction Decoction)

Original Source: *Yi Xue Xin Wu* (according to *Chinese Herbal Medicine Formulas and Strategies*)

Ingredients:

Quantity (Grams)	Chinese Herbs	English Translation
6	Qiang Huo	Notopterygium Rhizome
6	Du Huo	Self-Reliant Existence Root
6	Qin Jiao	Gentiana Qinjiao
18	Sang Zhi	Mulberry Twigs
18	Hai Feng Teng	Sea Wind Vine Stem
18	Dang Gui	Tangkuei
4	Chuan Xiong	Szechuan Lovage Root
5	Ru Xiang	Frankincense Resin
5	Mu Xiang	Costus Root

| 3 | Rou Gui | Saigon Cinnamon Inner Bark |
| 3 | Zhi Gan Cao | Honey-Cooked Licorice Root |

Description: This formula is used for relief from joint pain that increases in cold, damp weather and is also useful for osteoarthritis, rheumatoid arthritis, gout, and bursitis.

Analysis: The two chief herbs in this formula, Qiang Huo and Du Huo, used together relieve painful joints in both the upper and lower extremities of the body. Qin Jiao, Sang Zhi, and Hai Feng Teng all effectively expel dampness from the bones and joints. Dang Gui and Chuan Xiong improve circulation, which helps to eliminate pain. Ru Xiang assists in circulation and helps to reduce localized pain, Mu Xiang benefits the spleen and improves fluid metabolism, Rou Gui improves circulation and directs the action of the other herbs in this formula, and Zhi Gan Cao harmonizes their actions and improves the taste of the decoction.

Dosage and Method of Preparation: Make a decoction. Drink four ounces of Juan Bi Tang tea at room temperature three times daily, or drink six ounces twice daily.

Jian Bu Hu Qian Wan (Walk Vigorously [Like] a Tiger Stealthily Pill); also known as Chen Pu Hu Chien Wan

Description: This patent formula benefits the tendons and bones and is appropriate for chronic arthritis, lumbago, and sciatica.

Dosage: It comes in bottles of two hundred pills, with complete instructions on dosage.

Feng Shih Hsiao Tung Wan (Wind Damp Dispel Pain Pill); also known as Feng Shi Xiao Tong Wan

Description: This patent formula is excellent for rheumatism that causes lower backache, chronic sciatica, or pain in the joints, including fingers, shoulders, knees, and hips.

Dosage: It comes in bottles of two hundred pills, with complete instructions on dosage.

Guan Jie Yan Wan (Close Down Joint Inflammation Pill)

Description: This patent formula is for arthritis, rheumatism, and aching joints and is useful for a periodic flare-up of the sciatic nerve as well as rheumatoid arthritis.

Caution: This patent formula is prohibited for use during pregnancy.

Dosage: It comes in bottles of three hundred pills, with complete instructions on dosage.

Ta Huo Lo Tan (Chinese Old Man Tea); also known as Da Huo Lou Dan

Description: This patent formula is useful for joint pain, back pain, stiff muscles, and difficulty walking or sitting.

Caution: This formula is prohibited for use during pregnancy.

Dosage: It comes in bottles of forty pills, with complete instructions on dosage.

Tian Ma Hu Gu Wan (Gastrodia Tiger Bone Pill)

Description: This patent formula is useful for dampness that has affected bones, muscles, and the lower back. It is excellent for chronic or acute arthritis and rheumatism that causes pain and numbness in the arms and legs.

Dosage: This patent medicine comes in bottles of sixty pills, with complete instructions on dosage.

Tu Zhung Feng Shi Wan (Eucommia Bark Wind Damp Pills); also known as Du Zhong Feng Shi Wan

Description: This patent formula strengthens the bones and tendons as well as stops pain. It is useful for rheumatic and arthritic aching joints and the lower back, including pain that moves from joint to joint, inflammations, and gout.

Caution: This formula is prohibited for use during pregnancy.

Dosage: It comes in bottles of 60 or 120 pills with complete instructions on dosage.

Asthma

The Chi Kung exercises (a type of breath therapy) that are at the root of all Chinese physical therapies rank above martial arts and all other classical exercises in terms of their contribution to overall health. Chi Kung combined with herbal therapy provides substantial benefits for those who suffer from chronic respiratory diseases. Chi Kung is considered in traditional Chinese medicine to be an essential part of treatment.

One of the more common respiratory diseases is bronchial asthma; the two main types of asthma are extrinsic, in which an allergy, usually to something inhaled, triggers the attack, and intrinsic, which has no apparent external cause.

The most common allergens responsible for triggering extrinsic bronchial asthma are pollens, house dust, dust mites, animal fur, dander, and feathers. It can also be the result of a respiratory infection from such triggers as a cold, cough, bronchitis, or by exercising in cold air, inhaling tobacco smoke or other air pollutants, or by an allergic reaction to a particular food or drug (most commonly aspirin).

Intrinsic asthma tends to develop later in life than extrinsic asthma, and an attack is most often triggered by emotional factors such as stress, anxiety, or depression.

The main symptoms of asthma are breathlessness, wheezing, a dry cough, and tightness in the chest. During a severe attack breathing becomes increasingly difficult, causing sweating, rapid heartbeat, great distress, and anxiety. The sufferer cannot lie down or sleep, may be unable to speak, wheezes loudly, and breathes rapidly. In a very severe attack the low amount of oxygen in the blood can cause facial cyanosis (blue-purple skin discoloration), in which case the lips and the skin may become pale and clammy. Such attacks can be fatal; it is therefore advisable to seek emergency professional help!

Although there is no known cure for asthma, attacks can to a large extent be prevented. For sufferers of extrinsic asthma, allergy tests are available to discover which common allergens trigger attacks. When a specific cause is discovered, steps can be taken to avoid the allergen. For example, if pollen is the cause, the sufferer will need to avoid parks and gardens during the pollen season; he or she might also consider wearing a surgical mask to filter out the pollen. If the dust mite is responsible, mattresses and pillows should be stored in airtight plastic covers, and the home should be kept as dust-free as possible.

Many Western doctors recommend using a bronchodilator (a type of drug that widens the airways) to control asthma attacks. In addition, Chinese herbs can be used during high-pollen seasons or during exposure to other known allergens to minimize attacks and treat related symptoms such as cough, phlegm and mucus, and wheezing. All of the following formulas can be used to treat asthma.

Xiao Qing Long Tang (Minor Blue Green Dragon Decoction)

Original Source: *Shang Han Lun* (according to *Chinese Herbal Medicine Formulas and Strategies*)

Ingredients:

Quantity (Grams)	Chinese Herbs	English Translation
9	Ma Huang★	Yellow Hemp
9	Gui Zhi	Saigon Cinnamon Twig
3	Gan Jiang	Dried Ginger Root
3	Xi Xin	Chinese Wild Ginger Plant
3	Wu Wei Zi	Schizandra Fruit
9	Bai Shao	White Peony Root
9	Ban Xia	Half Summer
9	Zhi Gan Cao	Honey-Cooked Licorice Root

★Persons with high blood pressure should not use Ma Huang; instead substitute 9 grams of Bai Qian (White Before Rhizome).

Description: This is an excellent formula for the relief of asthma with fever, chills, coughing, wheezing, thick sputum, difficulty expectorating, a tight sensation in the chest, or difficulty breathing when lying down.

Analysis: The chief herb, Ma Huang, is frequently used for treating asthma. It effectively arrests wheezing and sweats out viruses or toxins while strengthening the lungs. Gui Zhi assists in this action. Gan Jiang and Xi Xin relieve congestion and phlegm and also stop coughing. Wu Wei Zi fortifies lung Chi, Bai Shao nourishes the blood, Ban Xia settles the stomach, and Zhi Gan Cao harmonizes the actions of the other herbs and improves the taste of the decoction.

Dosage and Method of Preparation: Make a decoction. Drink four ounces of Xiao Qing Long Tang tea at room temperature three times daily, or drink six ounces twice daily, as needed.

Ding Chuan Tang (Arrest Wheezing Decoction)

Original Source: *Fu Shou Jing Fang* (according to *Chinese Herbal Medicine Formulas and Strategies*)

Ingredients:

Quantity (Grams)	Chinese Herbs	English Translation
9	Ma Huang★	Yellow Hemp
6	Su Zi	Purple Perilla Fruit
3	Gan Cao	Licorice Root
9	Kuan Dong Hua	Tussilago Flower
4.5	Xing Ren	Almond Kernel
9	Sang Bai Pi	Bark Mulberry Root
4.5	Huang Qin	Baical Skullcap Root
9	Ban Xia	Half Summer
21 pieces	Yin Xing	Gingko Nut Seed

★Persons with high blood pressure should not use Ma Huang; instead substitute 9 grams of Bai Qian (White Before Rhizome).

Description: For those who suffer from asthma, this formula will relieve coughing and wheezing accompanied by thick copious sputum and labored breathing.

Analysis: Ma Huang will arrest wheezing and strengthen the lungs while it opens the pores and causes sweating. Yin Xing clears phlegm and assists in controlling wheezing. Xing Ren reinforces the action of the first two herbs, Ban Xia calms the stomach and, with the assistance of Su Zi and Kuan Dong Hua, arrests wheezing and expels phlegm. Sang Bai Pi and Huang Qin drain heat from the lungs and stop coughing, while Gan Cao harmonizes the actions of the other ingredients and improves the taste.

Dosage and Method of Preparation: Make a decoction. Drink four ounces of Ding Chuan Tang tea at room temperature three times daily, or drink six ounces twice daily, as needed.

Chuan Ke Ling (Asthma Cough Efficacious Remedy)

Description: For those with symptoms of asthma, this patent medicine strengthens the lungs, resolves phlegm, assists labored breathing, and stops coughing. It is useful for asthma, bronchitis, or emphysema.

Dosage: It comes in bottles of one hundred tablets, with complete instructions on dosage.

Ping Chuan Wan (Calm Asthma Pill); also known as Ping Chuan Pills

Description: This patent formula is useful for chronic asthma, bronchitis, and emphysema. It strengthens the lungs, stops coughing, resolves phlegm, and relieves labored breathing.

Dosage: It comes in bottles of 120 pills, with complete instructions on dosage.

San She Dan Chuan Bei Ye (Three Snake Gallbladder with Fritillaria Liquid)

Description: This liquid patent formula is useful for asthma, bronchitis, or emphysema. It is particularly helpful in resolving stubborn phlegm; it also clears lung heat and stops coughing.

Dosage: It is a liquid extract that comes in a package containing six vials (10cc each), with complete instructions on dosage.

Athlete's Foot (see also Fungal Infections/Fungal Diseases; Ringworm)

Caused by a fungal infection known as tinea pedia, athlete's foot is commonly contracted by walking barefoot in pubic showers and locker rooms. It is most often treated with topical salves, creams, and lotions or by bathing the feet in antifungal washes.

Chinese herbology takes a somewhat different approach to treating athlete's foot by offering pills that can be used to eliminate it. They may also prevent initial infection if taken preventively.

Peng Sha (Borax)

Ingredient:

Quantity (Grams)	Chinese Herb	English Translation
10–15	Peng Sha (buy it powdered)	Borax, Mineral Salt

Description: This one-herb raw formula is used directly on the infected area to destroy the bacterial fungus found in athlete's foot. It prevents putrefaction, detoxifies poison, reduces swelling, and kills bacteria.

Analysis: It clears pathogens, toxins, and fungi from the body.

Method of Preparation: This powder can be sprinkled between the toes and on the infected area or mixed with water to make a paste and applied to the infected area. Use as needed until the infection clears up.

Note: This formula is for use externally—do not use internally!

Mi Tuo Seng (Galena)

Ingredient:

Quantity (Grams)	Chinese Herb	English Translation
10–15	Mi Tuo Seng (buy it powdered)	Galena

Description: This one-herb raw formula is excellent for athlete's foot; it absorbs fluids, reduces swelling, drains sores, ulcers, and damp skin eruptions, and eliminates leukoderma (deficiency of pigmentation in the skin, especially in patches).

Analysis: Mi Tou Seng drains pus and eliminates ulcers and various forms of leukoderma.

Method of Preparation: It can be used topically as a powder; sprinkle it onto the infected area, or add water and make it into a paste to apply to the infected area. Use as needed.

Note: This formula is for external use only—do not use internally!

San She Jie Yang Wan (Three Snake Dispel Itching Pill); also known as Tri-Snake Itch Removing Pills

Description: This patent formula dispels toxins, relieves itching, and is useful for a variety of pruritus dermatitis, eczema, and fungal infections.

Caution: This formula is prohibited for use during pregnancy.

Dosage: It comes in bottles of thirty pills, with complete instructions on dosage.

Hua She Jie Yang Wan (Pit Viper Dispel Itching Pill); also known as Kai Yeung Pills

Description: This patent formula counteracts the itch caused by athlete's foot and relieves various forms of pruritus and fungal infections.

Dosage: It comes in bottles of sixty pills, with complete instructions on dosage.

Back Pain

Back pain has many possible causes; therefore, it is advisable to seek medical advice to determine whether it is caused by an injury to the supporting tissues (muscles, spine, nerves) or due to a disease of the internal organs.

Most people at some time in their lives suffer from what is called nonspecific back pain. Nonspecific back pain is thought to be caused by mechanical disorders affecting one or more of the body's structures. The disorder can be a ligament strain, a muscle tear, or damage to a spinal disk. In addition to the pain created by the damaged structure, spasms from surrounding muscles can create pain and tenderness over a broader area. People most likely to suffer from this type of back pain are those whose jobs involve heavy lifting and carrying or those who spend long periods of time sitting in one position or bending awkwardly.

Other possible causes of back pain are abnormalities of a joint or a prolapsed disk (dislocation of a disk), which can cause sciatica (pain in the buttocks and down the back or side of the leg); osteoarthritis, which can cause persistent back pain; ankylosing spondylitis (arthritis in the spine), which causes pain and stiffness with loss of back mobility; fibrositis, or pain and tenderness in the large back muscles; and coccygodynia or pain in the base of the spine (coccyx or tailbone).

Once a specific cause for back pain has been established, traditional Chinese medicine offers several different treatment options.

Back pain caused by muscle strains, tears, or weakness is treated with *tui na* massage, herbs, ointments and liniments, and moxabustion (heat therapy). Osteoarthritis is treated with acupuncture, herbal therapy, hot herbal compresses and plasters. Fibrositis is treated with *tui na* massage, herbal therapy, ointments and liniments, hot compresses (for strains), and cold compresses (for inflammation and swelling). Ankylosing spondylitis and coccygodynia are treated with acupuncture, herbal therapy, plasters, cold compresses (for inflammation and swelling), and hot compresses (when there is no swelling).

In cases of sciatica, which is often caused by a slipped or prolapsed intervertebral disk pressing on a spinal root of the sciatic nerve, two recommendations are offered: consultation with an osteopathic physician or consultation with a chiropractor, whose adjustments can often remedy the problem.

The following herbal formulas can be used to treat back pain:

Du Huo Ji Sheng Tang (Angelica Pubescens and Sang Ji Sheng Decoction)

Original Source: *Qian Jin Yao Fang* (according to *Chinese Herbal Medicine Formulas and Strategies*)

Ingredients:

Quantity (Grams)	Chinese Herbs	English Translation
9	Du Huo	Self Reliant Existence Root
6	Xi Xin	Chinese Wild Ginger Root
6	Fang Feng	Guard Against the Wind Root
6	Qin Jiao	Gentiana Qinjiao
15	Sang Ji Sheng	Mulberry Parasite Stem
6	Du Zhong	Eucommia Bark
6	Niu Xi	Ox Knee Root
6	Rou Gui	Saigon Cinnamon Inner Bark
6	Dang Gui	Tangkuei
6	Chuan Xiong	Szechuan Lovage Root
6	Sheng Di Huang	Chinese Foxglove Root, Raw

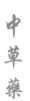
中
草
藥

6	Bai Shao	White Peony Root
6	Ren Shen	Ginseng
6	Fu Ling	Tuckahoe Root
6	Zhi Gan Cao	Honey-Cooked Licorice Root

Description: This raw herb formula relieves fixed pain in the lower back that is accompanied by weakness, stiffness, and/or numbness.

Analysis: The chief herb in this formula, Du Huo, expels wind and dampness from the lower extremities. Xi Xin assists in expelling wind-damp from the bones and also reduces pain. Fang Feng and Qin Jiao relax the sinews. Sang Ji Sheng, Du Zhong, and Niu Xi all expel dampness and benefit the liver and kidneys. Rou Gui unblocks the meridians and is an important herb for treating lower back pain. Dang Gui, Chuan Xiong, Bai Shao, and Sheng Di Huang serve the important function of enriching and circulating the blood. Ren Shen and Fu Ling combine to strengthen the body by increasing energy (Chi) and also benefit the spleen. Zhi Gan Cao harmonizes the other herbs in the formula and improves the taste of the decoction.

Dosage and Method of Preparation: Make a decoction. Drink four ounces of Du Huo Ji Sheng Tang tea at room temperature three times daily, or six ounces twice daily.

Kang Gu Zeng Sheng Pian (Combat Bone Hyperplasis Pill)

Description: This patent medicine tonifies the bones and is useful for ankylosing spondylitis (inflammation of the spine) and for back pain with accompanying numbness.

Dosage: It comes in bottles of one hundred tablets, with complete instructions on dosage.

Hu Gu Gao (Tiger Balm)

Description: This salve relieves muscle strain and sprain, alleviates stiffness, and reduces pain.

Dosage: It comes in bottles of 0.63 ounces, with complete instructions on dosage.

Die Da Zhi Tong Gao (Traumatic Injury Stop Pain Plaster); also known as Plaster for Bruise and Analgesic

Description: This is a medicated plaster adhesive used to stimulate healing and stop pain. It is used for bruises, sprains, fractures, muscle strain, and neuralgia.

Caution: Pregnant women should not apply this patent medicine to the lower abdomen.

Dosage: It comes in boxes of ten pieces or in a single long piece, with complete instructions on dosage.

Yao Tong Pian (Antilumbago Tablets); also known as Yao Tong Wan

Description: This patent formula strengthens the tendons and bones, alleviates pain, and is useful for lumbago, lower back pain, and sciatica.

Dosage: It comes in bottles of one hundred tablets, with complete instructions on dosage.

Shen Xian Jin Bu Huan Gao (Magic Plaster Not to Be Exchanged for Gold)

Description: A topical plaster that is used for muscle strain or sprain, numbness, or weakness in the muscle. It is known to invigorate the blood and relieve pain.

Caution: Pregnant women should not use this formula on the abdomen or lower back.

Dosage: It comes in a box containing a single cloth, with complete instructions on dosage.

Baldness

Baldness, clinically known as alopecia, is the loss or absence of hair. It is usually noticeable only on the scalp, but it can occur anywhere on the body. Hereditary alopecia (the most common type of baldness) is more commonly called male pattern baldness. It primarily affects men, although young women and women who have passed menopause are occasionally affected.

Generalized alopecia is a rare form of baldness wherein the hair falls out in large amounts. Such hair loss occurs because all the hairs simultaneously enter the resting phase and then fall out about three months later. Regrowth occurs when the cause is corrected. Causes for generalized alopecia include stress, fever, prolonged illness, or chemotherapy.

Localized alopecia is caused by permanent damage to the skin, by burns, or by radiation therapy.

Other possible causes of hair loss are trauma to the roots from excessive pulling when styling the hair, a nervous disorder in which sufferers pull out their own hair, fungal infection of the scalp (tinea), or other skin diseases such as lichen planus, lupus erythematosus, or skin tumors.

Alopecia universalis, a rare, permanent form of baldness, causes all of the hair on the head and body to fall out, including eyelashes and brows. Some forms of temporary baldness are treatable, such as scalp infections (tinea, ringworm, and dandruff), which can be treated with antifungal herbal preparations and by regularly massaging the scalp with almond oil to improve circulation.

Chinese medicine also recommends the use of tonic medicines, including a decoction of Ren Shen (Ginseng), with Gou Qi Zi (Matrimony Vine Root) and Hu Ma Ren (Black Sesame Seeds) that has been sweetened with Feng Wang Jiang (Royal Jelly) to provide the scalp with nutrients. The most effective Chinese herbs for promoting hair growth are Han Lian Cao (Eclipta Plant) and Nu Zhen Zi (Privet Fruit). Sang Shen Jiu (Mulberry Wine) is also considered helpful for hair loss.

Traditional Chinese medicine cites anemia, deficiencies in the thyroid hormones, contraceptive pills, antibiotics, and steroids as the greatest contributing factors to temporary hair loss. The following formulas are said to combat baldness:

Tong Qiao Huo Xue Tang (Unblock the Orifices and Invigorate the Blood Decoction)

Original Source: *Yi Lin Qai Cuo* (according to *Chinese Herbal Medicine Formulas and Strategies*)

Ingredients:

Quantity (Grams)	Chinese Herbs	English Translation
3	Chi Shao	Red Peony Root
3	Tao Ren	Peach Kernel
3	Chuan Xiong	Szechuan Lovage Root
3	Hong Hua	Safflower Flower
3	Cong Bai	Scallion
9	Sheng Jiang	Fresh Ginger Root
.15	She Xiang	Musk Deer Gland Secretions
7 pieces	Da Zao	Jujube Fruit

Description: This formula invigorates the blood, opens up the orifices, repairs hair loss, and improves dark-purple complexion and darkness around the eyes.

Analysis: Chi Shao and Chuan Xiong combine to open the pores (orifices) and increase blood circulation. Tao Ren and Hong Hua assist in circulating the blood. Cong Bai increases vital energy (Chi), and Sheng Jiang settles the stomach and corrects nutritional impairment. She Xiang supports the actions of all the previous herbs, while Da Zao harmonizes the other herbs in the formula.

Dosage and Method of Preparation: Make a decoction. Drink four ounces of Tong Qiao Huo Xue Tang tea at room temperature three times daily, or drink six ounces twice daily.

Qi Bao Mei Ran Dan (Seven Treasure Special Decoction for Beautiful Hair and Whiskers)

Original Source: *Yi Fang Ji Jie* (according to *Chinese Herbal Medicine Formulas and Strategies*)

Ingredients:

Quantity (Grams)	Chinese Herbs	English Translation
30	He Shou Wu	Polygonum Shouwu
15	Fu Ling	Tuckahoe Root
15	Niu Xi	Ox Knee Root
15	Dang Gui	Tangkuei
15	Gou Qi Zi	Matrimony Vine Fruit
15	Tu Su Zi	Dodder Seeds
12	Bu Gu Zhi	Scuffy Pea Fruit

中
草
藥

Description: This raw herb formula is excellent for hair loss and to prevent premature graying of hair.

Analysis: He Shou Wu is used here for strengthening the bones and sinews; this herb is also know for its ability to benefit the hair. Gou Qi Zi and Tu Su Zi nourish the liver and kidneys. Niu Xi assists in strengthening the bones and sinews. Dang Gui is added to enrich the blood and assist the chief herb (He Shou Wu) in nourishing the hair. Bu Gu Zhi strengthens the energy (Chi), while Fu Ling strengthens the spleen and resolves dampness.

Dosage and Method of Preparation: Make a decoction. Drink four ounces of Qi Bao Mei Ran Dan tea at room temperature three times daily, or drink six ounces twice daily.

Belching

Belching is not a disease but instead is usually a symptom of other disorders or diseases such as liver disease, gallbladder disease, heartburn, indigestion, dyspepsia, or hyperacidity. Some of the more common causes for belching are excessive acidity in the stomach, excessive use of alcohol, insufficient bile secretion, eating or drinking too quickly or too much, and insufficient mastication (chewing of food).

Chinese herbal remedies are mostly geared toward neutralizing the stomach acids with calcium-based ingredients (such as powdered cuttlefish bone), restoring gastrointestinal balance, and quelling stomach heat. The following herbal formulas can be used to relieve belching; however, in chronic or recurring cases refer to the entries in this chapter for the diseases and disorders listed above:

Ping Wei San (Calm the Stomach Decoction)

Original Source: *Tai Ping Hui Min He Ji Ju Fang* (according to *Chinese Herbal Medicine Formulas and Strategies*)

Ingredients:

Quantity (Grams)	Chinese Herbs	English Translation
15	Cang Zhu	Atractylodes Cangzhu
12	Huo Po	Magnolia Bark
12	Chen Pi	Ripe Tangerine Peel

6	Zhi Gan Cao	Honey-Cooked Licorice Root

Description: This raw herb formula will relieve stomach distention and fullness, diarrhea, belching, nausea, and acid regurgitation.

Analysis: Cang Zhu is one of the most important herbs in Chinese herbology for dispelling dampness and strengthening the spleen. Huo Po also dispels dampness and corrects abdominal bloating by strengthening the spleen. Chen Pi calms the stomach and eliminates belching. Zhi Gan Cao harmonizes the herbs in the formula.

Dosage and Method of Preparation: Make a decoction. Drink four ounces of Ping Wei San tea at room temperature three times daily, or as needed.

Wei Te Ling "204" (Stomach Especially Effective Remedy)

Description: This patent formula is useful for acute gastritis, excessive stomach acid, bloating, belching, and flatulence with pain.

Dosage: It comes in bottles of 120 pills, with complete instructions on dosage.

Mu Xiang Shun Qi Wan (Saussurea Smooth Chi Pills); also known as Aplotaxis Carminative Pills

Description: This patent formula is for upset stomach caused by liver congestion, belching, abdominal distention (bloating), and nausea.

Dosage: This patent medicine comes in a bottle of two hundred pills, with complete instructions on dosage.

Shen Ling Bai Zhu Pian (Codonopsis Poria Atractylodes Pills); also known as Shenling Baizhupian

Description: This patent formula is for belching, bloated stomach, indigestion, and loose stools.

Dosage: It comes in bottles of 150 pills, with complete instructions on dosage.

中草藥

Shu Kan Wan/Condensed (Smooth Liver Pill); also known as Shu Gan Wan Nong Suo

Description: This patent formula relieves abdominal gas, hiccups, belching, flatulence, abdominal pain, and indigestion.

Dosage: It comes in a bottle of 120 pills, with complete instructions on dosage.

Bell's Palsy (Facial Paralysis)

In spite of the fact that sufferers of herpes zoster (shingles) occasionally experience Bell's palsy (more commonly called facial paralysis), the occurrence is so infrequent that no positive connection can be made, and the exact cause remains a mystery to Western medicine. Traditional Chinese medicine, on the other hand, cites the effect on facial nerves of wind and dampness as the cause and recommends that sufferers of Bell's palsy undergo remedial facial exercises and combine acupuncture treatment with herbal therapy.

Symptoms, which include drooping of the eyelid and mouth on one side of the face with an inability to close the eye, can be severe, but normally it is a temporary condition, and sufferers can expect complete recovery. Traditional Chinese medicine has found some success treating Bell's palsy with the following formulas:

Bell's Palsy Formula

Ingredients:

Quantity (Grams)	Chinese Herbs	English Translation
6	Chuan Wu Tou	Aconitum Appendage
6	Cao Wu	Aconite Beiwutou
6	Ban Xia	Half Summer
6	Wei Ling Xian	Chinese Clematis Root
6	Bai Ji	Blettilla Rhizome
6	Chen Pi	Ripe Tangerine Peel

Description: This raw herb formula provides relief from the symptoms of Bell's palsy, including facial paralysis and involuntary muscle twitching.

Analysis: The chief herb, Chuan Wu Tou, warms the meridians and relieves cold and dampness. Cao Wu strengthens the function of the chief herb, and Ban Xia clears dampness. Wei Ling Xian is antirheumatic; it circulates Chi and also dispels dampness. Bai Ji reduces inflammation, and Chen Pi activates the Chi.

Method of Preparation: Powder the above herbs and mix them with enough ginger juice to form a paste. Apply the paste topically to the affected area. (Ginger juice is available commercially in Asian-food or health-food stores, or it can be made by blending ginger-root pieces in a blender on medium and then placing the ginger in a five-by-five-inch square of cheesecloth and squeezing out the juice.)

Qian Zheng Tang (Lead to Symmetry Decoction)

Original Source: *Yang Shi Jia Zang Fang* (according to *Chinese Herbal Medicine Formulas and Strategies*)

Ingredients:

Quantity (Grams)	Chinese Herbs	English Translation
6	Bai Fu Zi	White Appendage Rhizome
6	Jiang Can	Dead Body of Sick Silkworm
6	Quan Xie	Scorpion

Description: This formula is for relief of sudden facial paralysis with deviation of the eye and mouth and a muscle twitch.

Analysis: Bai Fu Zi dispels wind, stops spasms, and is especially effective for treating the head and face. Jiang Can extinguishes internal wind and dispels external wind. Quan Xie is very effective for stopping spasms, unblocking the meridians, and alleviating facial paralysis.

Dosage and Method of Preparation: Make a decoction. Drink four ounces of Qian Zheng Tang tea at room temperature three times daily, or drink six ounces twice daily.

Ren Shen Zai Zao Wan (Ginseng Restorative Pills); also known as Tsai Tsao Wan

Description: This patent formula provides relief from hemiplegia (paralysis on one half of the body), contractive facial muscles, and numbness or tingling of muscles and is useful in Bell's palsy (wind-induced facial paralysis).

Caution: This formula is prohibited for use during pregnancy.

Dosage: It comes in bottles of fifty pills, with complete instructions on dosage.

Tian Ma Chu Feng Pu Pien (Gastrodia Dispel Wind Tablets); also known as Tian Ma Qu Feng Bu Pian

Description: This patent formula is for relief from facial paralysis, earache, headache, and joint and muscle stiffness.

Dosage: This patent medicine comes in bottles of sixty tablets, with complete instructions on dosage.

Bladder Cancer

Bladder cancer, which accounts for approximately 4 percent of all cancers diagnosed in the United States, affects a disproportionate number of Americans compared to the number of cases reported among the Chinese population. For unknown reasons men are three times more likely to suffer from bladder cancer than women. Certain groups have been shown to be at increased risk, notably smokers and workers in the dye and rubber industries. Exposure to tobacco smoke and to carcinogenic substances used in these industries is presumed to be the cause. Recent research has shown an increased incidence of bladder cancer occurring in tropical areas, where the parasitic infection schistosomiasis is prevalent.

The main symptom of bladder cancer is blood in the urine. Ordinarily, passing urine is painless with bladder cancer; however, a bladder infection can develop, causing painful and frequent urination. Occasionally, a tumor may obstruct the urethral exit, making urination difficult (see also Cystitis; Urine Retention). While some progress has been made in treating bladder cancer, like all cancers it is a condition more easily prevented than cured. Traditional Chinese medicine offers a wide range of preventive medicines as well as dietary and lifestyle recommendations. These for the most part emphasize avoiding suspected carcinogens and strengthening the immune system. Chinese physicians believe that strengthening the immune system (called the Wei Chi) through the use of herbal therapy, along with a sound diet, stress reduction, and moderate habits (avoiding too much sex, alcohol, and processed foods), can do much to prevent cancer.

Dietary recommendations include the use of garlic, Chinese yams, mandarin oranges, and Chinese mushrooms. Practitioners also point out that a lower incidence of all cancers occurs when olive oil, cereal, fresh fruit and vegetables, fish, and whole grains are featured prominently in the diet. Stress is considered a contributing factor to cancer and can be reduced by practicing Chi Kung (breathing exercises) and meditation, which includes standing and sitting meditations, and the form of moving meditation known as Tai Chi Chuan.

An excellent book on Chinese medicines used to fight cancer is *Treating Cancer with Chinese Herbs,* by Hong-Yen Hsu. According to the author, the following formula has been used to treat bladder cancer:

Chia Wei Tao Jen Cheng Chi Tang (Modified Persica and Rhubarb Combination)

Source: *Treating Cancer with Chinese Herbs*
Ingredients:

Quantity (Grams)	Chinese Herbs	English Translation
12	Zhi Zi	Gardenia Fruit
15	Gan Cao	Licorice
9	Tao Ren	Peach Kernel
9	Mang Xiao	Mirabilite
9	Da Huang	Rhubarb Root
9	Dang Gui	Tangkuei
9	Feng Wei Cao	Phoenix Tail Fern
7.5	Rou Gui	Saigon Cinnamon Inner Bark
6	Xi Jiao	Rhinoceros Horn
6	Jin Sha Teng	Climbing Japanese Fern

Description: This formula is for the treatment of cancer of the urinary bladder.

Analysis: Zhi Zi clears pathogenic heat from the blood, reduces inflammation, and eliminates toxins. Tao Ren improves blood circulation and eliminates blood clots. Mang Xiao, another anti-inflammatory, softens the stool and assists Da Huang, which removes intestinal heat and promotes bowel movement. Dang Gui nourishes the blood and relieves pain. Feng Wei Cao and Jin Sha Teng, combined, clear infection, promote urination, and detoxify poisons in the urinary bladder. Rou Gui benefits the kidneys and urinary bladder and is useful for treating boils or nodules in either organ. Xi Jiao cools the blood and eliminates toxicity while Gan Cao moves the vital energy (Chi) and harmonizes the other herbs in the formula.

Dosage and Method of Preparation: Make a decoction. Drink four ounces of Chia Wei Tao Jen Cheng Chi Tang tea at room temperature three times daily, or drink six ounces twice daily.

Bladder Infection—see Cystitis

Blood Poisoning—see Septicemia

Blood Pressure—see Hypertension

Bloody Nose—see Nosebleed

Boils—see Carbuncles

Bones: Brittle, Broken, Fractured, and Cancer

Under normal circumstances healthy bone must be subjected to repeated stress or trauma for a fracture or break to occur. In some cases, however, bones' strength and rigidity is undermined due to nutritional deficiency (lack of calcium and vitamin D) or diseases such as osteoporosis (softening of the bones), osteogenesis imperfecta (fragile or brittle bones, where fractures occur with minimal trauma), or bone cancer (when a malignant growth replaces bone, causing pain and increasing the risk of fracture without a preceding injury).

I find it interesting that some of the Chinese herbal formulas most effective for healing and strengthening fractured and broken bones have a long history of use in Chinese martial arts. This is due, of course, to the somewhat higher incidence of bone injuries suffered by full-contact sparring or practicing *shiwara,* better known as "breaking technique." These same formulas are also used extensively in geriatric medicine for treating bone breaks and fractures that occur as a result of osteoporosis, which is quite common among the elderly.

Treating osteosarcoma (bone cancer) is a bit more complicated and depends on whether the disease has originated in the bone itself (primary bone cancer) or whether it has spread to the bones from elsewhere in the body (secondary bone cancer).

Primary bone cancer, which most often affects the femur (thigh bone), is most treatable when it is confined to the bone. In such cases, amputation is usually recommended, although radiation therapy to control the tumor is sometimes an option. Secondary or metastatic bone cancer is cancer that has spread to the bone from the breasts, lungs, prostate, thyroid, or kidneys, with metastasis (spreading of the cancer) occurring in the pelvis, vertebrae, ribs, and skull. Secondary bone cancers from the breast and prostate often respond to hormone therapy; in other cases removal of the endocrine glands (ovaries, testes) is the most effective treatment.

Antitumor herbal formulas can be used as an adjunct to conventional treatment, along with herbs to reduce the negative side effects of radiation therapy, such as nausea. While both primary and secondary bone cancer are serious and can be life threatening, generally the prognosis for primary bone cancer, when it is confined to the bone, is more encouraging than for secondary bone cancer, since it has already spread or metastasized from the original site of the cancer.

An excellent book on Chinese medicines used to fight cancer is *Anticancer Medicinal Herbs,* by Chang Minyi. According to the author, the following herbal formula has been used to treat osteocancer (bone cancer):

Bone Cancer Formula

Source: *Anticancer Medicinal Herbs*
Ingredients:

Quantity (Grams)	Chinese Herbs	English Translation
30	Shan Zha	Hawthorne Fruit
30	Huang Qi	Milk-Vetch Root
30	Fu Ling	Tuckahoe Root
30	Yi Yi Ren	Seeds of Job's Tears
30	Bai Hua She She Cao	White Patterned Snake's Tongue
10	Dang Gui	Tangkuei
10	Tian Hua Fen	Heavenly Flower Root
12	Gou Ji	Lamb of Tartary Rhizome
12	Xu Duan	Teasel Root
12	Huang Yao Zi	Dioscorae Tuber
10	Wu Mei	Dark Plum Fruit
15	Shan Yao	Chinese Yam Root

Description: This formula is used for the treatment of bone cancer.

Analysis: Shan Zha strengthens the stomach; Fu Ling benefits the stomach and spleen and resolves dampness. Huang Qi fortifies the Chi, increases immunity, and benefits the lungs. Yi Yi Ren eliminates inflammation and toxins. Bai Hua She She Cao clears heat, neutralizes toxins, and is useful for treating various cancers. Dang Gui nourishes the blood; Tian Hua Fen reduces inflammation and discharges pus. Gou Ji benefits the bones, and Xu Duan heals the bones by strengthening the liver and kidneys. Huang Yao Zi detoxifies poisonous swellings and is used for various kinds of cancer. Wu Mei generates fluids, and Shan Yao benefits the spleen and stomach.

Dosage and Method of Preparation: Make a decoction. Drink four ounces of the decocted tea at room temperature once daily.

Traditional Chinese medicine has experienced some success treating brittle bones or bones that have fractures or breaks with the following herbal formulas:

Die Da Jiu (Trauma Wine)

Original Source: *Quan Guo Zhong Cheng Yao Chu Fang Ji* (according to *Chinese Herbal Medicine Formulas and Strategies*)

Ingredients:

Quantity (Grams)	Chinese Herbs	English Translation
30	Dang Gui	Tangkuei
30	Chuan Xiong	Szechuan Lovage Root
60	Ru Xiang	Frankincense Resin
30	Mo Yao	Resin of Myrrh
30	Xu Jie	Dragon's Blood Resin
30	Tu Bie Chong	Wingless Cockroach
30	Ma Huang★	Yellow Hemp
30	Zhi Ran Tong	Pyrite

★Sufferers of high blood pressure or hypertension should not use Ma Huang; instead, substitute thirty grams of Bai Qian (White Before Rhizome).

Description: The formula reduces swelling and alleviates pain caused by brittle, broken, or fractured bones. It is useful for recovery from traumatic injury.

Analysis: Dang Gui nourishes the blood; Chuan Xiong, Ru Xiang, Mo Yao, Xu Jie, and Tu Bie Chong circulate the blood and dispel blood clots. Ma Huang guides the other herbs in the formula to invigorating the muscles. Zhi Ran Tong is well known for its ability to benefit broken or fractured bones.

Dosage and Method of Preparation: Have the above ingredients ground into a fine powder and make a medicinal wine. Drink one ounce of wine at room temperature three times daily (in the morning, afternoon, and evening). You can dilute the medicinal wine in four ounces of tepid water or drink it straight up.

Chin Koo Tieh Shang Wan (Muscle and Bone Traumatic Injury Pill); also known as Jin Gu Die Shang Wan

Description: This patent medicine is used in cases of brittle, broken, and fractured bones. It stops internal bleeding, bruising, and swelling, eases pain, and promotes healing. It is useful for acute traumatic injuries, including fractures with accompanying pain and swelling.

Caution: This formula is prohibited for use during pregnancy.

Dosage: This patent medicine comes in bottles of 120 pills, with complete instructions on dosage.

Gu Zhe Cuo Shang San (Broken Bones Capsules with Powder); also known as Fractura Pulvis

Description: This patent medicine is used in the healing of brittle, broken, or fractured bones, especially those associated with trauma and sports injuries.

Dosage: It comes in a box of sixty capsules, with complete instructions on dosage.

Botulism

*C*lostridium botulinum bacterium, better known as botulism, is unquestionably the deadliest of all forms of food poisoning. Symptoms such as weakness, nausea, vomiting, double vision, muscular paralysis, and difficulty swallowing usually appear between eight and thirty-six hours after eating contaminated food. If left untreated, botulism will cause death in about 70 percent of its victims.

The botulinum bacteria, found in soil and untreated water in most parts of the world, is also present in the intestinal tract of many animals, including fish. Usually harmless, the bacteria produce spores that multiply only in the absence of air and resist boiling, salting, smoking, and some forms of pickling. These spores do not normally infect humans but thrive in improperly preserved or canned foods. Foods most susceptible to botulism are canned vegetables, cured pork and ham, and smoked or raw fish. Infection can also occur when the bacterium enters the intestinal tract during bathing or immersion in untreated water (mostly affecting infants this way). Botulinum bacteria present in soil most often enters the body through skin already broken from an injury. If infection occurs, prompt treatment with an antitoxin reduces the risk of death to less than 25 percent.

Traditional Chinese and Western medicine make similar preventive recommendations:

- Preserved food should be sterilized by pressure-cooking at 250°F (120°C) for thirty minutes.
- Food in bulging cans should not be tasted or eaten; it should be immediately discarded.

If after taking the antitoxin, milder symptoms still exist, the following herbal formula should prove helpful:

Yu Zhen Tang (True Jade Decoction)

Original Source: *Wai Ke Zheng Zong* (according to *Chinese Herbal Medicine Formulas and Strategies*)

Ingredients:

Quantity (Grams)	Chinese Herbs	English Translation
3	Bai Fu Zi	White Appendage Rhizome
3	Tian Nan Xing	Jack in the Pulpit Rhizome
3	Qiang Huo	Notopterygium Rhizome
3	Bai Zhu	Atractylodes Rhizome
3	Fang Feng	Guard Against the Wind Root
3	Tian Ma	Gastrodia Rhizome

Description: For sufferers of the effects of botulism, including spasms and paralysis, this formula relieves the body of toxins.

Analysis: The chief herb, Bai Fu Zi, dries dampness and stops muscle spasms; Tian Nan Xing assists the chief herb. Qiang Huo, Fang Feng, and Bai Zhu disperse wind and dispel pathogenic influences, while Tian Ma unblocks the meridians and relieves spasms.

Dosage and Method of Preparation: Make a decoction. Drink four ounces of Yu Zhen Tang tea at room temperature three times daily, as needed.

Breasts, Disorders of: Infections; Cysts; Abscesses; Cancers

Hormonal disorders, infections, cysts, and abscesses are all minor breast disorders that are easily treated and normally pose no real threat to health. However, because of the risk of malignancy (breast cancer), whenever there is any real concern, medical advice should be sought. Hormonal imbalances affecting the breasts, which are usually associated with menstruation, are probably the most common and recurrent complaint. Occasionally, the breasts become larger and lumpy as a result of swollen milk glands, which shrink or return to normal when menstruation is over. More commonly, they become painful and tender as part of what has come to be known as PMS (premenstrual syndrome).

Infection or mastitis (inflammation of the breast), far less common than hormone-induced swelling and tenderness, usually occurs during breastfeeding and is caused by a clogged or blocked milk duct. If left untreated, an abscess with localized pain and swelling is likely to develop.

Breast lumps, one of the greatest causes for concern in gynecology, are most often caused by cysts (fluid-filled sacs), a fibroadenoma (thickening of the glandular tissue), or in a small number of cases a malignant tumor. Malignant breast tumors are usually felt rather than seen and in the great majority of cases are not painful. Other symptoms of malignant breast tumors may include a discharge from the nipple and a dimpled texture to the skin over the lump.

When a lump is discovered, it should be reported to a physician immediately. A mammogram, followed by a biopsy, is usually recommended if the physician suspects that the lump may be malignant. If cancer is discovered, further tests are carried out to determine whether the disease has spread to other parts of the body. The high mortality rate from breast cancer is usually due to its being discovered in the advanced stages, after it has spread from the breast to other parts of the body.

Both Western and Chinese medicine agree on the importance of early detection and the preventive role of a low-fat diet and exercise. Chinese medicine also contends that stress (negative emotions) and lifestyle seem to play a role in the incidence of breast cancer. Finally, even in the absence of hard scientific data, it is highly suspected throughout the Chinese medical community (myself included) that a connection exists between the use of birth control pills, hormone supplements (estrogen), and the high incidence of "female cancers."

An excellent book on Chinese medicines used to fight cancer is *Treating Cancer with Chinese Herbs,* by Hong-Yen Hsu. According to the author, the following herbal formula has been used to treat breast cancer and may actually reduce or eliminate tumors.

What follows are formulas that can be used for treating minor breast disorders as well as breast malignancy:

Tzu Ken Mu Li Tang (Oyster Shell and Lithospermum Combination)

Source: *Treating Cancer with Chinese Herbs*
Ingredients:

Quantity (Grams)	Chinese Herbs	English Translation
3	Dang Gui	Tangkuei
3	Chi Shao	Red Peony
3	She Chuang Zi	Cnidium Fruit Seed
3	Zi Cao	Groomwell Root
1.5	Da Huang	Rhubarb Root
1.5	Jin Yin Hua	Honeysuckle Flower
2	Sheng Ma	Black Cohosh Rhizome
2	Huang Qi	Milk-Vetch Root
4	Mu Li	Oyster Shell
1	Gan Cao	Licorice

Description: This herbal formula is useful for treating cancer of the breasts and suspected cancerous tumors.

Analysis: Dang Gui nourishes the blood; Chi Shao circulates the blood and resolves abscesses, boils, and tumors. She Chuang Zi benefits the kidneys and is useful for dissolving lumps. Zi Cao reduces fever and detoxifies poison. Da Huang increases the actions of Zi Cao. Jin Yin Hua resolves sores and swellings in various stages of development. Sheng Ma reduces fever and eliminates toxicity. Huang Qi increases immunity and circulates Chi. Mu Li dissipates nodules and lumps. Gan Cao harmonizes the other herbs in the formula and improves its flavor.

Dosage and Method of Preparation: Make a decoction. Drink four ounces of this herbal tea at room temperature three times daily, as needed.

Wu Wei Xiao Du Yin (Decoction to Eliminate Toxin)

Original Source: *Yi Zong Jin Jian* (according to *Chinese Herbal Medicine Formulas and Strategies*)

Ingredients:

Quantity (Grams)	Chinese Herbs	English Translation
15	Jin Yin Hua	Honeysuckle Flower
12	Yei Ju Hua	Wild Chrysanthemum Flower
15	Zi Hua Di Ding	Yedeon's Violet Root
15	Pu Gong Ying	Dandelion Herb
9	Chi Shao	Red Peony Root
12	Gua Lou Pi	Trichosanthes Fruit Seed's Husk
12	Zhe Bei Mu	Fritillaria Zhebei Bulb
12	Mu Dan Pi	Tree Peony Root, Bark of

Description: This herbal formula will relieve swollen lymph nodes in the armpits, breast abscess, carbuncles, mastitis, fibrocystitis, pain, and swelling.

Analysis: The chief herb, Jin Yin Hua, clears heat and infection and reduces swelling. Pu Gong Ying, Zi Hua Di Ding, Yei Ju Hua, and Zhe Bei Mu all clear heat and cool the blood and are useful for treating poisonous lesions. Chi Shao circulates blood and reduces blood clots. Gua Lou Pi circulates the vital energy (Chi), and Mu Dan Pi removes pathogenic heat from the blood, improves circulation, and softens nodules.

Dosage and Method of Preparation: Make a decoction. Drink four ounces of Wu Wei Xiao Du Yin tea at room temperature three times daily, or drink six ounces twice daily.

Tong Chi Tang (Unblock Chi Decoction)

Original Source: *Yi Lin Geri Cuo* (according to *Chinese Herbal Medicine Formulas and Strategies*)

Ingredients:

Quantity (Grams)	Chinese Herbs	English Translation
9	Wang Bu Liu Xing	Vacarria Seed
9	Dan Shen	Salvia Root
9	Qing Pi	Green Tangerine Peel

Description: This is an herbal formula that eliminates breast tenderness and pain and breast distention associated with premenstrual syndrome (PMS).

Analysis: Wang Bu Liu Xing circulates the blood and is useful for treating nonmalignant breast tumors; Dan Shen also circulates the blood and reduces clots and abscesses. Qing Pi circulates the vital energy (Chi).

Dosage and Method of Preparation: Make a decoction. Drink four ounces of Tong Chi Tang tea at room temperature three times daily, or drink six ounces twice daily.

Lien Chiao Pai Tu Pien (Forsythia Defeat Toxin Tablet); also known as Lian Qiao Bai Du Pian

Description: This patent formula dispels toxins and infections in the breast. It is also useful for ulcerated abscesses and carbuncles with pus.

Caution: This formula is prohibited for use during pregnancy.

Dosage: It comes in boxes of twelve vials, eight tablets per vial, with complete instructions on dosage.

Chuan Xin Lian-Antiphlogistic Pills (Penetrate Heart, Repeatedly Fighting Heat Pills); also known as Chuan Xin Lian Kang Yan Pian

Description: This patent medicine is for women suffering from breast abscesses and inflammations. It will purge toxic heat and inflammation and is also used for furuncles and mastitis and for resolving abscesses.

Dosage: It comes in bottles of sixty pills, with complete instructions on dosage.

Xi Huang Wan (West Gallstone Pills)

Description: This patent formula is for women suffering from breast abscess. It stops pain, promotes circulation, reduces swelling, and reduces carbuncles in the breast.

Caution: This formula is prohibited for use during pregnancy.

Dosage: The patent medicine comes in vials of 10cc each, with complete instructions on dosage.

Brittle Bones—see Bones: Brittle, Broken, Fractured, and Cancer

Bronchitis

Inflammation of the bronchial tubes, which connect the windpipe to the lungs, can either be acute (coming on suddenly and clearing up within a few days) or chronic (recurring and lasting for more than three months). Both are more common in smokers and in regions with high levels of atmospheric pollution.

Acute bronchitis is usually a complication of a viral infection such as a cold or influenza, but it may also be caused by the effects of air pollution. Chronic bronchitis often coexists with and can contribute to the development of emphysema. It is not uncommon for suffers of chronic bronchitis to also suffer from emphysema. When both diseases are present, together they are called chronic obstructive pulmonary disease.

Although air pollution is a contributing factor in bronchitis, in an overwhelming majority of cases the main cause is cigarette smoking. Symptoms include a cough with phlegm (mucus), shortness of breath, and, in rare instances, chest pain. Symptoms may be relieved by humidifying the lungs, either by using a humidifier in the house or by inhaling steam directly, and drinking plenty of warm herbal teas, which act as an expectorant (a medicine that promotes the discharge of mucus from the lungs). Developing the complications of pneumonia or pleurisy is possible but uncommon.

Chinese medicine has had some success treating bronchitis with the following formulas:

Xiao Qing Long Tang (Minor Bluegreen Dragon Decoction)

Original Source: *Shang Han Lun* (according to *Chinese Herbal Medicine Formulas and Strategies*)

Ingredients:

Quantity (Grams)	Chinese Herbs	English Translation
9	Ma Huang★	Yellow Hemp
9	Gui Zhi	Saigon Cinnamon Twig
3	Gan Jiang	Dried Ginger Root
3	Xi Xin	Chinese Wild Ginger Plant
9	Wu Wei Zi	Schizandra Fruit
9	Bai Shao	White Peony Root
9	Ban Xia	Half Summer
9	Zhi Gan Cao	Honey-Cooked Licorice Root

★Persons with hypertension (high blood pressure) should not use Ma Huang; instead substitute 9 grams of Bai Qian (White Before Rhizome).

Description: This is an excellent formula for the relief of bronchitis with symptoms of coughing, shortness of breath, phlegm, mucus, and difficulty expectorating. It is useful for chronic bronchitis as well as bronchial asthma.

Analysis: The chief herb, Ma Huang, arrests wheezing and opens the pores. Gui Zhi assists the chief herb. Gan Jiang and Xi Xin warm the interior and resolve congested fluids. Wu Wei Zi and Bai Shao benefit the lungs and nourish (or enrich) the blood. Ban Xia transforms congested fluids, and Zhi Gan Cao harmonizes the herbs in the formula.

Dosage and Method of Preparation: Make a decoction. Drink four ounces of Xiao Qing Long Tang tea at room temperature three times daily, or drink six ounces twice daily.

Hsiao Keh Chuan (Special Medicine For Bronchitis); also known as Xiao Ke Chuan Zhuan Zhi Qi Guan Yan

Description: This syrup is a patent formula for weak lungs indicated in acute and chronic bronchitis and for cough with phlegm.

Dosage: It comes in bottles of 100ml, with complete instructions on dosage.

San She Dau Chuan Bei Ye (Three Snake Gallbladder with Fritillaria Liquid)

Description: This patent formula resolves phlegm and stops chronic or acute cough with phlegm. It is useful for bronchitis, emphysema, or asthma and is notably valuable for stubborn phlegm that is hard to cough up.

Dosage: This patent medicine comes in boxes of six glass vials (10cc each), with complete instructions on dosage.

Chi Kuan Yen Wan (Bronchitis Cough, Phlegm, Labored Breathing Pill); also known as Qi Guan Yan Ke Sou Tan Chuan Wan

Description: This patent formula is used for sticky phlegm that is difficult to cough up due to heat in the lungs. It is appropriate for chronic lung diseases, including bronchitis and asthma.

Dosage: The patent medicine comes in bottles of two hundred pills, with complete instructions on dosage.

Ping Chuan Wan (Calm Asthma Pill); also known as Ping Chuan Pills

Description: This patent formula stops cough and resolves phlegm. It is used for cough with difficulty breathing and for chronic asthma, emphysema, and bronchitis.

Dosage: This patent medicine comes in bottles of 120 pills, with complete instructions on dosage.

Fu Fang Qi Guan Yan Wan (Medicinal Compound for Bronchitis Pill); also known as Bronchitis Pills/Compound

Description: This patent formula resolves phlegm and stops cough and is useful in acute and chronic bronchitis and chronic asthma.

Dosage: This patent medicine comes in bottles of sixty capsules, with complete instructions on dosage.

Bruise

A bruise is a contusion or discolored area caused by trauma, with bleeding under the skin. Bruises are normally treated topically with ointments, lotions, salves, compresses, and poultices. Chinese physicians will sometimes release the blood from under the skin, using a technique called bleeding, which involves breaking the skin and draining out the bruised blood. This is believed to hasten the healing process and reduce soreness and pain. The following patent medicines are also used to treat bruises:

Hsiung Tan Tieh Ta Wan (Bear Gallbladder Traumatic Injury Pill); also known as Xiong Dan Die Dan Wan

Description: This patent medicine breaks up blood, swelling, and stagnation; it promotes healing and reduces swelling and bruising. It is popular in China for injuries from sports and martial arts.

Dosage: It comes in a box of ten pills, with complete instructions on dosage.

Tieh Ta Yao Gin (Traumatic Injury Medicine); also known as Die Da Yao Jing

Description: This patent medicine promotes healing, stops pain, and is useful for a wide variety of traumatic injuries, including bruising of the skin.

Dosage: This patent medicine comes in bottles of 10ml, 30ml, and 100ml, with complete instructions on dosage.

Die Da Zhi Tong Gao (Traumatic Injury Stop Pain Plaster); also known as Plaster for Bruise and Analgesic

Description: This patent formula is for bruises, sprains, and swelling. It stimulates healing and stops pain.

Caution: Pregnant women should not apply this medicine to the lower abdomen.

Dosage: It comes in boxes of ten pieces, with complete instructions on dosage.

Bulimia—see Anorexia and Bulimia

Bunion—see Bursitis

Burns

Burns result when tissue is destroyed by heat, chemicals, electricity, scalding, or radiation. The severity of the burn is measured in intensity. A first-degree burn causes reddening of the skin and only affects the epidermis (the top layer of the skin). A second-degree burn damages the skin more deeply, causing blisters. Second-degree burns usually heal without scarring. A third-degree burn destroys all layers of the skin; the affected area appears white or charred. Muscle and bones may be exposed, and skin grafting will be required to prevent scarring.

Electrical burns can cause extensive internal damage with only a minimal amount of damage to the surface of the skin. They can cause heart damage and should be evaluated by a physician.

Although first-degree burns can be painful, they are not life threatening. Second- and third-degree burns are much more serious. Burns affecting more than 10 percent of the body's surface will send the victim into shock, with low blood pressure and a rapid pulse, caused by loss of fluids from the burned areas. This can be fatal if not treated by intravenous fluid replacement. Along with fluid replacement, attention must be given to protecting the victim from infections that can occur in the absence of the protective layer of skin. Infection can be controlled through the use of antibiotics; however, if left unattended, infection can be fatal.

Traditional Chinese medicine uses the following patent formula to treat burns:

Jing Wan Hong (Capitol City [Beijing] Many Red Colors); also known as Ching Wan Hung

Description: This patent medicine is used to stop pain, decrease inflammation, control infection, and promote regeneration of damaged tissue (skin). It is used to treat burns caused by steam, flame, hot oil, chemicals, radiation, sunburn, or electrical burn. It is useful for first-, second-, and third-degree burns. Pain usually stops immediately upon application.

Dosage: This patent medicine comes in tubes of thirty grams and five hundred grams, with complete instructions on dosage.

Bursitis

Bursitis is the inflammation of a bursa (a fluid-filled sac) usually resulting from pressure, friction, or an injury to the membrane surrounding a joint. The most common sites are the elbow, knee, shoulder, and foot (a bunion is a bursa near the toe).

Usually bursitis will subside after a few days, with the fluid being reabsorbed into the bloodstream. Applying an ice pack may help relieve the pain. Infection can be treated with herbal antibiotics, which also help to drain or release the fluid.

Juan Bi Tang (Remove Painful Obstruction Decoction)

Original Source: *Yi Xue Xin Wu* (according to *Chinese Herbal Medicine Formulas and Strategies*)

Ingredients:

Quantity (Grams)	Chinese Herbs	English Translation
3	Qiang Huo	Notopterygium Rhizome
3	Du Huo	Self-Reliant Existence Root
3	Qin Jiao	Gentiana Qinjiao
9	Sang Zhi	Mulberry Twigs
9	Hai Feng Teng	Sea Wind Vine Stem
9	Dang Gui	Tangkuei
2.1	Chuan Xiong	Szechuan Lovage Root
2.4	Ru Xiang	Frankincense Resin
2.4	Mu Xiang	Costus Root
1.5	Rou Gui	Saigon Cinnamon Inner Bark
1.5	Zhi Gan Cao	Honey-Cooked Licorice Root

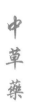

Description: This raw herb formula is used to treat gout and bursitis.

Analysis: Qiang Huo and Du Huo together treat the upper and lower body for wind dampness, which causes arthritis and bursitis. Qin Jiao, Sang Zhi, and Hai Feng Teng all expel wind dampness. Dang Gui enriches the blood. Chuan Xiong circulates the blood. Ru Xiang assists in circulating the blood and reduces blood clots. Mu Xiang benefits the spleen. Rou Gui directs the other herbs toward the extremities. Zhi Gan Cao harmonizes the other herbs in the formula and improves the flavor.

Dosage and Method of Preparation: Make a decoction. Drink four ounces of Juan Bi Tang tea three times daily, or drink six ounces twice daily, as needed.

Cancer—see specific entries, e.g., Breasts, Disorders of; Liver, Disorders of; etc.

Candidiasis (see also Leukorrhea; Trichomoniasis; Vaginal Discharge)

Candida albicans—also known as thrush, yeast infection, candidiasis, and moniliasis—is a fungal infection that most often affects the vagina. Less commonly it can affect other areas of the mucus membrane, such as inside the mouth or on moist skin. The penis can also be infected, causing inflammation of the head of the penis, after intercourse with an infected partner. The condition can spread from the genitals or mouth to other moist areas of the body, such as the skin folds in the groin or beneath the breasts.

Vaginal candidiasis normally produces a thick discharge, similar to cottage cheese, accompanied by itching and irritation, which may cause discomfort when urinating. Certain conditions—notably diabetes, hormonal changes that occur during pregnancy, and taking birth control pills—are believed to encourage growth of the fungus, creating a higher degree of susceptibility.

Traditional Chinese medicine has had some success treating this disease with patent medicines and the following herbal douche, for external use:

Vaginal Douche

Ingredients:

Quantity (Grams)	Chinese Herbs	English Translation
9	Chuan Lian Zi	Fruit of Szechuan Pagoda Tree
12	Gou Qi Gen	Matrimony Vine Root
9	Huang Bai	Amur Cork Tree Bark
12	Ku Shen	Bitter Root
9	She Chuang Zi	Cnidium Fruit Seed
9	Ku Fan★	Alum, Mineral Salt

★See special instructions for preparation below.

Description: This vaginal douche is useful for all vaginal infections with discharge, foul odor, itching, irritation, lower abdominal discomfort, and discomfort when urinating.

Caution: Do not ingest this formula; use only as a douche.

Analysis: Chuan Lian Zi circulates the vital energy (Chi) and relieves pain. Gou Qi Gen and Huang Bai eliminate heat, detoxify poisons, and clear infection. Ku Shen also effectively clears infection. She Chuang Zi, which is antiparasitic, also benefits the kidneys. Ku Fan dries dampness and eliminates itching.

Dosage and Method of Preparation: Make a decoction. Ku Fan should not be cooked with the other herbs but added after the normal cooking procedure, then allowed to steep with the decoction for thirty minutes before straining. Douche with eight ounces of this decocted tea at room temperature two times daily, as needed.

Chien Chin Chih Tai Wan (Thousand Pieces of Gold Stop Leukorrhea Pill); also known as Qian Jin Zhi Dai Wan

Description: This patent medicine, which detoxifies, is a special prescription for vaginal discharge due to infection. It is useful for all forms of vaginal infections, including yeast infection and trichomoniasis.

Dosage: It comes in bottles of 120 pills, with complete instructions on dosage.

Yu Dai Wan (Heal Leukorrhea Pill); also known as Yudai Wan

Description: This classical patent formula is used to clear vaginal infection and vaginal discharge with odor, itching, and irritation.

Dosage: It comes in bottles of one hundred pills, with complete instructions on dosage.

Canker Sores—see Fever Blister; Herpes (Oral); Stomatitis; Ulcer

Carbuncles

Carbuncles, also called boils or furuncles, are pus-filled, inflamed hair roots usually caused by the bacterium *Staphylococcus aureus.* Common sites for carbuncles are the back of the neck and the buttocks. Less common than single boils, carbuncles mainly affect people who have a lowered resistance to infection, in particular those with diabetes. Carbuncles are normally treated with applications of a hot compress (a cloth soaked in antibacterial herbal tea), which usually causes the pus-filled boils to burst, relieving the pain and discomfort. The formula used to treat carbuncles is a single-herb tea made from the antibacterial herb Jin Yin Hua (Honey-suckle).

Jin Yin Hua Tang (Antibacterial Honeysuckle Tea)

Ingredient:

Quantity (Grams)	Chinese Herb	English Translation
12	Jin Yin Hua	Honeysuckle Flower

Description: This formula is to be used externally as a hot compress to bring pus-filled boils to bursting. It will relieve pain.

Analysis: Jin Yin Hua clears heat and resolves toxins. It is both anti-bacterial and anti-inflammatory and is useful for treating infection caused by boils, carbuncles, furuncles, and abscess.

Dosage and Method of Preparation: Brew a decoction. Make a hot compress by soaking a small cloth or square of cotton fabric in the tea and applying it to the affected area three times daily, or as needed.

Cataract

A cataract is a condition causing the lens of the eye to become opaque, impairing vision. Although cataracts cannot cause complete blindness, because even a densely opaque lens will still transmit light, a loss of transparency causes the clarity and detail of images to be progressively lost.

Cataracts, which are occasionally caused by direct injury to the eye, occur most often in old age. In fact, they are so common among the elderly they are almost considered normal. Much less often, cataracts are associated with prolonged intake of corticosteriod drugs; poisoning from substances such as naphthalene (found in mothballs); severe diabetes with consistently high blood-sugar levels; and most forms of radiation, including X-rays, infrared, and microwave. There also appears to be a genetic predisposition for developing cataracts.

Cataracts are entirely painless, but they do cause visual symptoms including color-value disturbance (dulling of blue; accentuation of red, yellow, and orange), progressive loss of visual acuity, impairment of night vision, and discomfort from glare or extremely bright light sources.

The use of Chinese herbs in the early stages of the cataract's development has been reported as helpful in stopping the progressive loss of vision, and in some cases improvement has occurred; however, once a cataract has reached the advanced stages, surgery appears to be the most viable option. The following patent formulas have been used to treat cataracts.

Shi Hu Ye Guang Wan (Dendrobrium Leaf Night Sight Pills); also known as Dendrobrium Moniliforme Night Sight Pills

Description: This patent formula benefits the eyes and improves vision, especially eyesight that is beginning to diminish, accompanied by blurring. It is valuable in the early stages of cataract development and for hypertensive pressure behind the eyes.

Dosage: It comes in boxes of ten pills, with complete instructions on dosage.

Nei Zhang Ming Yan Wan (Cataract Vision Improving Pills)

Description: This formula benefits clarity of vision for those suffering from symptoms of cataract, glaucoma, impaired day or night vision; it is also useful for recovery following eye surgery.

Dosage: This patent medicine comes in bottles of 120 pills, with complete instructions on dosage.

Huang Lian Yang Gan Wan (Rhizoma Coptidis Goat Liver Pills)

Description: This patent formula is useful for eye disorders such as poor vision (especially at night), photophobia, pterygium (thickening of tissue) of the eye extending over part of the cornea, glaucoma, cataracts, and night blindness.

Dosage: It comes in box of ten pills, with complete instructions on dosage.

Chest Pain—see Angina

Chicken Pox (see also Herpes [Zoster])

Chicken pox is also called varicella and is caused by the *Varicella zoster* virus. It is an infectious disease that normally only affects children. When it does occur in adults, it is usually more severe. The varicella virus is spread from person to person in airborne droplets. Carriers of the virus are highly infectious from about two days before the virus surfaces until approximately a week after the rash appears.

Most children throughout the world have had chicken pox by age ten. Adults who have never had the disease should avoid becoming infected by staying away from children who have it. Women in the final stages of pregnancy should be particularly careful, as newborn infants can develop a severe attack. Herpes zoster (shingles) also has been associated with the varicella virus when the dormant virus contracted as a child resurfaces later.

Approximately a week after contracting chicken pox, but in some cases as long as three weeks later, a rash appears on the trunk and face, under the armpits, on the upper arms and legs, inside the mouth, and occasionally in the windpipe, causing a dry cough. In rare cases encephalitis (inflammation of the brain) occurs as a complication.

Traditional Chinese medicine treats chicken pox with a decoction of a single-herb tea made from Zi Cao (Groomwell Root/Purple Herb). As a tea, the herb is used both internally and externally to provide relief from chicken pox.

Zi Cao Tang (Groomwell Root Tea)

Ingredient:

Quantity (Grams)	Chinese Herb	English Translation
9	Zi Cao	Groomwell Root (a.k.a. Purple Herb)

Description: Used internally, the tea clears the heat and reduces the fever, as well as detoxifying while drawing rashes to the surface. Used externally, it is applied topically with a cloth to the rashes to reduce itching and heal the rash.

Analysis: Zi Cao circulates the blood and eliminates blood heat, and it is useful for treating febrile diseases with accompanying rash such as that occurring in measles or chicken pox; it is also useful for other forms of dermatitis and eczema.

Dosage and Method of Preparation: Make a decoction. For internal use: drink four ounces of Zi Cao tea at room temperature two times daily, as needed. For external use: using a soft cotton cloth, apply eight ounces of room temperature Zi Cao tea to the rash, as needed.

Cholera

Cholera is a serious and potentially fatal disease that results from infection by the *Vibrio cholerae* bacteria. In every instance, infection is the result of ingesting food or water that has been contaminated with feces. The two most common sources are drinking water and shellfish from polluted water.

Symptoms, occurring one to five days after infection, include profuse diarrhea, often accompanied by vomiting. The fluid loss caused by the diarrhea can lead to rapid dehydration, and death can occur within a few hours. When antibiotics are administered along with adequate rehydration (by consuming copious amounts of water containing the correct balance of salts and glucose), patients usually make a full recovery.

The best way to avoid infection is to be vaccinated before entering a cholera-infected area and to pay strict attention to hygiene. The following Chinese formulas can be used to combat the symptoms of cholera, including nausea, diarrhea, and vomiting:

Xiang Ru Tang (Elsholtzia Decoction)

Original Source: *Tai Ping Hui Min He Ji Ju Fang* (according to *Chinese Herbal Medicine Formulas and Strategies*)

Ingredients:

Quantity (Grams)	Chinese Herbs	English Translation
12	Xiang Ru	Aromatic Madder Plant
9	Bai Bian Dou	Hyacinth Bean
9	Huo Po	Magnolia Bark

Description: This raw herb formula is useful for gastroenteritis with vomiting, diarrhea, headache, and abdominal pain and also for cholera.

Analysis: The chief herb, Xiang Ru, opens the pores and causes sweating to release the toxins; it also benefits the spleen while settling the stomach. Bai Bian Dou assists the chief herb by reinforcing the spleen and strengthening its function. Huo Po eliminates dampness and disperses (or relieves) abdominal bloating.

Dosage and Method of Preparation: Make a decoction. Drink four ounces of Xiang Ru Tang tea at room temperature three times daily, as needed.

Huo Hsiang Cheng Chi Pien (Pogostemon Normalize Chi Pills); also known as Huo Xiang Zheng Qi Pian, or Lophanthus Antifebrile Pills

Description: This formula relieves nausea, vomiting, dizziness, and diarrhea. It is traditionally used for treating cholera.

Dosage: It comes in bottles of one hundred pills, with complete instructions on dosage.

Fu Zi Li Zhong Wan (Aconite Regulate the Center Pills); also known as Fu Tzu Li Chung Wan or Carmichaeli Tea Pills

Description: This patent formula is used for vomiting, diarrhea, and abdominal pain and is useful for acute gastroenteritis and cholera.

Dosage: It comes in boxes of ten honey pills or in bottles of one hundred smaller pills, both with complete instructions on dosage.

Cholesterol, High

In recent years concern about cholesterol levels has become a predominant health issue in the United States, mainly because of its relationship to the number one cause of death, coronary heart disease. It is not surprising that as the general public becomes more informed about health, diet, and physiology, there has occurred what I regard as a preoccupation with the much-discussed issue of good cholesterol versus bad cholesterol. Although it is basically true that saturated dietary fat is "bad" and polyunsaturated dietary fat is "good," such a statement is somewhat of an oversimplification. Its merits, however, lie in the fact that it causes us to refocus on diet. As current health issues fade into and out of prominence, we are reminded that the important role played by diet in every aspect of health remains unchanged. The dietary recommendations for maintaining acceptable cholesterol levels promoted by the American Heart Association and traditional Chinese dietetics are remarkably similar. Chinese health practitioners, however, have been touting these recommendations since long before the obsession with cholesterol developed. The shared opinion concerning the benefits of a low-fat diet is supported by overwhelming evidence that it is often possible to lower cholesterol levels significantly by simply reducing the amount of saturated fat in the diet.

In addition to being affected by diet, blood-cholesterol levels are also influenced by hereditary factors and certain diseases, for example, diabetes mellitus. It is well known that high blood-cholesterol levels increase the risk of developing atherosclerosis (accumulation of fatty tissues in the arteries) and with it the risk of coronary heart disease or stroke.

Recent research has shown that the risk of developing atherosclerosis can be assessed more accurately by measuring the proportions of different types of lipoproteins in the blood. Generally speaking, cholesterol in the form of high-density lipoproteins (HDL) seems to protect against arterial disease; cholesterol in the form of low-density lipoproteins (LDL) seems to increase the risk of arterial disease. People with relatives who have suffered a heart attack or stroke before age fifty have been shown to be at greater risk and should have their blood-cholesterol levels checked regularly.

The most effective preventive or corrective measures for high cholesterol are

- A low-fat diet, especially avoiding saturated oils, red meat, and too many dairy products.
- Regular exercise.
- Herbal therapy.

For high cholesterol levels, traditional Chinese medicine uses a decoction of a single-herb tea made from the herb Shan Zha (Hawthorne Berries), which is famous for its ability to affect cholesterol levels.

Shan Zha Tang (Hawthorne Berry Tea)

Ingredient:

Quantity (Grams)	Chinese Herb	English Translation
6	Shan Zha	Hawthorne Fruit

Description: This raw herb formula will bring down cholesterol levels.

Analysis: Shan Zha improves digestion and circulation of the blood. It removes lipids (fats) from the arterial walls and benefits hypertension and coronary heart disease.

Dosage and Method of Preparation: Make a decoction, observing the following special steps: place six grams of berries into a cup.

Add boiling water to the brim of cup, then cover the cup with a saucer, allowing the berries to steep for fifteen to twenty minutes. Drink the tea when it is tepid or slightly warm. You can eat the berries or discard them. Drink eight ounces of Shan Zha tea at room temperature two times daily. In order to experience its full effects, this formula should be taken regularly for at least six months to a year.

Chinese medicine also treats hypertension and high cholesterol with the following patent formulas:

Jing Ya Ping Pian (Hypertension Repressing Tablets); also known as Jiang Ya Ping Pian

Description: This patent medicine softens blood vessels while also strengthening them, and it decreases high cholesterol levels in the blood.

Dosage: It comes in boxes of twelve bottles, twelve tablets per bottle, with complete instructions on dosage.

Fu Fang Dan Shen Pian (Medicinal Compound With Salvia Root Tablet); also known as Dan Shen Tablets

Description: This patent formula reduces blood cholesterol and lowers blood lipids.

Dosage: It comes in bottles of fifty pills, with complete instructions on dosage.

Du Zhong Pian (Cortex Eucommine Tablets); also known as Compound Cortex Eucommiae

Description: This patent formula decreases cholesterol, lowers blood pressure, reduces hardening of the arteries, and calms the spirit.

Dosage: It comes in bottles of one hundred tablets, with complete instructions on dosage.

Cirrhosis (see also Liver, Disorders of)

Cirrhosis is a liver disease most commonly caused by alcoholism. It impairs the liver's ability to effectively remove toxic substances from the blood. The risk of developing cirrhosis relates to the amount of alcohol consumed rather than the type. Women are more susceptible to it than men. Other possible causes are hepatitis (inflammation of the liver) and, in rare instances, diseases or defects of the bile ducts. This can cause primary or secondary biliary cirrhosis and cystic fibrosis, in which the bile ducts become obstructed by mucus, or cardiac cirrhosis, in which heart failure has led to long-standing congestion of blood in the liver.

Common symptoms are jaundice (yellowing of the skin), edema (fluid collection in the tissues), mental confusion, hematemesis (vomiting blood), ascites (collection of fluid in the abdominal cavity), esophageal varices (enlarged veins in the wall of the esophagus), confusion, and coma (from the accumulation of toxins poisonous to the brain that would normally be detoxified by a healthy liver).

Chinese medicine has had some success treating cirrhosis with the following patent formulas:

Mu Xiang Shun Qi Wan (Saussurea Regulate Chi Pills); also known as Aplotaxis Carminative Pills

Description: This patent formula is useful for abdominal distention, belching, abdominal pain, and for cirrhosis in the early stages.

Dosage: It comes in bottles of two hundred pills, with complete instructions on dosage.

Shi Lin Tong Pian (Stone Dysuria Open Tablets); also known as Te Xiao Pai Shi Wan

Description: This patent formula treats hepatitis with symptoms of jaundice, liver ascites, and cirrhosis.

Dosage: It comes in bottles of one hundred tablets, with complete instructions on dosage.

Colds and Flu

Despite advances in medical research and modern medicine's ability to solve complex problems using sophisticated procedures and high-tech equipment, we still have not found a cure for the common cold. Even though a variety of so-called cold remedies exists, they mostly treat only the symptoms—after infection has occurred. A more prudent course of action is to avoid becoming infected by the more than two hundred different viruses known to cause colds.

Undoubtedly one of the main concerns in any preventive effort is developing a strong immune system to guard against what traditional Chinese medicine refers to as perverse energies. Additionally, Chinese medicine's contention that wind is the major factor in causing colds and flu should prompt us to take strong precautionary measures to protect ourselves from what the Chinese call wind invasion (as part of an overall preventive strategy).

According to Chinese medical theory, cold and flu viruses are ever present in the air we breathe, and it is the wind blowing into our faces that drives the virus into the body at the most common points of entry: the nose and the mouth. Protecting these portals is considered so important in China that instead of wrapping a scarf around the neck, people usually wear it across the face, covering the nose and mouth.

Along with vigilantly protecting the points of entry (nose and mouth), another effective preventive measure is the regular use of Chinese herbs to build up the immune system. If regular use of herbs is not possible, some comfort can be had in knowing that certain herbs have proven miraculous in their ability to prevent infection by fighting off viruses when they are taken immediately after the onset of initial symptoms. Traditional Chinese medicine attributes this to the fact that upon entering the body—usually through the mouth or nose—the virus remains on the surface (just beneath the skin) for a short time before entering the lungs. This is the "critical time" when quick action must be taken if there is any hope of successfully preventing the virus from advancing beyond the surface and entering deeper into the body's **organ** system (the lungs).

Once the virus has entered the lungs, one can expect full-blown cold or flu symptoms. Typically, the initial symptoms are sore throat, chills, or perspiration, which is the body's attempt to repel the invading virus.

In addition to using Chinese herbs as needed for preventing colds and flu, the systemic immune-enhancing effects of regular herbal use also provide protection in high-risk situations such as exposure to large crowds in poorly ventilated areas (shopping malls, movie theaters, schools); visits to hospitals, clinics, or other infectious environments; and during airline travel, when the traveler is breathing recirculated air.

One of the most famous, effective, and highly regarded cold remedies in the Chinese herbal system is the formula known as Yin Chiao. Well known among the Chinese population for centuries, Yin Chiao has recently begun to develop a reputation in the United States. Although Yin Chiao can be used to ease the discomfort of a cold, it is most famous for its ability to prevent infection by the virus—if it is taken during the "critical time" when the virus is still on the surface of the body.

This famous formula is available in two forms: a raw herb decoction and a pill.

Yin Chiao (Honeysuckle Forsythia Dispel Heat Decoction)

Original Source: *Wen Bing Tiao Bian* (according to *Chinese Herbal Medicine Formulas and Strategies*)

Ingredients:

Quantity (Grams)	Chinese Herbs	English Translation
15	Jin Yin Hua	Honeysuckle Flower
6	Jie Geng	Balloon Flower Root
6	Bo He★	Peppermint
9	Jing Jie	Schizonepeta Stem/Bud
30	Xian Lu Gen	Reed Root
15	Lian Qiao	Forsythia Fruit
12	Niu Bang Zi	Great Burdock Fruit
6	Dan Dou Chi	Prepared Blackbean
6	Dan Zhu Ye	Bland Bamboo Leaves
6	Gan Cao	Licorice Root

★See special instructions for preparation on the next page.

Description: This is an excellent remedy for the symptoms of cold and flu such as fever, slight chills, headache, thirst, cough, and sore throat.

Analysis: The chief herbs, Jin Yin Hua and Lian Qiao, clear heat and relieve toxicity. Jie Geng and Niu Bang Zi benefit the throat and lungs by spreading the vital energy (Chi). Bo He and Dan Dou Chi assist the chief herbs in clearing heat. Jing Jie nourishes the fluids, preventing dryness. Dan Zhu Ye, Xian Lu Gen, and Gan Cao all generate fluids and eliminate thirst.

Dosage and Method of Preparation: Make a decoction. The Bo He (Peppermint) should only be added to the simmering herbs during the last five minutes of cooking time. Overcooking Bo He will cause it to lose its effectiveness. Drink four ounces of Yin Chiao tea at room temperature three times daily, or drink six ounces twice daily, as needed.

Yin Chiao in pill form can be used several ways:

- Take one to two tablets per day for prevention, particularly during the cold and flu season.
- Take six to eight tablets during the "critical time" when the virus is still on the surface of the body and you have just begun to experience symptoms.
- Take three to four tablets when entering "high-risk" environments.

Yin Chiao Chien Tu Pien (Honeysuckle Forsythia Dispel Heat Tablets); also known as Yin Qiao Jie Du Pian

Dosage: Yin Chiao Chien Tu Pien comes in boxes containing twelve vials, eight tablets per vial, with complete instructions on dosage.

Although Chinese medicine emphasizes prevention, herbal therapy is also used for treating the full range of symptoms that are experienced once infection has occurred. The following herbal patent medicines can be used without concern about the side effects that accompany the use of chemical drugs (such as dizziness, ear-ringing, and drowsiness):

For Cough

Description: These formulas contain cough suppressants that stop the cough and expectorants that loosen and bring up phlegm mucus.

Mi Lian Chuan Bei Pi Pa Gao (Natural Herb Loquat Flavored Syrup); also known as Chuan Bei Pi Pa Gao
Dosage: This syrup comes in bottles of ten or twenty-five ounces, with complete instructions on dosage.

Lo Han Kuo Infusion (Momordica Fruit Instant Medicine); also known as Luo Han Guo Chong Ji
Dosage: This patent medicine comes in twelve small boxes with two cubes per box; the cubes must be dissolved in a cup of hot water. The package contains complete instructions on dosage.

Chuan Bei Jing Tang Yi Pian (Fritilleria Extract Sugar Coated Pills); also known as Chuan Bei Jing Pian
Dosage: This patent medicine comes in bottles of one hundred tablets, with complete instructions on dosage.

For Stuffy Nose

Description: This formula is useful for mucus congestion of the sinuses, sneezing, and sinus infections. It contains herbs that decongest and resolve phlegm/mucus.

Bi Yan Pian (Nose Inflammation Pill)
Dosage: It comes in bottles of one hundred tablets, with complete instructions on dosage.

For Sore Throat—see main entry on Sore Throat

Cold Sores—see Fever Blister; Herpes (Oral); Stomatitis; Ulcer

Colitis

Colitis, also known as nervous bowels, is an inflammation of the colon (large intestine) that causes toxins to irritate the lining of the intestines. It results in diarrhea with blood and mucus and, sometimes, abdominal pain and fever. The condition may come from infection by a virus, ameba (parasite), or bacteria. Antibiotics taken over a long period of time can provoke a form of colitis by killing the bacteria that normally live within the intestine, allowing another type of bacteria to proliferate and produce an irritating toxin.

Ischemia (impairment of the blood supply to the intestinal wall) is a rare cause of colitis seen in the elderly. Another disorder that can cause symptoms similar to colitis is proctitis (inflammation of the rectum, which may be due to a form of ulcerative colitis (chronic inflammation and ulceration of the lining of the colon and rectum) or gonorrhea or another sexually transmitted disease). Additionally, areas of the colon that are affected by diverticular disease and intestinal cancers are also known to exhibit symptoms similar to those associated with colitis. (See also Ulcer.)

Therefore, if you experience unexplained rectal bleeding, it is advisable to seek professional help. Traditional Chinese medicine has had some success treating the symptoms of colitis with the following herbal formulas:

Tong Xie Yao Fang (Important Formula for Painful Diarrhea)

Original Source: *Jing Yue Quan Shu* (according to *Chinese Herbal Medicine Formulas and Strategies*)

Ingredients:

Quantity (Grams)	Chinese Herbs	English Translation
12	Chao Bai Zhu	Dry-Fried Atractylodes Rhizome
9	Bai Shao★	White Peony Root
9	Chen Pi★	Ripe Tangerine Peel

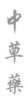

6	Fang Feng	Guard Against the Wind Root
9	Bai Tou Weng	Chinese Anemone Root
6	Huang Qin	Baical Skullcap Root

★See special instructions for preparation below.

Description: This formula is used for abdominal pain and diarrhea with blood and pus.

Analysis: Chao Bai Zhu strengthens the spleen and dries dampness. Bai Shao has a minor function in nourishing the blood and alleviating pain. Chen Pi transforms dampness and benefits the stomach and spleen. Fang Feng focuses the actions of the other herbs in the formula. Bai Tou Weng is both anti-inflammatory and astringent and is often used for bleeding and diarrhea. Huang Qin eliminates infection.

Dosage and Method of Preparation: Make a decoction. To increase the action of Bai Shao and Chen Pi, it is recommended that you dry-fry them for five minutes before cooking. (Dry-fry simply means to stir-fry in a frying pan with no oil.) Drink four ounces of Tong Xie Yao Fang tea at room temperature three times daily, as needed.

Fu Zi Li Zhong Wan (Aconite Regulate the Center Pills); also known as Fu Tzu Li Chung Wan

Description: This patent formula is for loose stools, diarrhea, and abdominal pain and for acute gastroenteritis and colitis.

Dosage: It comes in a box of ten honey pills or in a bottle with one hundred smaller pills, with complete instructions on dosage.

Yu Nan Bai Yao (Yunnan Province White Medicine); also known as Yunnan Paiyao

Description: This patent medicine is used for gastrointestinal bleeding including vomiting blood or intestinal bleeding with blood in the stool due to colitis.

Dosage: It comes in a box of sixteen capsules per package, with complete instructions on dosage.

Colon-Rectal Cancer

Colon-rectal cancer is the second most common cancer (after lung cancer) in the United States, where it accounts for 20 percent of all cancer deaths. It frequently occurs in association with other diseases such as ulcerative colitis and familial polyposis (intestinal polyps). Blood in the feces and an inexplicable change in bowel habits (either constipation or diarrhea) are often warning signs of its presence, as are pain and tenderness in the lower abdomen. Sometimes, however, no symptoms occur at all.

There are two types of colon-rectal cancer: carcinoid tumors and lymphomas. Carcinoid tumors are very slow-growing and usually occur without symptoms. They may spread to the liver, leading to carcinoid syndrome. Lymphomas, which damage the walls of the intestines and nearby lymph nodes, cause malabsorption of food, producing symptoms like diarrhea and rapid weight loss.

Although no single cause of colon-rectal cancer exists, Western medicine believes that environment and diet are the main contributing factors. While experts are less specific about possible environmental causes, they express little doubt that a diet high in meat and fat and low in fiber encourages the production and concentration of carcinogens. Genetics are also suspected of playing a role; brothers, sisters, and children of people suffering from colon cancer are more likely to acquire the disease later in life.

Traditional Chinese medicine for the most part supports the theory that genetics, diet, and environment play a significant role in colon cancer. The list of suspected environmental factors put forth by Chinese experts, however, is far more extensive and includes chemical and mechanical irritants, radioactivity, drugs, certain synthetic additives in food, alcohol, electromagnetic fields, tobacco, pesticides, fertilizers, fumes from automobile exhaust and from industrial processes, overuse of detergents, microwave ovens, and low-level radiation from electronic devices, among others. The Chinese system holds that colon-rectal and other cancers are by-products of modern civilization and that a sound diet, exercise, moderate habits, and natural living can do much to prevent cancer.

An excellent book on Chinese medicines used to fight cancer is *Anticancer Medicinal Herbs,* by Chang Minyi. According to this book, the following two herbal formulas are used to treat cancer of the rectum and the colon:

Colon-Rectal Cancer Formula Number 1

Ingredients:

Quantity (Grams)	Chinese Herbs	English Translation
15	Dong Gua Zi	Wintermelon Seed's Pulp
12	Da Huang	Rhubarb Root
9	Mu Dan Pi	Tree Peony Root, Bark of
9	Tao Ren	Peach Kernel
6	Mang Xiao★	Mirabilite

★See special instructions for preparation below.

Description: This formula is used to treat symptoms of colon-rectal cancer.

Analysis: Dong Gua Zi clears heat, infection, and abscesses from the large and small intestines. Da Huang also clears heat and resolves intestinal or rectal bleeding. Mu Dan Pi clears heat, cools the blood, improves circulation, and resolves firm masses, lumps, and tumors. Tao Ren circulates the blood and is useful for treating intestinal abscesses or immobile lower abdominal masses. Mang Xiao clears heat and reduces swelling and softens and moves the bowels.

Dosage and Method of Preparation: Make a decoction with all the ingredients except Mang Xiao. After the decoction has been cooked and the herbs have been removed, add six grams of Mang Xiao. The decoction in now ready to be used. Drink four ounces of the decocted tea at room temperature twice daily.

Colon-Rectal Cancer Formula Number 2

Ingredients:

Quantity (Grams)	Chinese Herbs	English Translation
30	Ban Zhi Lian	Scutellaria Barbatae
30	Bai Hua She She Cao	White Patterned Snake's Tongue
15	Hong Teng	Sargentodoxa Stem

12	Bai Jiang Cao	Herba Baijiangcao
12	Yi Yi Ren	Seeds of Job's Tears
12	Jin Yin Hua	Honeysuckle Flower
12	Bai Tou Weng	Chinese Anemone Root
9	Ci Wei Pi	Hedgehog Skin
9	Ku Shen	Bitter Root
9	Chuan Shan Jia	Pangolin Scales

Description: This formula is a treatment for the symptoms of rectal cancer.

Analysis: Bai Zhi Lian clears heat, eliminates infection, and stops bleeding. Bai Hua She She Cao and Hong Teng also clear heat and toxins and are often used for treating various kinds of cancer. Bai Jiang Cao clears heat and circulates blood. Yi Yi Ren strengthens the spleen, stops diarrhea, and is useful for treating intestinal abscesses. Jin Yin Hua clears infection and dissipates lumps and swelling in various stages of development. Bai Tou Weng clears heat and infection, especially in the stomach or intestines. Ci Wei Pi is astringent and stops bleeding. Ku Shen clears intestinal infection. Chuan Shan Jia circulates the blood and reduces nodules and poisonous swellings.

Dosage and Method of Preparation: Make a decoction. Drink four ounces of the decocted tea at room temperature three times daily, or drink six ounces twice daily.

Ji Xue Teng Qin Gao Pian (Millettia Reticulata Liquid Extract Tablets); also known as Caulis Millentiae

Description: This patent medicine has special effects for increasing the white blood cell count in cancer patients who have undergone chemotherapy or radiation. Research in China has shown an increase in the white blood cell count following three to four days of treatment with this herbal medicine.

Dosage: It comes in bottles of one hundred tablets, with complete instructions on dosage.

Conception—see Infertility

Concussion

A concussion is a jarring injury of the brain, resulting in disturbance of cerebral function (usually a result of a violent blow to the head). Symptoms include confusion, inability to remember events immediately preceding the injury, dizziness, blurred vision, and vomiting. Repeated concussion can cause brain damage with symptoms such as slurred speech, impaired concentration, and slow thinking. Anyone who has been knocked out should be resuscitated and examined by a physician. Symptoms such as drowsiness, difficulty breathing, visual disturbances, and repeated vomiting may be signs of extradural hemorrhage (bleeding between the skull and the outside of the brain).

The Chinese herbal formulas for resuscitation have been used in traditional Chinese martial arts. They are safe and effectively restore consciousness and mental clarity.

Er Wei Fu Sheng San (Two Flavor Recover Life Powder)

Source: *Shaolin Secret Formulas for the Treatment of External Injury*
Ingredients:

Quantity (Grams)	Chinese Herbs	English Translation
30	Ban Xia	Half Summer
30	Da Huang	Rhubarb Root

Description: This formula, for resuscitation after a concussion or knockout, is used by blowing the fine powder into the patient's nostril.
Analysis: Ban Xia circulates the vital energy (Chi) in the upper body and eliminates nausea. Da Huang circulates blood and clears orifices.
Dosage and Method of Preparation: Have the herbs mixed together and ground into a fine powder. Take a pinch and blow it into the patient's nostril. Use the right nostril for females, the left for males. Nasal pain may be felt when the patient regains consciousness; if so, apply ginger juice to relieve it. Ginger juice is available commercially in Asian-food or health-food stores, or it can be made by blending ginger root pieces in a blender on

medium and then placing the blended ginger into a five-by-five-inch square of cheesecloth and squeezing out the juice.

Shaolin Zhen Yu San (Shaolin Precious Jade Powder)

Source: *Shaolin Secret Formulas for the Treatment of External Injury*

Ingredients:

Quantity (Grams)	Chinese Herbs	English Translation
15	Fang Feng	Guard Against the Wind Root
15	Ming Tian Ma	Gastrodia-Heavenly Hemp Root
15	Nan Xing★	Jack in the Pulpit Rhizome
15	Bai Zhi	Angelica Dahuricae Root
3	Bai Fu Zi	White Appendage Rhizome

★See special instructions for preparation below.

Description: This formula is used for concussion with symptoms of confusion, inability to remember, dizziness, blurred vision, and vomiting.

Analysis: Fang Feng is used for treating headache; Ming Tian Ma is used for headache and/or dizziness. Nan Xing helps restore mental clarity. Bai Zhi also relieves headache, and Bai Fu Zi relieves headache and is an anticonvulsive.

Dosage and Method of Preparation: Have the herbs mixed together and ground into a fine powder. (Stir-fry Nan Xing in ginger juice before it is ground into a powder.) Mix .2 to .3 grams of powder with 4 ounces of sweet rice wine or boiled water. Drink it at room temperature, as needed.

Conjunctivitis

中
草
藥

An inflammation of the conjunctiva (the mucus membrane lining the inner eyelid and the front of the eyeball), conjunctivitis causes redness, discomfort, and a discharge. The most common causes are infection and allergies. Infection usually comes from staphylococci bacteria spread by hand-to-eye contact or from a virus associated with a cold, sore throat, or an illness such as measles. Allergic reactions are usually provoked by cosmetics, contact lens cleaning solutions, or pollen. Regular hand washing is a good measure for preventing infection, and most allergic reactions can be prevented by avoiding the causative substances or by replacing cosmetics and contact lens solutions regularly.

Traditional Chinese medicine treats conjunctivitis with a decoction of a single-herb tea made from Xia Ku Cao (Prunella Spike-Self-Heal).

Xia Ku Cao Tang (Prunella Spike-Self-Heal Decoction)

Ingredient:

Quantity (Grams)	Chinese Herb	English Translation
9	Xia Ku Cao	Self-Heal Spike Prunella

Description: This formula is useful for red, painful, and swollen eyes.

Analysis: Xia Ku Cao is antibacterial and specific for treating conjunctivitis.

Dosage and Method of Preparation: Make a decoction. Drink four ounces of Xia Ku Cao Tang tea at room temperature three times daily, as needed.

Huang Lian Su Yan Gao (Rhizoma Coptidis Extract Eyes Ointment)

Description: This patent formula is used to treat red, inflamed eyes with swelling and infection such as occurs with conjunctivitis and keratitis.

Dosage: It comes in tubes of 2.5 grams, with complete instructions on dosage.

Constipation

Eliminating waste material through regular bowel movements is surpassed only by diet and nutrition on traditional Chinese medicine's list of prerequisites for maintaining good health. While daily bowel movements are preferable, the frequency varies from person to person depending on dietary habits and lifestyle. A bowel movement every other day might be acceptable, but general consensus exists that any length of time beyond two days without the elimination of fecal matter is cause for concern.

Chronic constipation can result from a number of serious health problems such as diverticular disease, bowel obstruction, and colon-rectal cancer. However, constipation much more often results from simple factors like inadequate fiber in the diet, inadequate fluid intake, and a lack of regular exercise. Other contributing factors are an excess of meat and dairy products in the diet (notably cheese), food allergies, and the side effects of certain medications. Care must be taken in using laxatives because of the tendency of the bowels to become inactive when laxatives are used regularly over an extended period of time.

Bowel movements should occur naturally, without pain or discomfort, except where problems exist that are associated with bowel movement, such as hemorrhoids, colitis, and anal fissures. In both Western and Chinese medicine, strict monitoring of bowel habits is recommended for detecting many potentially serious illnesses in their early stages. It is important to pay attention to the frequency of the bowel movement as well as the texture (soft or hard; solid or liquid), size (long and thin like a pencil, or slightly thicker like a hot dog, or as thick as a polish sausage), and color (blond, tan, medium brown, dark brown or black).

Excavation of the bowels, which is the final stage in the digestive process, can benefit from attention given to good intestinal maintenance, which means:

- A diet high in fiber (oats, whole wheat, nuts, grains, fresh vegetables and fruits).
- Herbal enemas (recommended once or twice a year).
- Intestinal cleansing (recommended every ninety days).
- Drinking plenty of water (a minimum of four eight-ounce glasses daily).
- Regular exercise (walking, running, swimming, cycling, or other aerobic exercise for a minimum of thirty minutes daily).

Intestinal maintenance plays such an important role in preventive health care that traditional Chinese medicine refers to the intestines as the "source of 10,001 diseases." All of the following herbal formulas can be used to treat both chronic and acute constipation.

Run Chang Tang (Moisten the Intestines Decoction)

Original Source: *Shen Shi Zun Sheng Shu* (according to *Chinese Herbal Medicine Formulas and Strategies*)

Ingredients:

Quantity (Grams)	Chinese Herbs	English Translation
15	Huo Ma Ren	Cannabis Seed
9	Tao Ren	Peach Kernel
9	Dang Gui	Tangkuei
15	Sheng Di Huang	Chinese Foxglove Root, Raw
9	Zhi Ke	Bitter Orange Fruit Ripe

Description: This raw herb formula moistens the intestines and unblocks the bowels.

Analysis: Huo Ma Ren and Tao Ren contain volatile oils that lubricate the intestine and unblock the bowels. Dang Gui and Sheng Di Huang nourish the blood and moisten the intestines. Zhi Ke reinforces the laxative effect of the formula and also benefits the spleen and stomach.

Dosage and Method of Preparation: Make a decoction. Drink four ounces of Run Chang Tang tea at room temperature, allow eight hours for a bowel movement to occur, then take another four ounces if needed.

Ma Zi Ren Tang (Hemp Seed Tea)

Original Source: *Shang Han Lun* (according to *Chinese Herbal Medicine Formulas and Strategies*)

Ingredients:

Quantity (Grams)	Chinese Herbs	English Translation
50	Huo Ma Ren	Cannabis Seed (Hemp)
15	Xing Ren	Almond Kernel

15	Bai Shao Yao	White Peony Root
15	Zhi Shi	Green Bitter Orange Fruit
9	Huo Po	Magnolia Bark
15	Da Huang	Rhubarb Root

Description: This raw herb formula moistens the intestine, clears heat, and unblocks the bowels. This formula is for more serious constipation, with a hard stool that is difficult to expel.

Analysis: Huo Ma Ren moistens the intestines and unblocks the bowels. Xing Ren directs the energy of the other herbs downward. Bai Shao Yao nourishes the body fluids. Zhi Shi breaks up accumulation, especially in the intestines. Huo Po reduces abdominal bloating. Da Huang is a purgative that cools the intestinal heat and moves the bowels.

Dosage and Method of Preparation: Make a decoction. Drink four ounces of Ma Zi Ren Tang tea at room temperature. Allow eight hours for a bowel movement to occur; if necessary, take another four ounces, as needed.

Run Chang Wan (Moisten the Intestines Pill); also known as Fructus Persica Compound Pills

Description: This patent formula moistens the intestines, reduces heat, and stimulates peristalsis. It is recommended to treat chronic constipation in older people and for new mothers after childbirth.

Dosage: It comes in bottles of two hundred pills, with complete instructions on dosage.

Tao Chih Pien (Guide Away Red Pills); also known as Dao Chi Pian

Description: This patent medicine stimulates the bowels, clears heat, and relieves constipation. It is an excellent formula for small children and babies.

Dosage: It comes in boxes containing twelve small bottles (eight tablets per bottle), with complete instructions on dosage.

Cough

Coughing is an involuntary reflex action to clear the airways of mucus phlegm, irritants, blockages, or a foreign body. It is not a disease, but a symptom with a number of possible causes. When inexplicable coughing occurs, it should be investigated to determine the underlying cause. Possible causes include the common cold or flu, upper respiratory tract infection (viral), bronchitis, asthma, pneumonia, tuberculosis, pertussis (whooping cough), or pulmonary edema. (For more thorough discussions of these conditions, see their individual entries in this chapter.) Other causes of coughing include lung cancer and histoplasmosis (fungal infection).

Coughing Up Blood (Hemoptysis)

The underlying causes of this condition can range from persistent coughing that ruptures a blood vessel to a serious disorder such as cancer. It is therefore advisable to seek professional help. The most common cause of coughing up blood is infection as a result of any of the following diseases or conditions: pneumonia, bronchitis, tuberculosis, or stomach ulcer. (For more thorough discussion of these conditions, see their individual entries in this chapter.) Other underlying causes resulting in infection that may lead to coughing up blood are pulmonary embolism (a blood clot lodged in an artery in the lungs), tracheitis (inflammation of the wind pipe), and hemophilia.

Cramps, Menstrual—see Dysmenorrhea

Crohn's Disease

Crohn's disease is a painful inflammatory disease that can affect any part of the gastrointestinal tract. It most often occurs at the end of the small intestine, where it joins the large intestine at what is known as the ileum. Typical symptoms are pain, diarrhea (sometimes bloody), fever, and loss of weight. It can also cause chronic anal abscesses, fissures, fistulas, and intestinal obstruction. Although the cause of Crohn's disease is unknown, there is a slight genetic predisposition. A person may be affected at any age, but the peak ages are adolescence and early adulthood and after sixty years of age. Complications from Crohn's disease have been known to cause inflammation of various parts of the eye, severe arthritis affecting various joints, and skin disorders including eczema. Crohn's disease is chronic, with symptoms fluctuating over many years.

Traditional Chinese medicine recommends herbal therapy consisting of anti-inflammatory and antibiotic herbal formulas. Additionally, tonics are often prescribed to resolve the anemia that results from malabsorption of nutrients in the large intestines. Dietary modifications can also help by omitting certain foods that exacerbate the condition.

Zhen Ren Yang Zang Tang (True Man's Decoction to Nourish the Organs)

Original Source: *Tai Ping Hui Min He Ji Ju Fang* (according to *Chinese Herbal Medicine Formulas and Strategies*)

Ingredients:

Quantity (Grams)	Chinese Herbs	English Translation
6	Ren Shen	Ginseng
12	Bai Zhu	Atractylodes Rhizome
5	Rou Gui	Saigon Cinnamon Inner Bark
15	Wei Rou Dou Kou	Dry-Fried Nutmeg Seeds
15	He Zi	Myrobalan Fruit
20	Zhi Ying Su Ke	Honey-Fried Opium Poppy Husk
15	Bai Shao	White Peony Root
12	Dang Gui	Tangkuei
9	Mu Xiang	Costus Root
9	Zhi Gan Cao	Honey-Cooked Licorice Root

Description: This herbal formula is used to tonify deficient organs (in this case, the intestines). It is very useful for Crohn's disease, as it stops diarrhea, resolves bleeding with pus, and the accompanying abdominal pain, loss of appetite, and fatigue.

Analysis: Ren Shen and Bai Zhu combined are very effective for strengthening the stomach and spleen. Rou Gui and Wei Rou Dou Kou dispel cold and benefit the kidneys and spleen. He Zi and Zhi Ying Su Ke are both effective for arresting diarrhea. Bai Shao and Dang Gui enrich the blood to offset the anemia that is often a result of chronic diarrhea. Mu Xiang supports digestion and relieves abdominal pain. Zhi Gan Cao harmonizes the other herbs in the formula and improves taste.

Dosage and Method of Preparation: Prepare a decoction. Drink four ounces of Zhen Ren Yang Zang Tang tea three times daily, as needed.

Xiang Sha Liu Jun Wan (Saussurea Amomum Six Gentlemen Pills); also known as Aplotaxis-Amomum Pills, or Six Gentlemen Tea Pills

Description: This patent formula is used for Crohn's disease with poor digestion, stomachache, chronic diarrhea, gastritis, nausea, and vomiting.

Dosage: It comes in bottles of one hundred pills, with complete instructions on dosage.

Cyst—see Breasts, Disorders of (Cysts); Ovarian Cyst

Cystitis (Bladder Infection)

Cystitis, or urinary bladder infection, is sometimes mistakenly thought to be a gynecological disorder because it is so rarely seen in men. Even though bladder infection is one of the most preventable infections, it ranks second after the common cold as the most common illness among women. Improper cleaning or wiping with toilet tissue from the anus forward spreads *Escherichia coli* (a bacterium that lives in the intestines) to the urethra and subsequently to the bladder; this occurrence is cited as the cause of 90 percent of bladder infections. This unnecessary bacterial contamination can be avoided by simply wiping from the front to the back, away from the urethra.

In a relatively small number of cases, cystitis can also occur as a result of bacteria being transported from the anal area to the urethra during sexual activity. This infection can be easily avoided by paying strict attention to hygiene before moving sexual contact from the anal to the vaginal area.

The following herbal formulas can be used for treating cystitis, both chronic and acute:

Ba Zheng Tang (Eight Herb Decoction for Rectification)

Original Source: *Tai Ping Hui Min He Ji Ju Fang* (according to *Chinese Herbal Medicine Formulas and Strategies*)

Ingredients:

Quantity (Grams)	Chinese Herbs	English Translation
6	Mu Tong	Wood with Holes
12	Hua Shi	Talcum, Mineral
15	Che Qian Zi	Plantago Seed
12	Qu Mai	Fringed Pink Flower Plant
12	Bian Xu	Knotweed Plant
9	Zhi Zi	Gardenia Fruit
9	Da Huang	Rhubarb Root
6	Deng Xin Cao	Rush Pith
9	Gan Cao	Licorice Root

Description: This raw herbal formula is excellent for clearing up urinary tract and bladder infections, with difficult urination, burning sensation, and lower abdominal tenderness.

Analysis: The chief ingredient, Mu Tong, clears heat and resolves infection. Hua Shi, Che Qian Zi, Qu Mai, and Bian Xu clear infection by promoting urination. Zhi Zi clears heat and also promotes urination. Da Huang moves the bowels. Deng Xin Cao directs the action of the other herbs downward, and Gan Cao harmonizes them.

Dosage and Method of Preparation: Make a decoction. Drink four ounces of Ba Zheng Tang tea at room temperature three times daily, as needed.

Bei Xie Fen Qing Yin (Dioscorea Hypoglauca Decoction to Separate the Clear)

Original Source: *Dan Xi Xin Fa* (according to *Chinese Herbal Medicine Formulas and Strategies*)

Ingredients:

Quantity (Grams)	Chinese Herbs	English Translation
6	Bei Xie	Fish-Poison Yam Rhizome
1.5	Huang Bai	Amur Cork Tree Bark
1.5	Shi Chang Pu	Sweet Flag Rhizome
3	Fu Ling	Tuckahoe Root
3	Bai Zhu	Atractylodes Rhizome
4.5	Dan Shen	Salvia Root
4.5	Che Qian Zi	Plantago Seed

Description: This formula is useful for bladder infections with cloudy urine, lower abdominal pain, and urine that continues to drip after urination ceases.

Analysis: Bei Xie, the chief herb, eliminates infection and is specific for use in bladder infections. Huang Bai assists and strengthens this function in addition to dispersing heat. Shi Chang Pu dispels dampness and benefits the stomach. Fu Ling benefits the stomach and spleen. Bai Zhu assists in this function. Dan Shen circulates the blood. Che Qian Zi reinforces the actions of the chief herb by eliminating pathogenic heat and infection.

Dosage and Method of Preparation: Make a decoction. Drink four ounces of Bei Xie Fen Qing Yin tea at room temperature three times daily, as needed.

Chuan Xin Lian-Antiphlogistic Tablets (Penetrate Heart, Repeatedly Fighting Heat Pills); also known as Chuan Xin Lian Kang Yan Pian

Description: This patent formula is for urinary tract and bladder infections. It is useful as a preventive measure against urinary tract infection when traveling.

中草藥

Dosage: It comes in bottles of sixty pills, with complete instructions on dosage.

Dandruff

Dandruff is a condition in which dead skin is shed from the scalp. It is usually caused by a rash called seborrheic dermatitis. Although dandruff is most often confined to the head or scalp, it can also occur on the face, chest, and back. Western medicine recommends using antidandruff shampoos and corticosteroid creams and lotions that are applied to the scalp. By contrast, traditional Chinese medicine advises dandruff sufferers to use a scalp rinse made from thyme, Niu Bang Zi (Great Burdock Fruit), and watercress. Additionally, it recommends that the following be avoided: shampoos (which tend to dry the scalp); wearing hats (which create a moist, humid condition in which seborrheic dematitis flourishes), using sharp combs or brushes (which can inflame rather than stimulate the scalp).

Chinese medicine holds that the scalp should be kept meticulously clean with surgical spirit (alcohol) or gin and that the diet should be low in fat and carbohydrates and high in fruits and vegetables. Chinese medicine recommends a decoction made from the following herbs as a scalp rinse:

Niu Bang Zi Tang (Burdock Scalp Rinse)

Ingredients:

Quantity (Grams)	Chinese Herbs	English Translation
10	Niu Bang Zi	Great Burdock Fruit
12	★	Thyme
10	★	Watercress

★These are Western herbs; therefore they have no Chinese name.

Description: Used as a scalp rinse, this formula will relieve dry, itchy scalp and dandruff.

Analysis: The chief ingredient, Niu Bang Zi, is anti-inflammatory, antibacterial, and antifungal. Thyme and watercress assist in these actions, but mainly they circulate the blood.

Dosage and Method of Preparation: Make a decoction. Rinse scalp with room-temperature decoction, as needed.

Depression—see Anxiety; Stress

Diabetes (see also Hypoglycemia; Pancreas, Disorders of)

There are two forms of diabetes: diabetes insipidus, caused by failure of the pituitary gland to secrete an antidiuretic hormone (ADH), and diabetes mellitus, a disorder in which the pancreas produces either insufficient amounts of insulin or none at all. In diabetes insipidus, the rarer form, the failure of the pituitary gland to produce ADH causes the sufferer to experience extreme thirst and pass enormous quantities of urine (ten to forty pints per day), creating a condition known as polyuria. Several reasons can exist for the pituitary gland's inability to secrete the antidiuretic hormone, including diseases of the pituitary gland, damage from injury, a tumor, or in some cases a disease known as nephrogenic diabetes insipidus. This rare condition is usually congenital (present from birth), but it may result from a kidney disease called pyelonephritis (inflammation of the kidneys; see also Pyelonephritis).

Excessive urination and thirst are also symptoms of diabetes mellitus but to a much lesser degree. Apart from these symptoms, the two forms of diabetes have nothing in common.

Diabetes mellitus, which is more common, results from insufficient insulin production, resulting in high blood-sugar levels, degeneration of small blood vessels, and problems with lipid (fat) metabolism. The two types of diabetes mellitus are type I (insulin dependent), the more severe form, and type II (non-insulin dependent). Sufferers of type I require regular injections of insulin, without which the sufferer eventually lapses into a coma and dies. In type II, insulin is produced but in insufficient quantities to meet the body's needs. With type II, in most cases insulin-replacement injections are not required; the combination of dietary measures, weight control, and oral medication can keep the condition under control. The onset of type II diabetes is often associated with obesity. Diabetes mellitus tends to run in families.

One of the side effects of diabetes mellitus is poor circulation, especially in the lower extremities (legs and feet). Poor circulation can cause cramping and accompanying pain, a fairly common problem among diabetic patients. Several herbal blood tonic formulas are available that are used to cool the blood and improve circulation, bringing the patient relief from the discomfort of poor circulation.

Si Wu Tang (Four Substance Decoction)

Original Source: *Tai Ping Hui Min He Ji Ju Tang* (according to *Chinese Herbal Medicine Formulas and Strategies*)

Ingredients:

Quantity (Grams)	Chinese Herbs	English Translation
9	Sheng Di Huang	Chinese Foxglove Root, Raw
6	Bai Shao	White Peony Root
9	Dang Gui	Tangkuei
9	Chuan Xiong	Szechuan Lovage Root
9	Hong Hua	Safflower Flower
9	Tao Ren	Peach Kernel

Description: This herbal blood tonic will provide relief from the discomfort of poor circulation and is used by those suffering from diabetes to cool the blood.

Analysis: Sheng Di Huang cools the blood and benefits both the liver and the kidneys. Bai Shao and Dang Gui enrich the blood. Chuan Xiong circulates the blood and is assisted by Hong Hua and Tao Ren.

Dosage and Method of Preparation: Make a decoction. Drink four ounces of Si Wu Tang tea three times daily, as needed. This formula can be taken over long periods of time; it can be used as an adjunct to daily insulin injections.

The following patent formulas should also be useful for treating what traditional Chinese medicine refers to as sugar urine disease:

Ci Wu Jia Pian (Acanthopanax Senticosus)

Description: This patent formula is used to treat the symptoms of diabetes. Research in China has suggested that this formula increases insulin production and decreases blood sugar if it is excessively high and increases endocrine function (ovaries, testes, and adrenal glands). It also has an antidiuretic property that will help prevent the patient from producing excess urine.

Dosage: It comes in bottles of one hundred tablets, with complete instructions on dosage.

Jin Kui Shen Qi Wan (Deficient Kidney Chi Pills); also known as Jin Gui Shen Qi Wan, or Sexotan

Description: This patent formula is useful for treating diabetes in cases with deficient kidney syndrome, with symptoms that include excess urination and thirst.

Dosage: It comes in bottles of two hundred pills, with complete instructions on dosage.

Yu Quan Wan (Jade Spring Pills); also known as Yeuchung Pills

Description: This patent formula is a classical prescription for the treatment of diabetes. It is used for both diabetes insipidus and diabetes mellitus.

Dosage: This patent medicine comes in bottles of 180 grams of powder, or boxes of twenty vials of pills, with complete instructions on dosage.

Diaper Rash—see Rash

Diarrhea

One of the most intriguing characteristics of traditional Chinese medicine is its ability to appeal to the rationale of people who have little or no experience in matters pertaining to health. While it should be remembered that the practice of medicine—or the art and science of treating disease—requires an in-depth study of the biological and medical sciences, it is Chinese medicine's ability to bring all of these complex subjects together and present them in the simplest terms that I appreciate. The uncomplicated way that diarrhea and its treatment are viewed by traditional Chinese medicine is a good case in point. Simply put, diarrhea is defined as having loose, watery stools.

Diarrhea can be mild or serious; it can be acute, sudden, and severe or it can be chronic, mild, and reoccurring. Acute diarrhea is usually caused by bacterial infection, food poisoning, lactose intolerance, allergic reaction to certain foods, ingesting bad or unripe fruit, or the side effects of certain medications. Chronic diarrhea is usually caused by Crohn's disease, irritable bowel syndrome, malnutrition, intestinal cancers, or an imbalance of the stomach and spleen.

Acute diarrhea, which is usually not a serious health threat to a reasonable healthy adult, can be dangerous in infants and small children. Therefore, the following rules of thumb should be strictly adhered to:

- Adults: If diarrhea lasts more than three or four days and shows no signs of ending, seek professional help.
- Infants and Small Children: Diarrhea should be taken seriously. If it lasts throughout one full day and persists to a second day, seek immediate professional help.

The chief symptoms of diarrhea are (1) dehydration, which is caused by fluid loss; (2) general weakness, which is a result of a lack of nutrient absorption; and (3) bacterial infection, which is only present when unclean food has been eaten.

Treatment should include (1) rehydration, to replenish the lost fluid with broth, soup, and water and (2) controlling the infection. In cases of bacterial infection, herbal formulas should be used that contain antibiotic herbs, which will reestablish the balance between the small and large intestines and end the diarrhea.

Unlike most over-the-counter remedies that act like a plug to stop the diarrhea—and thereby keep the infected material inside the body instead of allowing it to come out—the herbal formulas that follow are based on principals compatible with this treatment plan.

Zhen Ren Yang Zang Tang (True Man's Decoction to Nourish the Organs)

Original Source: *Tai Ping Hui Min He Ji Ju Fang* (according to *Chinese Herbal Medicine Formulas and Strategies*)

Ingredients:

Quantity (Grams)	Chinese Herbs	English Translation
6	Ren Shen	Ginseng
12	Bai Zhu	Atractylodes Rhizome
4	Rou Gui	Saigon Cinnamon Inner Bark
15	Wei Rou Dou Kou	Dry-Fried Nutmeg Seeds
15	He Zi	Myrobalan Fruit
20	Zhi Ying Su Ke	Honey-Fried Opium Poppy Husk
15	Bai Shao	White Peony Root
12	Dang Gui	Tangkuei
9	Mu Xiang	Costus Root
9	Zhi Gan Cao	Honey-Cooked Licorice Root

Description: This raw herb formula settles the stomach and stops diarrhea. It is excellent for chronic long-term diarrhea. It relieves abdominal pain, short-term diarrhea, and reduced appetite.

Analysis: Ren Shen and Bai Zhu combined are very effective for strengthening the stomach and spleen. Rou Gui and Wei Rou Dou Kou dispel cold and benefit the kidneys and spleen. He Zi and Zhi Ying Su Ke are both effective for arresting diarrhea. Bai Shao and Dang Gui enrich the blood to offset the anemia that is often a result of chronic diarrhea. Mu Xiang supports digestion and relieves abdominal pain. Zhi Gan Cao harmonizes the other herbs in this formula.

Dosage and Method of Preparation: Make a decoction. Drink four ounces of Zhen Ren Yang Zang Tang tea at room temperature three times daily, or drink six ounces twice daily, as needed.

Po Chi Pill (Protect and Benefit Pill); also known as Bao Ji Wan, China Po Chi Pills, and Zhong Guo Bao Ji Wan

Description: This patent medicine is useful for a wide variety of digestive complaints and is especially effective to control acute or sudden onset of diarrhea, nausea, vomiting, stomach cramps, stomach flu, and motion sickness.

Dosage: It comes in a bottle of one hundred pills or a box containing ten vials, with complete instructions on dosage.

Ji Zhong Shui (Benefit Many Problems Liquid); also known as Liu Shen Shui, or Chi Chung Shui

Description: This patent medicine settles the stomach, dispels pathogenic heat, and neutralizes toxins. It can be used as an emergency remedy for travelers to treat a variety of stomach problems, such as stomach or intestinal cramping, nausea, vomiting, and diarrhea. A decreased dosage of this formula can be used for children—check the package instructions for correct dosage.

Caution: This formula is prohibited for use during pregnancy.

Dosage: This patent formula comes in boxes of twelve vials, with complete instructions on dosage.

Important Note: The presence of blood in the feces should never be ignored. While it can indicate non-life-threatening conditions such as dysentery, hemorrhoids, or bleeding ulcers, it can also indicate a more serious disease like cancer. It is strongly recommended that a physician be consulted so that a stool analysis can be performed and the cause determined before selecting an herbal formula for self-treatment.

Digestive System, Disorders of

The digestive system is a group of organs that break down food into chemical components so that it can be absorbed and used by the body for energy and for repairing and building cells and tissue. The digestive system's chief component is the digestive tract, also known as the alimentary canal, which is basically a tube through which food passes. It consists of the mouth, pharynx, esophagus, stomach, small intestine, large intestine, and anus. Associated digestive organs are the liver, gall bladder, and pancreas. For disorders of the digestive system, see the entry that deals with the specific organ in question.

Diuretics

Diuretics are medicines that stimulate or increase urination. For discussions of edema or urine retention, see either of those entries in this chapter.

Some commonly used diuretics in traditional Chinese medicine are listed below. A word of caution: many women use diuretics to relieve the swollen legs that are a result of water retention during pregnancy. The herbs Che Qian Zi, Yi Yi Ren, and Qu Mai should not be used by pregnant women.

Chinese herb: Fu Ling; Latin botanical: Poria cocos sclerotium; English translation: Tuckahoe Root; Indications: Promotes urination, used for difficulty urinating or edema.

Chinese herb: Ze Xie; Latin botanical: Rhizome alismatis orientalis; English translation: Water Plantain Rhizome; Indications: Strong diuretic, promotes urination, useful for difficult urination and edema.

Chinese herb: Che Qian Zi; Latin botanical: Semen plantaginis; English translation: Plantago Seed; Indications: For urinary dysfunction, promotes urination, clears heat, used for edema.

Chinese herb: Yi Yi Ren; Latin botanical: Coicis lachryma-jobi semen; English translation: Seeds of Job's Tears; Indications: Promotes urination, used for edema and for difficult urination.

Chinese herb: Qu Mai; Latin botanical: Diathus herba; English translation: Fringed Pink Flower Plant; Indications: Clears heat, promotes urination, and is useful for urinary dysfunction.

Chinese herb: Zhu Ling; Latin botanical: Polyporus umbellatus; English translation: Polyporous Fungu; Indications: Promotes urination, useful for edema and scanty urine.

Dizziness

Sometimes called vertigo, dizziness is a feeling of lightheadedness that is usually mild and brief and that is caused by a momentary fall in blood pressure to the brain, as can occur when getting up suddenly from a sitting or lying position (compare Vertigo). These occasional episodes of dizziness, called postural hypotension, are usually more common in the elderly and in people taking drugs to treat hypertension (high blood pressure). Similar symptoms may result from a temporary partial blockage in the arteries that supply blood to the brain; this is known as a transient ischemic attack. Other causes of dizziness include fatigue, stress, fever, anemia, hypoglycemia (low blood sugar), subdural hemorrhage, and hematoma (bleeding between the membranes that cover the brain). Certain disorders of the inner ear can cause dizziness, including labyrinthitis, Ménière's disease, and disorders of the acoustic nerve (such as acoustic neuroma and meningitis).

Severe, prolonged, or recurrent dizziness should be investigated by a physician, who will try to determine the cause from a description of the symptoms, an ear examination, and in some cases further diagnostic tests.

For herbal remedies to treat dizziness, see Anemia; Fever; Hypertension; Hypoglycemia; Stress.

Douche (see also Candidiasis; Leukorrhea; Trichomoniasis; Vaginal Discharge)

To douche is to introduce water, an herbal decoction, or any fluid solution into the vagina for cleansing or disinfecting. It is typically administered using a bag and tubing with a nozzle. Douches are often used to treat vaginal infection or itching or to provide cleansing beyond what a shower or bath can offer.

Two important points to observe about douching are (1) the nozzle must be cleaned properly before use to avoid the risk of introducing infection into the vagina, and (2) a douche is not effective as a contraceptive!

For normal vaginal cleaning, vinegar and water are commonly used. Suggested dosage: four ounces of distilled plain vinegar to one-half gallon of warm water.

For vaginal infections such as candidiasis (yeast infection), trichomoniasis, leukorrhea, see those specific entries for an herbal douche formula.

Drug Addiction—see Addiction to Drugs

Duodenal Ulcer—see Ulcer

Dysentery

Dysentery is a severe infection of the large intestines causing diarrhea that often contains blood, pus, and mucus. Two distinct forms exist. Shigellosis, also called bacillary dysentery, results from infection caused by the *Shigella* bacterium. Its major symptom is the sudden onset of watery diarrhea, sometimes with the presence of bacterial toxins in the blood. Amebic dysentery, the second form, is caused by a protozoan (single-celled) parasite. Although diarrhea is also a main symptom, it starts more gradually and often runs a chronic course.

As with all diarrhea, dehydration from the loss of fluids is a primary concern; so is eliminating parasitic and bacterial infection. Chinese medicine treats dysentery with the following herbal formulas:

Bai Tou Weng Tang (Pulsatilla Decoction)

Original Source: *Shang Han Lun* (according to *Chinese Herbal Medicine Formulas and Strategies*)

Ingredients:

Quantity (Grams)	Chinese Herbs	English Translation
6	Bai Tou Weng	Chinese Anemone Root

9	Huang Lian	Golden Thread Root
9	Huang Bai	Amur Cork Tree Bark
9	Qin Pi	Korean Ash Branches, Bark of

Description: This herbal formula is useful for bacillary dysentery, amebic dysentery, enteritis, and ulcerative colitis.

Analysis: Bai Tou Weng is the principle herb in Chinese herbology for treating dysenteric disorders. Huang Lian clears infection, especially from the stomach and intestines. Huang Bai assists in this function, and Qin Pi restrains the diarrhea and strengthens the actions of the other herbs in the formula.

Dosage and Method of Preparation: Make a decoction. Drink four ounces of Bai Tou Weng Tang tea at room temperature, as needed.

Huang Lian Su Pian (Coptidis Extract Tablets); also known as Superior Tabellae Berberini

Description: This patent formula is used to treat intestinal infection and inflammation, including amebic dysentery with pain, diarrhea, vomiting, and fever.

Dosage: It comes in vials containing twelve tablets, with complete instructions on dosage.

Jia Wei Xiang Lian Pian (Extra Ingredients Tablets); also known as Chia Wei Hsiang Lien Pian

Description: This patent formula is useful for treating acute bacillary dysentery, with fever, abdominal pain, and diarrhea with blood and pus.

Dosage: It comes in vials of eight tablets, with complete instructions on dosage.

Dysmenorrhea

The use of Chinese herbs for treating many serious female reproductive diseases is well documented, as is their use for treating what is by far the most common female complaint: painful menstruation, clinically known as dysmenorrhea. The mental anguish that develops in anticipation of menstrual pain along with hormonal imbalances is at the root of PMS (premenstrual syndrome).

There are two forms of dysmenorrhea: primary and secondary. Most women suffer to some degree from primary dysmenorrhea, which creates discomfort ranging from mild to severe pain and suffering. A long list of accompanying symptoms includes migraine headaches, bloating, lower abdominal pain (cramps), severe blood loss, anemia, and fatigue. Secondary dysmenorrhea is due to an underlying disorder such as endometriosis (a condition in which fragments of the lining of the uterus are found in other parts of the pelvic cavity), ovarian cysts, or pelvic inflammatory disease. See also Endometriosis; Ovarian Cyst; Pelvic Inflammatory Disease.

Traditional Chinese medicine treats primary dysmenorrhea with blood tonics, which contain herbs that eliminate the blood clots that cause cramps by thinning and cooling the blood. Other herbs in the blood-tonic formulas improve circulation, resolve anemia (which results from monthly blood loss), and regulate the menstrual cycle (which means controlling the duration of the period to no fewer than three and no more than five days). In cases of secondary dysmenorrhea, the underlying disorder must be corrected before blood tonics can be effectively used.

Ba Zhen Tang (Eight Treasure Decoction)

Original Source: *Zheng Ti Lei Yao* (according to *Chinese Herbal Medicine Formulas and Strategies*)

Ingredients:

Quantity (Grams)	Chinese Herbs	English Translation
9	Ren Shen	Ginseng
12	Bai Zhu	Atractylodes Rhizome
12	Fu Ling	Tuckahoe Root
3	Zhi Gan Cao	Honey-Cooked Licorice Root
15	Shu Di Huang	Chinese Foxglove Root, Wine-Cooked
12	Bai Shao	White Peony Root
12	Dang Gui	Tangkuei
9	Chuan Xiong	Szechuan Lovage Root

Description: This overall blood and Chi tonic improves circulation, reduces anemia, eliminates clots, and is eminently useful for women suffering from difficult menstruation.

Analysis: Ren Shen and Bai Zhu together increase the vital energy (Chi) throughout the entire body, while specifically benefiting the spleen. Fu Ling clears dampness. Shu Di Huang, Bai Shao, and Dang Gui all enrich the blood and eliminate pain. Chuan Xiong improves blood circulation. Zhi Gan Cao harmonizes the herbs in this formula and improves the taste.

Dosage and Method of Preparation: Make a decoction. Drink four ounces of Ba Zhen Tang tea at room temperature twice daily.

Wu Ji Bai Feng Wan (Black Chicken White Phoenix Pills/Condensed); also known as Wu Chi Pai Feng Wan, or Wu Ji Bai Feng Wan Nong Suo

Description: This patent formula enriches the blood, relieves anemia, and is useful for reproductive disorders including menstrual cramps, postpartum fatigue, and PMS.

Dosage: It comes in bottles of 120 pills, with complete instructions on dosage.

Bu Xue Tiao Jing Pian (Nourish Blood Adjust Period Tablets); also known as Bu Tiao Tablets

Description: This patent formula treats irregular periods, cramps, and excessive bleeding and is highly recommended for correcting menstrual disorders.

Dosage: It comes in bottles of one hundred tablets, with complete instructions on dosage.

To Jing Wan (Regulate Menses Pills)

Description: This patent formula is excellent for eliminating cramps.

Dosage: It comes in bottles of eighty pills, with complete instructions on dosage.

Ear, Disorders of: Ache; Infection; Tumors (see also Otitis Media)

Earaches can occur for a variety of reasons: an excess of ear wax, colds, infected sinuses, the presence of foreign objects, and changes in atmospheric pressure such as that experienced when ascending or descending in an aircraft. With most earaches there is generally little cause for concern, except in cases involving foreign objects and infections that become uncontrollable and persistent. In such instances a physician should be consulted.

Other possible causes of earache include labyrinthitis (inflammation of the fluid-filled chambers in the inner ear that sense balance), dental problems, tonsillitis, throat cancer, problems involving the lower jaw or neck (such as temporomandibular syndrome and on rare occasions herpes zoster infection), tumors in the ear, and certain drugs (in particular aminoglycoside antibiotics such as streptomycin and gentamicin).

Traditional Chinese medicine uses the following patent formulas to treat ear disorders:

Shuang Liao Hou Feng San (Double Ingredient Sore Throat Disease Powder); also known as Superior Sore Throat Powder Spray

Description: This patent formula clears heat and inflammation. Use it for sore throat, inflamed sinuses, and middle-ear infections.

Dosage: It comes in 2.2-gram bottles of spray, with complete instructions on dosage.

Niu Huang Jie Du Pian (Cow Gallstone Dispel Toxin Tablet); also known as Niu Huang Chieh Tu Pien, or Bezoar Antipyretic Pills

Description: This patent formula clears heat, reduces inflammation, eliminates infection, and is useful for tonsillitis, fever, and ear infection.

Caution: This formula is prohibited for use during pregnancy.

Dosage: It comes in bottles of twenty tablets, with complete instructions on dosage.

Eczema—see Rash

Edema

Edema, once popularly known as dropsy, is the abnormal accumulation of fluid in the body tissue, characterized by visible swelling. The two types of edema are local edema, which occurs following an injury, and general edema, seen with heart failure, kidney damage, cirrhosis of the liver, dietary protein deficiency (often associated with alcoholism), and thiamin (vitamin B1) deficiency leading to beriberi. Certain drugs can also cause edema, including corticosteroids, androgen, and high-estrogen contraceptives, which act on the kidneys to cause salt retention. In the early stages, often the only sign of edema is an increase in weight; however, once excess body fluid increases by more than 15 percent, visible swelling becomes evident. Although the swelling occurs most often in the lower part of the body (lower back and ankles), in severe cases fluid can accumulate in one or more of the large body cavities, as with ascites (accumulation of fluid in the abdomen) and pulmonary edema (fluid in the lungs).

Traditional Chinese medicine's approach to treating edema, which it calls dampness, is to determine the underlying cause. In cases that are not remediable, herbal diuretics are used to make the body excrete the excess fluid by increasing the urinary output of the kidneys. The following two formulas have proven helpful in reducing edema:

Wu Pi Tang (Five Peel Decoction)

Original Source: *Tai Ping Hui Min He Ji Jun Fang* (according to *Chinese Herbal Medicine Formulas and Strategies*)

Ingredients:

Quantity (Grams)	Chinese Herbs	English Translation
15	Di Gu Pi	Wolfberry Root Bark
6	Sheng Jiang Pi	Fresh Ginger Root, Skin
15	Fu Ling Pi	Tuckahoe Root Skin
9	Wu Jia Pi	Five Bark Root, Bark
15	Da Fu Pi	Betel Husk

6	Dong Gua Pi	Wintermelon Seed's Husk
6	Che Qian Cao	Plantago Plant
6	Huang Qi	Milk-Vetch Root

Description: This decoction can be used for generalized edema with a sensation of heaviness.

Analysis: Di Gu Pi, Sheng Jiang Pi, Fu Ling Pi, Wu Jia Pi, Da Fu Pi, and Dong Gua Pi all combine with the single purpose of eliminating edema by moving body fluids and promoting urination. Che Qian Cao's diuretic function is somewhat minor; it clears heat, and along with Huang Qi, it increases and promotes the movement of vital energy (Chi) and assists in the transportation of fluids.

Dosage and Method of Preparation: Make a decoction. Drink four ounces of Wu Pi Tang tea at room temperature twice daily.

Jin Kui Shen Qi Wan (Deficient Kidney Chi Pill); also known as Sexotan, or Jin Gui Shen Qi Wan

Description: For relief of edema with cold hands and feet, low backache, and poor circulation.

Dosage: This patent medicine comes in a bottle of 120 pills, with complete instructions on dosage.

Ejaculation, Disorders of

Ejaculatory disorders take on three forms: inhibited ejaculation, retrograde ejaculation, and premature ejaculation.

Inhibited ejaculation, a relatively rare condition, is when ejaculation does not occur at all even though erection is normal. Its cause can be psychological in origin (in which case counseling may help), or a complication of some physical disorder such as diabetes, or a side effect of certain drugs, particularly antihypertensives.

Retrograde ejaculation is when ejaculation is forced backward into the bladder. It is a physical disorder in which the valve at the base of the bladder fails to close during ejaculation, forcing the ejaculate (semen) back into the bladder. Retrograde ejaculation can occur as a result of neurological disease, after surgery on the neck of the bladder, after prostatectomy (surgery to remove part or all of the prostate gland), or after extensive pelvic surgery. Although no herbal treatment exists for this condition, engaging in intercourse with a full bladder can sometimes lead to normal ejaculation.

Premature ejaculation, by far the most common of the three ejaculatory disorders, is when ejaculation occurs before or very soon after penetration. It is the most common sexual problem in men and is especially common in adolescents. Most adult men occasionally experience premature ejaculation due to overstimulation or anxiety about sexual performance. If premature ejaculation occurs frequently, its causes may be psychological. Sexual counseling and techniques for delaying ejaculation are often effective remedies.

Traditional Chinese medicine offers several recommendations for treating premature ejaculation:

Meditation and breathing exercises serve two purposes: to calm down when overstimulated and to stop the mind from wandering (fantasizing) and make the person totally present so that ejaculation does not accidentally occur.

Reflexology, or the deer exercise, is an ancient Chinese practice for invigorating and strengthening the entire urogenital system as well as correcting premature ejaculation. In recent years it has been renamed the Kegel exercise after gynecologist Dr. Arnold Kegel, who has incorrectly been given credit for developing it. It is done by contracting the muscles that are used to cut off the flow of urine. Once you squeeze, try to hold the contraction for a full five seconds before you release. Do this procedure ten to twenty-five times daily.

Manual interruption of the seminal flow involves using the index and second fingers to find the spot called the perineum (between the scrotum and the anus). When ejaculation is eminent press the area firmly and hold. This will stop ejaculation.

The following herbal remedy is available for ejaculatory disorders:

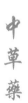

Chin So Ku Ching Wan (Golden Lock [Tea] Pills); also known as Jin Suo Gu Jing Wan, or Golden Lock Consolidate-Jing Pills

Description: This patent formula astringes seminal discharge and is useful for nocturnal emissions, premature ejaculation, and is used in Taoist sexual practices. A recent report by Jake Fratkin, who is a source for a number of the patent formulas in this book and the author of *Chinese Herbal Patent Formulas,* recommends limiting use of this formula to short periods of time.

Dosage: It comes in bottles of one hundred pills, with complete instructions on dosage.

Encephalitis—see Meningitis

Encephalitis is an inflammation of the brain, usually caused by a viral infection.

Endometriosis

Endometriosis, perhaps the most common cause of infertility, is the presence of fragments of the uterine lining in other parts of the pelvic cavity. Although the exact cause is uncertain, it is thought to occur when fragments of the uterine lining that are shed during menstruation do not leave the body with the menstrual flow. Instead, they travel up the fallopian tubes and into the pelvic cavity, where they may adhere to and grow on any of the pelvic organs. These displaced fragments continue to respond to the menstrual cycle as if they were still inside the uterus, bleeding each month. The blood, unable to escape, causes the formation of slow-growing cysts that can vary from the size of a pin head to the size of a grapefruit. The growth and swelling of the cysts are responsible for much of the pain associated with endometriosis.

The symptoms of endometriosis can include severe abdominal and/or lower back pain during menstruation, painful intercourse, and symptoms associated with digestive problems such as diarrhea, constipation, or painful defecation. The most common symptom, however, is abnormal or heavy menstrual bleeding.

The following formulas can be used to treat endometriosis:

Gui Zhi Fu Ling Tang (Cinnamon Twig and Poria Decoction)

Original Source: *Jin Gui Yao Lue* (according to *Chinese Herbal Medicine Formulas and Strategies*)

Ingredients:

Quantity (Grams)	Chinese Herbs	English Translation
12	Gui Zhi	Saigon Cinnamon Twig
12	Fu Ling	Tuckahoe Root
15	Chi Shao Yao	Red Peony Root
12	Mu Dan Pi	Tree Peony Root, Bark of
12	Tao Ren	Peach Kernel

Description: This raw-herb formula can be used for abdominal pain, blood clots, and heavy menstrual bleeding associated with endometriosis.

Caution: This formula is prohibited for use during pregnancy.

Analysis: Gui Zhi and Fu Ling unblock the meridians and promote blood circulation. Chi Shao Yao and Mu Dan Pi both promote circulation and dissolve blood clotting while removing heat. Tao Ren assists in this action.

Dosage and Method of Preparation: Make a decoction. Drink four ounces of Gui Zhi Fu Ling Tang tea at room temperature three times daily, or drink six ounces twice daily.

Fu Ke Wu Jin Wan (Gynecology Black Gold Pills); also known as Wu Jin Wan

Description: Use this patent medicine to treat endometriosis with fatigue, lower abdominal pain, back pain, and heavy menstrual flow.

Caution: This formula is prohibited for use during pregnancy.

Dosage: This patent medicine comes in a box of ten honey pills, with complete instructions on dosage.

Fu Ke Zhong Zi Wan (Gynecology Pregnancy Pills); also known as De Sheng Dan, or Zhong Zi Wan

Description: Use this patent medicine to treat irregular menstruation, sharp abdominal pain, heavy bleeding, and blood clots associated with endometriosis.

Caution: This formula is prohibited for use during pregnancy.

Dosage: This patent medicine comes in bottles of one hundred pills, with complete instructions on dosage.

Enema

Traditional Chinese medicine's assertion that the bowels are the "source of 10,001 diseases" powerfully reminds us of the wisdom in adopting a diet high in fiber. It should also cause us to consider using herbal enemas as an additional means of insuring gastrointestinal health.

Enema, a procedure in which fluid is passed through a tube into the rectum, can be used for promoting bowel movement (in case of constipation), removing impacted fecal matter (intestinal cleansing), and treating intestinal disorders such as inflammation and infection by introducing antibiotic and anti-inflammatory herbal tea into the intestinal tract. Important points to remember when administering an enema are (1) the nozzle should be thoroughly cleaned (to avoid infection) and well lubricated (to avoid discomfort) before inserting it into the rectum, (2) the fluid (herbal tea) used for the enema should be tepid (not cold) to prevent sudden contraction of the intestines, and (3) insertion should be done slowly and gently.

The formula used for enema is a single-herb tea made from Pu Gong Ying (Dandelion).

Pu Gong Ying Tang (Dandelion Decoction)

Ingredient:

Quantity (Grams)	Chinese Herb	English Translation
9	Pu Gong Ying	Dandelion

Description: This decoction can be used internally (as a drink) or externally (as an enema) for inflammation of the intestine, abscess, ulcerative colitis, and other intestinal disorders.

Analysis: Pu Gong Ying eliminates toxins in the blood, resolves pathogenic heat, and resolves infections.

Dosage and Method of Preparation: Make a decoction. Internal Use: drink four ounces of Pu Gong Ying Tang tea at room temperature twice daily, as needed. External Use: fill the enema bag with room temperature Pu Gong Ying Tang tea that has been thoroughly strained. Use as needed.

Epilepsy (see also Seizure)

The recurrent seizures that are the most recognizable feature of epilepsy can occur for a variety of reasons. They can be associated with head injuries, birth trauma, brain infections such as meningitis or encephalitis, brain tumors, stroke, a metabolic imbalance, or there may simply be an inherited predisposition. There are two main types of epileptic seizures: grand mal and petit mal. Grand mal, the more severe form, generally affects adults. During grand mal seizures, the person falls down unconscious and the body stiffens and jerks uncontrollably. Following the seizure, the muscles relax, and bowel or bladder control may be lost. Petit mal seizures are normally less severe and only affect children and teenagers. They are shorter in duration, usually lasting a few seconds to half a minute, and to the onlooker it may appear that the child is simply daydreaming or inattentive.

In almost every case, Western medicine treats epilepsy with anticonvulsant drugs. Occasionally, brain surgery may be considered if a single area of brain damage (usually the temporal lobe) is causing the seizures and medication proves ineffective. Traditional Chinese medicine takes a somewhat different approach. The fairly complicated treatment involves following a carefully planned diet and herbal therapy regimen and treating the heart, spleen, and liver with acupuncture.

Herbal formulas for the treatment of epilepsy are as follows:

Zhi Jing San (Stop Spasms Powder)

Original Source: *Fang Ji Xue* (according to *Chinese Herbal Medicine Formulas and Strategies*)

Ingredients:

Quantity (Grams)	Chinese Herbs	English Translation
9	Quan Xie	Scorpion
9	Wu Gong	Centipede

Description: This raw-herb formula stops muscle twitches, convulsions, rigidity, and spasms of the entire body.

Analysis: Both Quan Xie and Wu Gong are effective for relieving spasms and stopping pain; when combined, they have a strong synergistic action.

Dosage and Method of Preparation: Have the herbs ground into a fine powder or purchase them powdered. Use .9 grams (minimum dose) to 1.5 grams (maximum dose) of Zhi Jing San formula per dose; drink four ounces of warm water with the powdered formula two to four times daily depending on the severity of the seizures, as needed.

Tze Zhu Wan (Magnetite Cinnabar Pills); also known as Ci Zhu Wan

Description: This patent formula is useful for epilepsy and manic disorders.

Dosage: It comes in bottles of 120 pills, with complete instructions on dosage.

She Dan Chen Pi San (Snake Gallbladder Tangerine Peel Powder); also known as San She Tan Chen Pi Mo

Description: This formula is used to treat disharmonies, which lead to mania, uneasiness, hysteria, or epilepsy, including grand mal and petit mal seizures. It can be taken with Western medicine's seizure medications such as phenobarbital or Dilantin.

Dosage: It comes in small vials each containing .6 grams of powder, with complete instructions on dosage.

Yan Hu Suo Zhi Tong Pian (Yan Hu Extract, Stop Pain Tablets); also known as Corydalis Yanhusus-Analgesic Tablets, or Yan Hu Su Zhi Tong Pian

Description: Use this patent medicine to treat uneasiness and agitation; it is effective in relaxing striated muscle spasms and tremors. When combined with Dilantin, this medication has a synergistic effect in reducing seizures.

Dosage: It comes in vials containing twelve tablets, with complete instructions on dosage.

Tian Ma Mi Huan Pian (Gastrodia Name of a Fungus Extract); also known as Tien Ma Mi Huan Su

Description: This patent medicine is useful for treating epileptic seizures and numbness of the limbs.

Dosage: It comes in bottles of thirty-six capsules, with complete instructions on dosage.

Erection (Penile), Disorders of

Three conditions are considered erection disorders: chordee, priapism, and impotence (also called erectile dysfunction).

Chordee is a painfully bowed or curved erection. Chordee most often occurs in males with hypospadias, a congenital defect in which the urethral opening is on the underside of the penis instead of on the tip. Surgery usually corrects the condition and is often performed in early childhood. Untreated, chordee can make intercourse very difficult and in some cases impossible.

Priapism is an erection that persists without any sexual stimulation. It occurs when blood fails to drain from the penis, keeping it erect. This can result from nerve damage, from a blood disease like leukemia or sickle cell anemia that causes partial blood clotting, or in rare instances from a blockage of the normal outflow of blood from the penis as a result of an infection such as prostatitis (infection of the prostate gland) or urethritis (inflammation of the urethra). To avoid the risk of permanent damage to the penis, emergency treatment is recommended. Treatment may involve spinal anesthesia and then withdrawal of blood from the penis through a wide-bore needle.

Impotence, also called erectile dysfunction, is the total or partial failure to attain or maintain an erection. It is a common sexual disorder among men and affects most men at some time in their lives. In about 90 percent of cases impotence is caused by temporary or long-standing psychological factors such as stress, anxiety, or depression. Only about 10 percent of impotence cases are caused by physical disorders. Possible physical causes are diabetes mellitus or some other hormonal imbalance, neurological disorders such as spinal chord damage, chronic alcohol abuse, poor blood circulation to the penis, or lowered levels of the male sex hormone testosterone. Certain drugs can also cause impotence, particularly antipsychotics, antidepressives, antihypertensives, and diuretics. Impotence also becomes more common as men get older, probably due to altered circulation or lowered levels of the male sex hormone testosterone.

In addition to recognizing these physical complications as possible causes, traditional Chinese medicine also cites an excessive loss of semen (engaging in too much sex) and weak kidneys as possible causes or contributing factors to impotence. The following herbal formulas are recommended (1) for treating impotence by replenishing lost sperm when sexual excess is the suspected cause, (2) for improving blood circulation in the lower jiao (lower part of the body) when poor circulation is suspected, and (3) for strengthening the kidneys.

Zan Yu Dan Tang (Special Decoction to Aid Fertility)

Original Source: *Jing Yue Quan Shu* (according to *Chinese Herbal Medicine Formulas and Strategies*)

Ingredients:

Quantity (Grams)	Chinese Herbs	English Translation
6	Fu Zi	Accessory Root of Szechuan Aconite
6	Rou Gui	Saigon Cinnamon Inner Bark
12	Rou Cong Rong	Fleshy Stem of Broomrape
12	Ba Ji Tian	Morinda Root
12	Yin Yang Huo	Licentious Goat Work Leaf

6	She Chuang Zi	Cnidium Fruit Seed
12	Jiu Zi	Chinese Leek Seed
12	Xian Mao	Golden Eye Grass Rhizome
12	Shan Zhu Yu	Fruit Asiatic Cornelian Cherry
12	Du Zhong	Eucommia Bark
24	Shu Di Huang	Chinese Foxglove Root, Wine-Cooked
18	Dang Gui	Tangkuei
18	Gou Qi Zi	Matrimony Vine Fruit
24	Bai Zhu	Atractylodes Rhizome

Description: This herbal formula is used for impotence or infertility, to strengthen the kidneys, and improve energy levels.

Analysis: The chief ingredients in this formula are Fu Zi, Rou Gui, Ron Cong Rong, Ba Ji Tian, Yin Yang Huo, She Chuang Zi, Jiu Zi, Xian Mao, Shan Zhu Yu, and Du Zhong. Combined, their action for strengthening the kidneys becomes quite powerful. Shu Di Huang, Dang Gui, and Gou Qi Zi are supportive by enriching the blood and replenishing sperm levels. Bai Zhu is added to strengthen the spleen and eliminate dampness.

Dosage and Method of Preparation: Prepare a decoction. Drink four ounces of Zan Yu Dan Tang tea three times daily, as needed.

Kang Wei Ling (Excessively Limp Efficacious Remedy)

Description: This patent formula builds sperm, circulates blood, and is a strong male tonic for treating impotence and premature ejaculation. In China this formula has a high clinical effectiveness rating for impotence.

Dosage: It comes in bottles of 120 pills, with complete instructions on dosage.

Nan Bao (Strong Man Bao Capsules)

Description: This patent medicine is used to treat deficiency of kidneys and is useful for impotence, failure to obtain an erection, and lowered sexual drive.

Dosage: It comes in a package of twenty capsules, with complete instructions on dosage.

Tabellae Chuang Yao Tonic (Strengthen Kidney Tablets); also known as Zhuang Yao Jian Shen Pian

Description: This patent medicine strengthens the kidneys and treats problems arising from excessive sexual activity such as lowered sex drive and impotence.

Dosage: It comes in bottles of one hundred pills, with complete instructions on dosage.

Hai Ma Bu Shen Wan (Seahorse Genital Tonic Pills); also known as Seahorse Herb Tea

Description: This patent formula improves low sperm count and impotence, strengthens the kidneys, and treats spermatorrhea (involuntary loss of semen without orgasm).

Dosage: It comes in bottles of 120 pills, with complete instructions on dosage.

Eye, Disorders of—see Cataract; Conjunctivitis; Glaucoma

Fatigue—see Tonics (in chapter 2)

Fever

Fever is an abnormal rise in body temperature usually caused by bacterial or viral infections ranging from those associated with the common cold or a case of the flu to those much more serious such as typhoid. Clinically known as pyrexia, fever may also occur in noninfectious conditions such as dehydration or thyrotoxicosis (a condition resulting from overactivity of the thyroid gland), myocardial infarction (heart attack), and tumors of the lymphatic system. High fevers (100°F or above) can cause confusion or delirium, seizures, or coma (chiefly among the elderly). The average person's normal body temperature is 98.6°F, but this can vary by as much as a degree either way.

If the fever sufferer is elderly or is younger than six months, a physician should be consulted immediately. Additionally, any fever lasting longer than three days or exhibiting symptoms such as severe headache with stiff neck, abdominal pain, or painful urination should also be considered an emergency and a physician should be contacted right away.

Western medicine treats fever caused by infection with antipyretic (temperature-lowering) drugs; otherwise, treatment is directed toward resolving the underlying cause by, for example, administering the appropriate antibiotic for a bacterial infection. If it is determined that infection is the cause of the fever, traditional Chinese medicine similarly treats fevers using antipyretic and antibiotic herbs. Occasionally, the traditional Chinese physician will perform bloodletting. In the early stages of a fever, bathing the sufferer in lukewarm water is also recommended to help lower the body's temperature.

The following herbal formulas have been used successfully to fight infection and lower bodily temperature:

Lien Chiao Pai Tu Pien (Forsythia Defeat Toxin Tablet); also known as Lian Qiao Bai Du Pian

Description: This patent formula is used for acute infections causing fever, ulcerated carbuncles, and abscesses with rash.
Caution: This formula is prohibited for use during pregnancy.
Dosage: It comes in boxes of twelve vials, eight tablets per vial, with complete instructions on dosage.

An Kung Niu Huang Wan (Peaceful Palace Ox Gallstone Pill); also known as An Gong Niu Huang Wan

Description: This patent medicine clears heat from the body and treats restlessness, vertigo, delirium, and high fevers; it is also useful for measles.
Caution: This formula is prohibited for use during pregnancy.
Dosage: It comes in boxes of one pill, with complete instructions on dosage.

Fever Blister (see also Stomatitis; Herpes [Oral]; Ulcer)

The term fever blister dates back to the pre-antibiotic era when blisters often appeared on the body during feverish infectious diseases. Also known as cold sores, fever blisters usually appear on the face and are in many cases caused by the herpes simplex virus.

Chinese medicine uses the following patent medicine to treat fever blisters:

Lung Tan Xie Gan Wan (Gentiana Purge Liver Pills); also known as Long Dan Xie Gan Wan

Description: This patent medicine will relieve itchiness from a fever blister on the mouth and is helpful in cases of genital and oral herpes.

Dosage: It comes in bottles of one hundred pills, with complete instructions on dosage.

Fibroid Tumor

A fibroid is a benign tumor of the uterus. The cause is un-known, but it is suspected that fibroids are related to an abnormal response to estrogen. Fibroids are one of the most common tumors, occurring in about 20 percent of all women over age thirty. In many cases there are no symptoms, particularly if the fibroid is small. If the fibroid grows and erodes the lining of the uterine cavity, it may cause heavy or prolonged menstrual periods. Large fibroids can exert pressure on the bladder, causing discomfort or urinary frequency, or on the bowel, causing backache and constipation. Occasionally, fibroids attach to the wall of the uterus and become twisted, causing sudden pain in the lower abdomen. Fibroids that distort the uterine cavity are also likely to cause recurrent miscarriage or infertility.

Western medicine usually recommends surgical removal of the fibroid tumors or removal of the entire uterus (hysterectomy) when severe symptoms occur.

Although traditional Chinese medicine cannot claim a high success rate, some herbal remedies are offered as a possible option to surgery. Susan C. Chen, author of *Gynecology According to Traditional Chinese Medicine,* recommends a combination of the following formulas for treating uterine myoma (fibroid tumors):

Formula A for Uterine Myoma (Fibroid Tumors)

Ingredients:

Quantity (Grams)	Chinese Herbs	English Translation
3	Gui Zhi	Saigon Cinnamon Twig
5	Chi Shao	Red Peony Root
5	Fu Ling	Tuckahoe Root
4	Tao Ren	Peach Kernel
4	Mu Dan Pi	Tree Peony Root, Bark of
5	Dan Shen	Relative Root
5	Da Huang	Rhubarb Root
4	Dang Gui	Tangkuei
3	Ji Nei Jin	Chicken Gizzard Lining
4	San Leng	Bur Reed Rhizome
4	E Zhu	Zedoary Rhizome

Analysis: Gui Zhi opens the pores and activates the meridians. Chi Shao stops pain, eliminates blood clots, clears heat, and cools the blood. Fu Ling dries dampness. Tao Ren and Mu Dan Pi circulate the blood, dissipate heat, and reduce nodules and blood clots. Dan Shen circulates blood and eliminates heat. Da Huang removes toxins and moves the bowels. Dang Gui enriches the blood. Ji Nei Jin strengthens the stomach. San Leng circulates blood and energy (Chi). E Zhu circulates blood and resolves clots.

Formula B for Uterine Myoma (Fibroid Tumors)

Ingredients:

Quantity (Grams)	Chinese Herbs	English Translation
2	Dang Gui	Tangkuei
2	Di Long	Earthworm
3	Zhi Ke	Bitter Orange Fruit Ripe

3	Chi Shao	Red Peony Root
3	Mu Yao	Strychnifolia Root
3	Hong Hua	Safflower Flower
2	Mu Xiang	Costus Root
3	Chuan Xiong	Szechuan Lovage Root
3	Ze Lan	Marsh Orchid Aerial
3	San Leng	Bur Reed Rhizome
2	Ru Xiang	Frankincense Resin
4	Yi Mu Cao	Chinese Motherwort Plant

Analysis: Dang Gui enriches the blood. Di Long clears heat and opens the meridians. Zhi Ke circulates the vital energy (Chi). Chi Shao circulates the blood and dissolves clots. Mu Yao and Hong Hua assist in improving circulation and reducing clotting. Mu Xiang and Chuan Xiong circulate the blood and reduce pain. Ze Lan circulates the blood and reduces water retention. San Leng circulates blood and Chi. Ru Xiang circulates blood and treats painful menstrual periods. Yi Mu Cao circulates the blood, relieves blood clotting, and constricts the uterus.

Description: The combined use of these two formulas shrinks fibroid tumors that cause heavy menstruation or irregular and painful menstruation with a heavy sensation in the lower abdomen, frequent urination, or constipation.

Dosage and Method of Preparation: Make a decoction. Drink four ounces of Formula A tea two times daily for two weeks, then four ounces of Formula B tea two times daily for two and a half months. At the end of the three-month period, schedule a gynecological exam to confirm that the fibroids are shrinking.

Flatulence

Flatulence, also known by the earthier names passing wind or farting, is the expulsion of intestinal gas (flatus) through the anus. Gas is usually caused by the fermentation of food that is incompletely digested. The main culprits are heavily spiced foods, green vegetables, cucumbers, nuts, onions, garlic, and dried fruits. Flatulence can usually be prevented by eating a plain diet and exercising regularly. In addition to the following herbal remedies, traditional Chinese medicine also recommends other, rather unconventional remedies like chewing the seeds of mandarin oranges.

Wei Te Ling #204 (Stomach Especially Effective Remedy)

Description: This patent medicine is helpful with gastritis, abdominal bloating, and flatulence.

Dosage: It comes in bottles of 120 pills, with complete instructions on dosage.

Wei Yao (Gastropathy Capsules); also known as 707 Gastropathy Capsules

Description: For gastritis, with stagnant food in the stomach and flatulence.

Dosage: It comes in bottles of forty-two capsules, with complete instructions on dosage.

Flu—see Colds and Flu

Food Poisoning (see also Diarrhea; Nausea)

Food poisoning is a term used for any illness of sudden onset characterized by stomach pains, vomiting, and diarrhea that is suspected of being caused by food recently eaten. Food poisoning is normally classified according to cause: infective, which is caused by a viral or bacterial contamination, and noninfective, which is not.

The bacteria most often responsible for food poisoning belongs to a group called salmonella. Some farm animals (particularly poultry) commonly harbor this bacteria. Salmonella may be transferred to food from the excrement of infected animals or people either by flies or a food handler whose hands have not been washed after using the toilet. Other bacterial sources are staphylococcal bacteria, which can be spread from a septic abscess on the skin of a food handler, and botulism, a rare, life-threatening form of food poisoning caused by a bacterial toxin associated with home preservation of food (see also Botulism). Viruses responsible for food poisoning are the Norwalk virus, a common contaminant of shellfish, and rotavirus, associated with water contaminated by human excrement.

Noninfective causes of food poisoning include poisonous mushrooms and toadstools and fresh fruits or vegetables that have been contaminated with insecticides.

The onset of symptoms varies according to the cause of poisoning. Chemical poisoning triggers symptoms after about thirty minutes; bacterial poisoning takes one to twelve hours; viral poisoning takes twelve to forty-eight hours.

If severe vomiting and diarrhea develop, or if the sufferer collapses, medical assistance should be sought. Samples of any food remaining from a recent meal should be kept to help pinpoint the cause and possibly prevent a widespread outbreak of food poisoning.

The following herbal formula can be used in the early stages of nonchemical food poisoning, while food is still in the stomach, with symptoms such as abdominal distention, inability to belch or relieve bloating, an urge to vomit but an inability to do so, sweating, and difficulty breathing:

Gua Di Tang (Melon Pedicle Decoction)

Original Source: *Shang Han Lun* (according to *Chinese Herbal Medicine Formulas and Strategies*)

Ingredients:

Quantity (Grams)	Chinese Herbs	English Translation
3	Gua Di	Melon Pedicle
3	Chi Xiao Dou	Aduki Beans

Description: This herbal formula discharges food stagnation or stomach contents via vomiting.

Caution: Because this formula induces vomiting, it should not be used in cases of chemical poisoning. Regurgitation of chemicals can burn or irritate the esophagus and throat.

Analysis: Gua Di is a bitter substance that effectively induces vomiting to clear the stomach. Chi Xiao Dou eliminates stomach discomfort and fullness (distention).

Dosage and Method of Preparation: Make a decoction; however, do not cook the herbs in this formula for longer than ten minutes. Sip from a glass of Gua Di Tang slowly, and stop drinking as soon as vomiting begins.

Bai Shao Yao Tang (White Peony Decoction)

Source: *Handbook of Chinese Herbs and Formulas,* volume 2
Ingredients:

Quantity (Grams)	Chinese Herbs	English Translation
15	Bai Shao Yao	White Peony Root
6	Dang Gui	Tangkuei
4.5	Gan Cao	Licorice
4.5	Mu Xiang	Costus Root
6	Bing Lang	Betel Nut
6	Huang Lian	Golden Thread Root
9	Huang Qin	Baical Skullcap
6	Da Huang	Rhubarb Root
1.5	Guan Gui	Inner Bark of Saigon Cinnamon

Description: This formula is used for abdominal pain, diarrhea, burning in the anus, and food poisoning; it is useful for milder cases of food poisoning.

Analysis: Bai Shao Yao and Dang Gui enrich the blood and relieve pain. Mu Xiang benefits the spleen and stomach. Bing Lang benefits the stomach and moves the bowels. Huang Qin, Huang Lian, and Da Huang clear heat, reduce inflammation, and treat dysenteric symptoms. Guan Gui warms the center and promotes digestion. Gan Cao harmonizes the herbs in the formula and improves the taste.

Dosage and Method of Preparation: Make a decoction. Drink four ounces of Bai Shao Yao Tang tea at room temperature three times daily, or as needed.

Fractures—see Bones

Fungal Infections/Fungal Diseases (see also specific complaint, e.g., Athlete's Foot; Jock Itch; Ringworm)

Fungal infections, also known as mycoses, are diseases of the skin or organs caused by the spread of fungal organisms. Fungal infections can be either mild or severe and are sometimes fatal. They can trigger allergic reactions leading to serious disorders such as asthma.

The incidence of fungal infections is more frequent and more serious among people taking long term antibiotics, corticosteroids, or immunosuppressant drugs. Infections common among people with immune deficiency disorders (such as AIDS) are described as opportunistic because they take advantage of the victim's lowered defenses.

The different classifications of fungal infections include:

- superficial infections: those that affect the skin, hair, nails, genital organs, and the inside of the mouth.
- subcutaneous infections: those beneath the skin.
- deep infections: those affecting internal organs including the lungs, liver (more rarely), bones, lymph nodes, brain, heart, or urinary tract.

Chinese medicine has had success treating fungal infections with the following herbal formulas:

Hua She Jie Yang Wan (Pit Viper Dispel Itching Pill); also known as Kai Yeung Wan

Description: This patent formula counteracts skin itching and various pruritus, dermatitis, and fungal infections due to allergic and drug reactions.

Caution: This formula is prohibited for use during pregnancy.

Dosage: It comes in bottles of sixty pills, with complete instructions on dosage

San She Jie Yang Wan (Tri Snake Itch Removing Pills)

Description: This patent formula is used for all kinds of fungal infections; it resolves infections and relieves itch.

Caution: This formula is prohibited for use during pregnancy.

Dosage: It comes in bottles of thirty pills, with complete instructions dosage.

Hua Tuo Gao (Hua Tuo Chinese Physician Ointment)

Description: This patent formula is useful for superficial fungal infections, dermatitis, eczema with scaling, and itching.

Dosage: Hua Tuo Gao comes in .20-gram tubes, with complete instructions on dosage.

Fu Ling Tu Jin Pi Ding (Complex Tu Jin Bark Tincture); also known as Composita Tujin Ointment

Description: This patent is used to treat superficial skin infections caused by fungi.

Note: This formula is for external use only.

Dosage: It comes in bottles of 15cc, with complete instructions on dosage.

Furuncles—see Carbuncles

Gallbladder, Disorders of: Stones, Infection, Inflammation, Tumor

The gallbladder stores bile that is produced by the liver. Several disorders are associated with it.

Congenital and genetic defects are abnormalities present from birth—usually an oversized gallbladder—that rarely cause problems. In problem cases, however, because the digestive system can function without a gallbladder, it is usually surgically removed with little known long-term effect.

Gallstones, which are composed primarily of cholesterol and bile pigments such as chalk, develop when the liver produces bile containing too much cholesterol. This occurs most often with obesity. Once the bile is overloaded with cholesterol, tiny particles can form that gradually grow as additional material solidifies around them, eventually forming a stone. Rare in childhood, gallstones become progressively more common with age. Three times as many women as men are affected. High-risk groups include overweight people and women who have had many children.

Inflammation and infection occur when a gallstone gets stuck in the bile duct leading from the gallbladder. This causes pain in the upper right side of the abdomen or between the shoulder blades (biliary colic), creates symptoms such as nausea and vomiting, and can also lead to jaundice. In some cases antibiotics are given to treat the infection, and ursodeoxycholic acid can be taken over several months to dissolve the stones. However, stones reoccur in about 50 percent of cases after the drug is stopped, requiring surgical removal of the gallbladder (cholecystectomy).

Surgical removal of the gallbladder is one of the most frequently performed surgeries in Western medicine. Traditional Chinese medicine has used the following formulas with a reasonable amount of success to dissolve gallstones and eliminate inflammation and infection:

Hao Qin Qing Dan Tang (Artemsia Annua and Scutellaria Decoction to Clear the Gallbladder)

Original Source: *Chong Ding Tong Su Shang Han Lun* (according to *Chinese Herbal Medicine Formulas and Strategies*)

Ingredients:

Quantity (Grams)	Chinese Herbs	English Translation
6	Qing Hao	Wormwood (Artemsia Annua) Root
9	Huang Qin	Baical Skullcap (Scutellaria) Root
9	Zhu Ru	Bamboo Shavings
4.5	Zhi Shi	Green Bitter Orange Fruit

4.5	Chen Pi	Ripe Tangerine Peel
4.5	Ban Xia	Half Summer
9	Chi Fu Ling	Red Tuckahoe Root
9	Bi Yu San	Jasper Powder

Description: This raw herb formula reduces pain in the upper abdomen, relieves infection, stops vomiting, and treats the gallbladder.

Analysis: Qing Hao and Huang Qin drain heat from the gallbladder. Zhu Ru also drains heat and stops vomiting. Zhi Shi, Chen Pi, and Ban Xia assist in reducing heat and directing the energy downward to arrest vomiting. Chi Fu Ling and Bi Yu San clear heat, relieve toxicity, and expel dampness.

Dosage and Method of Preparation: Make a decoction. Drink four ounces of Hao Qin Qing Dan Tang tea at room temperature three times daily, as needed.

Lidan Paishi Wan (Benefit Gallbladder Discharge Stone Tablet); also known as Li Dan Pai Shi Pian, or Li Dan Tablets

Description: This formula benefits the liver and gallbladder; it is used to reduce inflammation, disintegrate and remove gallstones, and promote bile secretion.

Caution: This formula is prohibited for use during pregnancy.

Dosage: It comes in bottles of 120 pills, with complete instructions on dosage.

Li Gan Pian/Liver Strengthening Tablets (Benefit Liver Tablets)

Description: This patent medicine reduces infection in the liver and gallbladder, regulates bile, and treats jaundice, hepatitis, and gallstones. It is a good adjunct for the previous formula.

Dosage: It comes in bottles of one hundred tablets, with complete instructions on dosage.

Tumors in the gallbladder are a rare form of cancer, occurring mainly in older people. The cancer may cause jaundice and tenderness in the upper right side of the abdomen, or it can be symptomless. Occasionally, the cancer is discovered during surgery on the gallbladder. It is treated by removal of as much of the tumor as possible. In most cases the cancer has invaded the liver by the time it has been detected, making the outlook grim. However, an excellent book on Chinese medicines used to fight cancer, *Anticancer Medicinal Herbs,* by Chang Minyi, claims that the following herbal formula has been used to treat gallbladder cancer:

Gallbladder Cancer Formula

Ingredients:

Quantity (Grams)	Chinese Herbs	English Translation
15	Long Dan Cao	Chinese Gentiana Root
15	Xia Ku Cao	Self Heal Spike
30	Pai Ying	White Nightshade
9	Jing Da Zi	Peking Spurge Seed
9	Chuan Shan Jia	Pangolin Scales
9	Ji Nei Jin	Chicken Gizzard Lining
9	Kun Bu	Kelp Thallus
9	Hai Zao	Seaweed Plant
9	Fu Hai Shi	Pumice
9	Tong Cao	Rice Paper Pith
1.5	Ah Wei	Asafoetida Gum Resin
1.5	Bao Mao	Cantharides

Description: This raw herb formula is used for treatment of cancer of the gallbladder.

Analysis: Long Dan Cao is useful for treating infection in the gallbladder and liver. Xia Ku Cao clears heat and dissipates nodules. Jing Da Zi eliminates toxins. Pai Ying treats inflammation and tumors in the gallbladder. Chuan Shan Jia reduces poisonous swelling. Ji Nei Jin strengthens the spleen. Kun Bu reduces nodules and swellings. Hai Zao assists in strengthening these functions. Fu Hai Shi clears heat and softens nodules. Tong Cao clears infections. Ah Wei aids digestion, and Bao Mao detoxifies poisons and dissolves palpable masses.

Dosage and Method of Preparation: Make a decoction. Drink eight ounces of the decocted tea at room temperature once daily.

Gallstones—see Gallbladder, Disorders of

Gastric Ulcer—see Ulcer

Gastritis

Because of the organic nature of herbs and the fact that they are consumed and digested much like food, Chinese medicine looks upon them as an extension of nutrition. The embodiment of this rationale can clearly be seen in the use of what are called Chinese food cures, employed in combination with herbal therapy for treating gastritis (inflammation of the mucus membrane lining the stomach). Some of the common causes of gastritis include drugs such as aspirin or alcohol or infection caused by the *Campylobacter* bacterium. Occasionally, it is caused by extreme physical stress such as head injury, severe burns, or liver failure. Symptoms can include discomfort in the upper abdomen (often aggravated by eating), nausea, vomiting, abdominal bleeding (resulting in dark feces due to the presence of blood), and anemia characterized by fatigue and breathlessness.

For treatment of gastritis, traditional Chinese medicine recommends a bland, wholesome diet (rice, steamed vegetables, scrambled eggs, porridge), combined with herbal therapy and the food cure that follows:

Crack open four to six eggs, discard the yolk and egg whites, then break the shells into smaller pieces. Bake the eggshells in a 350-degree oven for approximately fifteen minutes until the shells are dried. In a blender, crush the shells into powder, the finer the better. Mix four grams of powdered eggshells with four ounces (one-half cup) of warm water; add honey to taste. Drink the mixture before meals three times daily to reduce stomach acid and gastric irritation. Store the unused powdered eggshells in a glass jar and refrigerate for later use.

Additional herbal formulas used to assist in healing gastric inflammation follow.

Wei Yao (Gastropathy Capsules); also known as 707 Gastropathy Capsules

Description: This patent formula reduces gas, burping, and acid regurgitation. It stops pain and promotes tissue regeneration of the stomach mucus.

Dosage: It comes in bottles of forty-two capsules, with complete instructions on dosage.

Sai Mei An (The Race Between Rot and Peaceful Health)

Description: This patent formula stops stomachache, promotes tissue regeneration, and is used for acute or chronic gastritis with hyperacidity in the stomach.

Dosage: It comes in bottles of fifty capsules, with complete instructions on dosage.

Wei Tei Ling #204 (Stomach Especially Effective Remedy)

Description: This patent formula neutralizes stomach acid, relieves stomachache, and strengthens the stomach.

Dosage: It comes in bottles of 120 pills, with complete instructions on dosage.

Geriatric Medicine—see Tonics (in chapter 2)

Gingivitis

Gingivitis is inflammation of the gums due to infection. It is usually caused by a buildup of plaque (a sticky deposit of bacteria mucus and food particles) around the base of the teeth. Gingivitis can also be the result of injury—from brushing too vigorously or from careless flossing. Mild gingivitis, very common in young adults, is sometimes also seen in pregnant women and persons with diabetes, due to changes in their hormone levels.

Good oral hygiene is the best way to prevent and treat gingivitis, combined with the following herbal formulas:

Qing Wei Tang (Clear Stomach Decoction)

Original Source: *Yi Zong Jin Jian* (according to *Chinese Herbal Medicine Formulas and Strategies*)

Ingredients:

Quantity (Grams)	Chinese Herbs	English Translation
6	Huang Lian	Golden Thread Root
6	Sheng Ma	Black Cohosh Rhizome
9	Mu Dan Pi	Tree Peony Root, Bark of
12	Sheng Di Huang	Chinese Foxglove Root, Raw
12	Dang Gui	Tangkuei

Description: This herbal formula is used to relieve toothache, facial swelling, bad breath, bleeding and sore gums, and gingivitis.

Analysis: Huang Lian reduces stomach heat. Sheng Ma assists in the reduction of stomach heat and also relieves toxicity. Mu Dan Pi and Sheng Di Huang cool the blood. Dang Gui reduces swelling and alleviates pain.

Dosage and Method of Preparation: Make a decoction. Drink four ounces of Qing Wei Tang tea at room temperature three times daily, or as needed.

Niu Huang Jie Du Pian (Cow Gallstone Dispel Toxin Tablet); also known as Niu Huang Chieh Tu Pien, or Bezoar Antipyretic Pills

Description: This patent medicine is used for those with low-grade fever, inflamed tooth or gums, toxic swelling or abscess, headache, or oral ulcers.

Caution: This formula is prohibited for use during pregnancy.

Dosage: It comes in bottles of eight or twenty tablets, with complete instructions on dosage.

Ching Fei Yi Huo Pien (Clear Lungs Restrain Fire Tablets); also known as Qing Fei Yi Huo Pian

Description: This patent medicine is used to relieve fever, mouth sores, bleeding gums, gingivitis, and toothache.

Dosage: It comes in boxes of twelve vials, eight tablets per vial, with complete instructions on dosage.

Glaucoma

The condition known as glaucoma is the result of abnormally high amounts of fluid in the eye, which create compression of blood vessels and the fibers of the optic nerve, leading to nerve-fiber destruction and causing partial or complete loss of vision. The most common form of glaucoma is open-angle glaucoma, which rarely occurs before middle age. Open-angle glaucoma tends to run in families and often exhibits no symptoms until there is a noticeable loss of vision. Other forms are acute closed-angle glaucoma, characterized by the sudden onset of impaired vision, and congenital glaucoma, caused by structural abnormalities in the drainage of the eye.

There are several possible causes of glaucoma, including injury to the eye, eye diseases such as uveitis, dislocation of the lens, and adhesions between the iris and the cornea.

Due to the lack of symptoms and the loss of peripheral vision occurring so gradually, sufferers of chronic glaucoma frequently experience irreversible damage before it is diagnosed. The opposite is true for acute glaucoma, whose list of symptoms includes a sudden loss or fogginess of vision, a dull, severe, aching pain above the eye, and the perception of halos or rainbow rings around light sources at night. Occasionally, nausea and vomiting occur. The eye can become red, with a partially dilated pupil, and a hazy or cloudy cornea can develop.

Western medicine's standard method for treating chronic open-angle glaucoma is to use eye drops that reduce the pressure in the eye. Acute closed-angle glaucoma, although treated similarly, is considered more of a medical emergency, calling for urgent treatment. The eye drops used by Western practitioners to treat both kinds of glaucoma, although relatively benign, have been known to produce hair loss, dry skin, and brittle nails.

Traditional Chinese medicine's approach to treating glaucoma is in many ways quite similar, with an emphasis on reducing fluid and eliminating pressure in the eye. However, use of the recommended herbal formulas does not have the reported side effects associated with the Western medication.

Huang Lian Yang Gan Wan (Rhizoma Coptidis Goat Liver Pills)

Description: This patent formula is used to treat eye disorders with symptoms of poor vision (especially at night), photophobia, glaucoma, cataracts, and night blindness.

Dosage: It comes in boxes of ten pills, with complete instructions on dosage.

Shi Hu Ye Guang Wan (Dendrobrium Leaf Night Sight Pills); also known as Dendrobrium Moniforme Night Sight Pills

Description: This patent formula is useful for treating diseases of the eye such as glaucoma, retinitis, choroiditis, optic neuritis, and night blindness.

Dosage: It comes in boxes of ten pills, six grams each, with complete instructions on dosage.

Qi Ju Di Huang Wan (Lycium Chrysanthemum Rehmannia Pill); also known as Lycci and Chrysanthemum Tea, or Lycium-Rehmannia Pills

Description: This patent medicine is used for symptoms of blurry vision, painful eyes, pressure behind the eyes, and poor night vision.

Dosage: It comes in bottles of one hundred pills, with complete instructions on dosage.

Goiter

Goiters are enlarged thyroid glands and are caused when excessive amounts of thyroid hormones are produced. They can range in size from a barely noticeable lump to an immense swelling. Goiters can occur at puberty, during pregnancy, as a result of taking birth-control pills, or due to a lack of sufficient iodine in the diet. Until recently, goiters were either totally or partially removed using a surgical procedure called thyroidectomy. Today, due to certain risks, surgery is usually performed only when large goiters press on the esophagus or the trachea, causing difficulty swallowing or breathing.

A toxic goiter, known as thyrotoxicosis and primarily associated with Graves' disease, is characterized by symptoms such as increased appetite, warm dry skin, weight loss, tremors, insomnia, and occasional muscle weakness and agitation.

In rare instances, damage to the thyroid gland may also be caused by a tumor, a nodule (lump), or thyroid cancer. Often goiters that are not caused by disease disappear naturally or become so small that treatment is unnecessary. When iodine deficiency is determined as the cause, an increase in dietary intake of the mineral iodine is recommended.

It is interesting to note the similarities in Western and traditional Chinese medicine's approach to treating such a deficiency, which involves recommending increased amounts of iodine-rich food. While Western medicine prescribes adding more fish and iodized salt to the diet, the ancient Chinese method was to administer iodine-rich black ash obtained from burnt seaweed. Although this ancient practice has been discontinued, ironically, modern Chinese physicians—much like their ancient predecessors—do continue to use herbal formulas in which seaweed (condensed in pills and capsules) is often a main ingredient.

Xiao Luo Tang (Reduce Scrofula Decoction)

Original Source: *Yi Xue Xin Wu* (according to *Chinese Herbal Medicine Formulas and Strategies*)

Ingredients:

Quantity (Grams)	Chinese Herbs	English Translation
12	Xuan Shen	Ningpo Figwort Root
12	Mu Li	Oyster Shell
12	Zhe Bei Mu	Fritillaria Zhebei Bulb

Description: This herbal formula is used to reduce nodules in the neck, to treat hyperthyroidism, and to shrink simple goiters.

Analysis: Zhe Bei Mu clears heat and dissipates nodules. Mu Li is also used to clear heat and dissipates nodules, and it is very effective for strengthening the activities of the chief herb, Xuan Shen. Xuan Shen is used here to clear heat and is often part of formulas used for treating problems involving the throat and neck.

Dosage and Method of Preparation: Make a decoction. Drink four ounces of Xiao Luo Tang tea at room temperature three times daily, or six ounces twice daily, as needed.

Hai Zao Yu Hu Tang (Sargassum Decoction for the Jade Flask)

Original Source: *Wau Ke Zheng Zong* (according to *Chinese Herbal Medicine Formulas and Strategies*)

Ingredients:

Quantity (Grams)	Chinese Herbs	English Translation
9	Hai Zao	Seaweed Plant
9	Kun Bu	Kelp Thallus
9	Hai Dai	Laminaria Plant
9	Zhe Bei Mu	Fritillaria Zhebei Bulb
9	Ban Xia	Half Summer
9	Du Huo	Self Reliance Existence Root
9	Chuan Xiong	Szechuan Lovage Root
9	Dang Gui	Tangkuei
6	Qing Pi	Green Tangerine Peel
4.5	Chen Pi	Ripe Tangerine Reel
9	Lian Qiao	Forsythia Fruit
3	Gan Cao	Licorice Root

Description: This herbal formula softens nodules, reduces and dissipates goiters, and is effective in removal of hard, large goiters.

Analysis: The chief ingredients, Hai Zao, Kun Bu, and Hai Dai, all effectively soften and dissolve masses. Zhe Bei Mu clears heat and assists the chief herbs. Ban Xia and Du Huo eliminate phlegm. Chuan Xiong and Dang Gui enrich and circulate the blood. Qing Pi and Chen Pi circulate the vital energy (Chi). Lian Qiao dissipates heat, and Gan Cao harmonizes the action of the other herbs in the formula and relieves toxicity.

Dosage and Method of Preparation: Make a decoction. Drink four ounces of Hai Zao Yu Hu Tang tea at room temperature three times daily, or drink six ounces twice daily, as needed.

Hai Zao Jing (Seaweed Extract); also known as Haiodin

Description: This patent formula reduces nodules, is useful for treating chronic lymphadenitis in the neck (swollen glands), and is used to treat goiters due to inadequate dietary intake of iodine.

Dosage: It comes in bottles of fifty pills, with complete instructions on dosage.

Gout—see Arthritis

Graves' Disease—see Goiter

Hangover—see specific complaint, e.g., Headache; Nausea; etc.

Hangovers are the effects experienced after overindulgence in alcohol. The most common symptoms are headache, nausea, vertigo, and depression. In most cases the severity of a hangover is determined by the amount and type of alcohol consumed. Because of their high concentrations of congeners, which is a secondary product of alcohol fermentation, brandy, bourbon, and red wine usually cause more severe hangovers. Normally, recovery takes eight to twelve hours. For treating hangover symptoms, refer to the entry for the specific complaint.

Hardening of the Arteries—see Arteriosclerosis

Hay Fever—see Allergies

Headache (see also Migraine)

Without a doubt, the most common type of pain is headache pain. It may be felt all over the head, or it may occur in only one area such as the forehead, the back of the neck, or on one side of the head. Headache pain, which may be dull, throbbing, or sharp, can cause varying degrees of discomfort. Some types of headaches are especially painful and persistent but despite their symptoms do not indicate any progressive or serious disorder.

The main causes of headaches are tension due to stress, improper diet, alcohol abuse, colds, sinus congestion, concussion, persistent noise, constipation, poor posture, menstruation, ear infections, toothache, and food additives. Recent research has also shown that certain foods such as chocolate, cheese, and red wine trigger migraine attacks in susceptible people. Rare and more serious causes of headache are brain tumors, hypertension, temporal arthritis (inflammation of the arteries of the brain and scalp), and aneurysm (localized swelling of a blood vessel).

Generally speaking, headaches fall into three categories: tension headaches, cluster headaches, and migraine headaches. The most common of the three, tension headaches, are caused by tightening in the muscles of the face, shoulders, and neck and usually result from stress or poor posture. Tension headaches can last for hours, days, or in some cases weeks. Cluster headaches, the rarest of the three forms, are characterized by intense pain behind one eye and insomnia. Cluster headaches can last for weeks or months. Migraine headaches, which are more serious and incapacitating and cause pain that has been described as excruciating, are often accompanied by visual or abdominal disturbances. Migraine headaches are normally periodic and can last for several days.

Preventing a headache is more important than treating one, and many of the known causes can be avoided, particularly if the sufferer knows what triggers the headache. If, however, headaches are persistent without an obvious cause and do not respond to self-treatment, medical advice should be sought, and appropriate tests should be performed to rule out the presence of a brain tumor or other serious disorder.

Traditional Chinese medicine has had some success treating headaches using the following formulas:

Zhi Jing San (Stop Spasms Powder)

Original Source: *Fang Ji Xue* (according to *Chinese Herbal Medicine Formulas and Strategies*)

Ingredients:

Quantity (Grams)	Chinese Herbs	English Translation
8	Quan Xie	Scorpion
8	Wu Gong	Centipede

Description: The synergistic effect of Quan Xie and Wu Gong is very strong and should only be used for cluster or severe migraine headaches.

Caution: (1) This formula should not be taken in large doses or over the long term, and (2) it is prohibited for use during pregnancy.

Analysis: Both Quan Xie and Wu Gong are effective for relieving spasms and stopping pain; when combined, they have a strong synergistic action.

Dosage and Method of Preparation: Grind the herbs together into a fine powder and store the powder in a glass container. Mix 1.5 grams of powdered Zhi Jing San with four ounces of warm water and drink two to three times daily, as needed. Or a 1.5-gram dose of Zhi Jing San can be placed into capsules and taken with warm water two to three times daily, as needed.

Pian Tou Tong Wan (Headache Stop Pain Pill)

Description: This patent formula is used for migraine headache, neurogenic pain, and tension.

Caution: This formula is prohibited for use during pregnancy.

Dosage: It comes in a bottle of thirty capsules, with complete instructions on dosage.

Yan Hu Su Zhi Tong Pian (Yan Hu Extract Stop Pain Tablets); also known as Corydalis Yanhusus-Analgesic Tablets

Description: This patent formula promotes circulation, stops pain, and is especially effective for chronic headaches associated with insomnia.

Dosage: It comes in vials containing twelve tablets, with complete instructions on dosage.

Chuan Xiong Cha Tiao Wan (Ligusticum Tea Adjust Pill); also known as Chuan Qiong Cha Tiao Wan

Description: This patent formula is useful for treating headache due to colds and sinus congestion. It is used for frontal headaches, as well as headaches on the side, top, and back of the head.

Dosage: It comes in a bottle of two hundred pills, with complete instructions on dosage.

Heart Attack—see Myocardial Infarction

Heartburn—see Acid Reflux; Indigestion

Heartburn is experienced as a burning pain in the center of the chest that usually travels from the tip of the breastbone to the throat. It may be caused by overeating, eating rich or spicy foods, or drinking alcohol. Recurrent heartburn, which is a symptom of esophagitis, is usually caused by acid reflux.

Heatstroke—see Sunstroke

Hemorrhoids

Even though there is a higher incidence of hemorrhoids during pregnancy and immediately following childbirth, it is generally agreed that the main causes of hemorrhoids are chronic constipation and lack of fiber in the diet Another interesting postulation, based on the fact that four-legged mammals do not have hemorrhoids, is traditional Chinese medicine's theory that humans' upright stance is also a contributing factor

Prolapsed hemorrhoids, which protrude outside of the rectum, produce a mucus discharge with itching around the anal opening. Certain complications of prolapsed hemorrhoids, such as thrombosis and strangulation (clot formation in the vein), can cause extreme pain. The most common symptoms include rectal bleeding and increased discomfort and pain during defecation.

Most cases of hemorrhoids can be controlled by increasing fluid intake, eating a high-fiber diet, and having regular bowel movements. The following herbal formulas should also prove useful for treating hemorrhoids, by arresting bleeding as well as reducing swelling and pain:

Huai Jiao Tang (Sophora Japonica Fruit Decoction)

Original Source: *Tai Ping Hui Min He Ji Ju Fang* (according to *Chinese Herbal Medicine Formulas and Strategies*)

Ingredients:

Quantity (Grams)	Chinese Herbs	English Translation
12	Huai Jiao	Fruit of the Pagoda Tree
9	Fang Feng	Guard Against the Wind Root
9	Di Gu	Wolfberry Root
9	Dang Gui	Tangkuei
9	Huang Qin	Baical Skullcap Root
9	Zhi Ke	Bitter Orange Fruit, Ripe

Description: This herbal formula is used to control the bleeding that accompanies hemorrhoids or rectal prolapse.

Analysis: Huai Jiao eliminates heat from the blood and stops bleeding and is often used for treating bleeding hemorrhoids. Fang Feng relieves pain. Di Gu clears heat and eliminates infection. Dang Gui enriches the blood and relieves pain. Huang Qin clears heat and infection. Zhi Ke benefits the stomach.

Dosage and Method of Preparation: Prepare a decoction. Drink four ounces of Huai Jiao Tang tea three times daily, or as needed.

Hua Zhi Ling Wan (Fargelin for Piles); also known as Qiang Li Hua Zhi Ling

Description: This patent formula reduces swelling and stops pain and bleeding from hemorrhoids. It is also used to treat prolapsed anus with swelling and bleeding.

Dosage: It comes in bottles of sixty pills (either regular or extra strength), with complete instructions on dosage.

Zhi Wan (Hemorrhoid Pills)

Description: This patent formula stops pain, discharges pus, and is used to treat infected hemorrhoids and anal abscesses with swelling, inflammation, bleeding, and pain.

Dosage: It comes in bottles of one hundred pills, with complete instructions on dosage.

Xiong Dan Zhi Ling Gao (Fel Ursi Hemorrhoid Effective Ointment); also known as Xiong Dan Zhi Chuang Gao

Description: This patent formula reduces inflammation, stops pain and bleeding, and is used to treat hemorrhoids with swelling, bleeding, inflammation, and itching.

Dosage: This treatment is used externally as a topical ointment. It comes in tubes of four or ten grams, with complete instructions on dosage.

Hepatitis: A, B, C (see also Liver, Disorders of)

Hepatitis is an inflammation of the liver that can be either acute (of limited duration) or chronic (continuing). Acute hepatitis, the most common form, is usually caused by infection from a virus (as in viral hepatitis type A or B; see below), a drug overdose, or exposure to certain chemicals. Acute hepatitis can also affect heavy drinkers who suffer from progressive liver disease. The most obvious symptom is jaundice, often preceded by nausea, vomiting, loss of appetite, aching muscles and joints, and tenderness in the upper right side of the abdomen.

Occasionally, a sufferer fails to recover from acute hepatitis, leading to further cell damage, which creates a chronic condition. Chronic hepatitis may also develop as a result of heavy alcohol consumption, from an autoimmune deficiency disorder (in which the body's defenses attack its own tissues), from a metabolic disorder affecting the liver, or from a reaction to certain medication. In still another type, known as chronic active hepatitis, cell destruction and scarring can (if untreated) lead to cirrhosis of the liver. The symptoms of chronic hepatitis are usually vague, although there is an overall feeling of being sick. In many cases the disease remains undetected until the enlarged liver is discovered during a routine medical examination.

There are three forms of viral hepatitis: type A, type B, and type C. Type A is often called infectious hepatitis because it is spread from an infected person's feces that have directly or indirectly contaminated food or drinking water. Type B is often referred to as serum hepatitis, because in the past it was mainly spread by blood transfusions and the use of blood products. Today, the development of tests have minimized the risk of infection via blood transfusion, making the most common forms of transmission sexual activity (particularly among male homosexuals) and needle sharing among drug abusers. There is also some degree of risk in razor sharing and body piercing. Viral hepatitis type B is in many ways more serious than type A. In a proportionate number of cases, the infectious virus persists for years after the initial infection occurs, possibly leading to chronic hepatitis, cirrhosis, or liver cancer—with the carrier of the virus experiencing few and in some cases no symptoms.

Although vaccines are available for viral hepatitis type B, most often they are only offered or recommended to those at high risk of infection such as health-care workers, children born to infected mothers, male homosexuals, and drug addicts. For all others, prevention of both type A and B is recommended. Avoidance of type A is aided by observing good hygiene practices regarding food and drink, particularly in certain parts of the world where sanitary standards are low and high incidence of infection has been reported. The chances of contracting hepatitis B can be reduced through the use of condoms, by not sharing needles, and by avoiding body piercing or tattooing unless the equipment used is verifiably sterile.

The hepatitis C virus, also known as HCV, was first isolated in 1988 and is usually the cause of all cases of non-A or non-B hepatitis. Between 150,000 and 250,000 new cases of hepatitis C are believed to occur in the United States each year. Although hemophiliacs and intravenous drug abusers are at the greatest risk, anyone in any walk of life is at risk of becoming infected with the virus.

For the majority of sufferers of hepatitis C, the illness begins with flu-like symptoms. Many other symptoms may also be present; however, they differ from patient to patient. The list of possible symptoms include fatigue, low-grade fever, headaches, slight sore throat, loss of appetite, nausea, vomiting, and stiff or aching joints. Many people develop a pain in the right side above the liver area. The urine often turns dark brown and is accompanied by pale feces. In severe acute infections, jaundice can develop in which the skin and the whites of the eyes become yellowish.

Most people with hepatitis C contracted it either through a transfusion of blood or blood products (plasma, etc.) contaminated with the virus or by sharing needles with infected intravenous drug users. It is also possible to contract the virus through body piercing, tattooing, an accidental needle prick, or the sharing of personal-care items (such as toothbrushes, razors, and nail clippers) with infected persons. Therefore, any sharing of these items is not recommended.

The risk of sexual transmission of the C virus has not been thoroughly investigated, but it appears to be minimal. However, people with acute undiagnosed illness or multiple sexual partners should use condoms to reduce the risk of acquiring or transmitting hepatitis C— or any other known sexually transmitted disease.

Currently, there exists no vaccine to prevent infection of hepatitis C, and similarly there is no cure. Consequently, the best approach to treatment appears to be the combined therapies offered by Western and traditional Chinese medicine for treating recurrent symptoms until hepatitis C's root cause can be determined and a cure found. Some of the herbal formulas used for treating hepatitis A or B can also be useful for treating hepatitis C when the symptoms are correspondent. For treating specific complaints such as vomiting, nausea, sore throat, loss of appetite, fatigue, fever, headache, or jaundice, refer to the appropriate entries in this chapter.

Hepatitis is commonly referred to in Chinese medicine as liver stagnation. Traditionally, Chinese physicians use herbal formulas containing fruits of the Gardenia (Zhi Zi) and Bupleurum Hare's Ear Root (Chai Hu) as main ingredients for treating it. The following herbal formulas should relieve symptoms in hepatitis sufferers. In addition, some of the antibiotic herbs that are part of these formulas are known to eliminate infection.

Da Chai Hu Tang (Major Bupleurum Decoction)

Original Source: *Shang Han Lun* (according to *Chinese Herbal Medicine Formulas and Strategies*)

Ingredients:

Quantity (Grams)	Chinese Herbs	English Translation
24	Chai Hu	Bupleurum Hare's Ear Root
9	Huang Qin	Baical Skullcap Root
9	Zhi Shi	Green Bitter Orange Fruit
6	Da Huang	Rhubarb Root
9	Bai Shao	White Peony Root
24	Ban Xia	Half Summer
15	Sheng Jiang	Fresh Ginger Root
12 pieces	Da Zao	Jujube Fruit
9	Zhi Zi	Gardenia Fruit
6	Huang Bai	Amur Cork Tree Bark

Description: This formula is used for hepatitis symptoms of fever, pain in the upper abdomen, nausea, yellow eyes; it is suggested for both chronic and acute jaundice.

Analysis: When the chief ingredient, Chai Hu, is combined with Huang Qin, its ability to clear heat from the liver and gallbladder is strengthened. Zhi Shi moves the vital energy, and Da Huang moves the bowels, which indirectly stimulates the flow of bile. Bai Shao nourishes the blood and reduces abdominal spasms. Ban Xia calms the stomach. Sheng Jiang and Da Zao also benefit the stomach by improving digestion. Zhi Zi clears pathogenic heat and infection from the gallbladder. Huang Bai assists the other herbs while benefiting the kidneys.

Dosage and Method of Preparation: Make a decoction. Drink four ounces of Da Chai Hu Tang tea at room temperature three times daily, as needed.

Li Gan Pian (Benefit Liver Tablets); also known as Liver Strengthening Tablets

Description: This patent formula clears heat and soothes the liver. It is used for acute hepatitis with or without jaundice to decrease pain and relieve symptoms.

Dosage: It comes in bottles of one hundred tablets, with complete instructions on dosage.

Ji Gu Cao Wan (Herba Abri Pills); also known as Jigucao Wan

combined with

Hsiao Yao Wan (Bupleurum Sedative Pills); also known as Xiao Yao Wan

Description: The combined use of these two patent formulas is very effective for acute hepatitis with or without jaundice and is also useful for chronic hepatitis or gallstones. It clears heat in the liver and bile ducts, providing relief from the symptoms of hepatitis.

Dosage: Ji Gu Cao Wan comes in bottles of fifty pills, and Hsiao Yao Wan comes in bottles of two hundred pills, both with complete instructions on dosage.

Hernia

A hernia is the protrusion of an organ through a weak area in the muscle or tissue that normally contains it. The two most common types are intestinal hernia (protrusion of the intestine through the abdominal wall) and hiatal hernia (protrusion of the stomach through the diaphragm into the chest). Common causes of hernia are a congenital weakness in the abdominal wall, which may appear following surgery; damage caused by lifting heavy objects; substantial weight gain; persistent coughing; and straining to defecate.

The first symptom is usually a bulge in the abdominal wall, which can in some cases be pushed back through the weak area, a procedure called replacement. If replacement is not possible, severe pain occurs. When an intestinal hernia bulges out and cannot be replaced, it may become twisted, impairing the blood supply and creating a condition known as strangulated hernia. This condition requires urgent treatment because of the possibility of gangrene developing as a result of a lack of blood flow to the bowel.

Western medicine often recommends a supportive garment (a truss) for hernias that are not particularly painful and can be easily pushed back into place. When hernias are painful and cannot be pushed back into place, surgery is usually recommended. Chinese physicians often treat hernias with manipulation and herbal therapy for managing related symptoms.

The herbal formulas that follow are among those commonly used:

Zuo Jin Tang (Left Metal Decoction)

Original Source: *Dan Xi Xin Fa* (according to *Chinese Herbal Medicine Formulas and Strategies*)

Ingredients:

Quantity (Grams)	Chinese Herbs	English Translation
18	Huang Lian	Golden Thread Root
3	Wu Zhu Yu	Evodia Fruit

Description: Use this formula for pain in the upper stomach or chest, vomiting, acid regurgitation, belching with a bitter taste in the mouth, or other symptoms associated with hiatal hernia.

Analysis: Huang Lian is assisted by Wu Zhu Yu, and together they drain fire from the liver and calm the stomach, thus clearing infection, arresting vomiting, stopping belching, reducing pain, and eliminating acid regurgitation.

Dosage and Method of Preparation: Make a decoction. Drink four ounces of Zuo Jin Tang tea three times daily, as needed.

Nuan Gan Jian (Warm the Liver Decoction)

Original Source: *Jing Yue Quan Shu* (according to *Chinese Herbal Medicine Formulas and Strategies*)

Ingredients:

Quantity (Grams)	Chinese Herbs	English Translation
9	Dang Gui	Tangkuei
9	Gou Qi Zi	Matrimony Vine Fruit
6	Xiao Hui Xiang	Fennel Fruit
6	Rou Gui	Saigon Cinnamon Inner Bark
6	Wu Yao	Lindera Root
3	Chen Xiang	Aloeswood

| 6 | Fu Ling | Tuckahoe Root |
| 3–5 slices | Sheng Jiang | Fresh Ginger Root |

Description: This formula is used to relieve lower abdominal pain and scrotal discomfort, to improve blood circulation, and by those suffering from intestinal hernia.

Analysis: The chief herb, Xiao Hui Xiang, benefits the kidneys and disperses cold. Wu Yao and Chen Xiang support the chief herb by promoting the movement of the vital energy (Chi) and reducing pain. Rou Gui and Gou Qi Zi, combined, benefit the liver and kidneys. Fu Ling eliminates dampness and strengthens the spleen. Dang Gui benefits the blood that supports the liver. Sheng Jiang harmonizes the stomach.

Dosage and Method of Preparation: Prepare a decoction. Drink four ounces of Nuan Gan Jian tea three times daily or as needed.

Bu Zhong Yi Qi Wan (Tonify Center to Invigorate Qi Pills); also known as Central Qi Pills, or Bu Zhong Yi Chi Wan

Description: This patent formula is useful for treating prolapse of an organ, including hernia, hemorrhoids, varicose veins, and prolapsed rectum.

Dosage: It comes in bottles of one hundred pills, with complete instructions on dosage.

Shen Xian Jin Bu Huan Gao (Magic Plaster Not to Be Exchanged for Gold)

Description: This patent formula is used for muscle and tissue weakness with protrusion as seen in hernia.

Caution: This formula is prohibited for use on the lower abdomen by pregnant women with intestinal or umbilical hernia.

Dosage: It comes in a topical plaster, which is applied externally to the herniated area.

Herpes: Genital, Oral, Zoster

Generally speaking, herpes is a condition in which small, particularly painful blisters erupt on the surface of the skin. More specifically, when a person is said to be suffering from herpes, it usually refers to infection by the herpes simplex virus, which exists in two forms. Herpes simplex I (known as oral herpes) is associated with infection and causes blisters (cold sores) on the lips, mouth, and face (see also Fever Blister; Stomatitis; Ulcer). More seriously, it is the virus most commonly responsible for causing encephalitis. Herpes simplex II (known as genital herpes) is associated with infection and causes painful blisters to erupt on the genitalia. Both types I and II are episodic, incurable, and contagious. Herpes is spread by direct contact with the blisters that develop when infected or with the infectious fluid contained inside of them.

If people with immune-deficiency disorders such as AIDS or those taking immunosuppressant drugs become infected with the herpes virus, they sustain a greater risk of developing a more severe, generalized infection that can be fatal.

After initial infection, recurrent episodes or attacks can be brought on by stress, illnesses that tax or lower the immune system, fever, and prolonged exposure to sun. Chinese physicians ascribe herpes to damp heat or chronic infection in the gallbladder duct. They treat it by recommending a diet free of red meat and gluten (the protein found in wheat and rye) and encouraging the consumption of chicken, fish, and fresh vegetables. Additionally, saline baths and douches can provide relief from blisters, along with herbal therapy to eliminate infection.

Even though they show certain similarities, herpes simplex I and II should not be confused with herpes zoster, the medical term for shingles. Herpes zoster gets its name from the *Varicella zoster* virus, which also causes chicken pox (see also Chicken Pox). Although all four varieties of herpes (herpes simplex I and II, shingles, and chicken pox) are characterized by a severe, painful rash, treatment differs somewhat for each. Herbal formulas for treating each form of the disease follow.

Sheng Ma Ge Gen Tang (Cimicifuga and Kudzu Decoction)

Original Source: *Xiao Er Yao Zheng Zhi Jue* (according to *Chinese Herbal Medicine Formulas and Strategies*)

Ingredients:

Quantity (Grams)	Chinese Herbs	English Translation
6	Sheng Ma	Black Cohosh (Cimicifuga) Rhizome
9	Ge Gen	Kudzu Root
3	Zhi Gan Cao	Honey-Cooked Licorice Root
9	Chi Shao	Red Peony Root
6	Zi Cao	Groomwell Root

Description: This formula reduces fever and resolves all types of rashes; it is especially useful for chicken pox/herpes zoster.

Analysis: Sheng Ma clears the stomach and effectively reduces rashes. Ge Gen assists by opening the pores of the skin and expels heat. Zhi Gan Cao relieves toxicity. Chi Shao moves blood and clears infection. Zi Cao is specific for effectively treating various kinds of rashes by cooling the blood.

Dosage and Method of Preparation: Prepare a decoction. Drink four ounces of Sheng Ma Ge Gen Tang tea three times daily, as needed.

Note: Do not cook this formula for more than twenty minutes.

Lung Tan Xie Gan Pill (Gentiana Purge Liver Pills); also known as Long Dan Xie Gan Wan

Description: This patent formula is useful for oral herpes and genital herpes with fever and blisters.

Dosage: It comes in bottles of one hundred pills, with complete instructions on dosage.

Niu Huang Shang Qing Wan (Cow Gallstone Upper Clear Pills); also known as Niu Huang Shang Ching Wan

Description: Use for inflammation or infection with fever and blisters on the lips and in the mouth (oral herpes).

Caution: This formula is prohibited for use during pregnancy.

Dosage: This patent medicine comes in bottles of fifty pills, with complete instructions on dosage.

中
草
藥

Hiatal Hernia—see Hernia

High Blood Pressure—see Hypertension

Hoarseness, Loss of Voice (see also Laryngitis)

Although hoarseness can be caused by pathologic interference with the normal working of the vocal cords or larynx, it is most often associated with a sore throat caused by the common cold. Most attacks are of short duration and clear up on their own. If it does persist, it is a good idea to investigate its cause, in order to exclude the possibility of serious disease.

Short-term hoarseness often results from overuse of the voice, leading to strain of the small muscles in the larynx and inflammation of the vocal cords, causing acute laryngitis. Teachers, speakers, and singers are susceptible. In young children hoarseness is one of the symptoms of croup (an inflammation and narrowing of the airways). Among the many possible causes of persistent or chronic hoarseness are irritation of the larynx caused by smoking, excessive consumption of alcohol, and chronic bronchitis. Irritation can also be caused by mucus constantly dripping on the larynx (postnasal drip) such as occurs with nasal polyps (harmless growths in the nose), hay fever, sinusitis, or a deviated nasal septum (crookedness in the cartilage separating the two nostril passages).

Occasionally, persistent hoarseness in adults has a more serious cause such as accidental damage to the vocal cords during thyroid gland surgery or from tissue forming on the vocal cords. On rare occasions, hoarseness is caused by cancers of the larynx or thyroid gland.

Traditional Chinese medicine generally concurs with Western medicine concerning the causes of hoarseness and offers the following herbal formulas for treating it:

San She Dan Chuan Bei Pi Pa Gao (Snake Gall and Loquat Extract)

Description: This patent formula sedates heat, moistens lungs and throat, and is used for hoarseness and acute bronchitis.

Dosage: It comes in seven-ounce bottles of syrup, with complete instructions on dosage.

Qiu Li Gao (Autumn Pear Syrup)

Description: This patent formula is used to treat asthma, dry throat with frequent thirst, and hoarseness associated with bronchitis and other lung diseases.

Dosage: It comes in twelve-ounce bottles of syrup, with complete diseases instructions on dosage.

Yang Yin Qing Fei Tang Jiang (Nourish Yin Clear Lung Sweet Syrup); also known as Yang Yin Ching Fei Tang Chiang

Description: This patent formula is used for treating hoarseness of the throat with thirst, pain, blood, or dryness in the throat.

Dosage: It comes in 120cc bottles, with complete instructions on dosage.

Qing Yin Wan (Clear Voice Pills)

Description: This patent medicine is used to treat sore throat associated with hoarseness due to bronchitis, laryngitis, or other problems causing dryness and pain, as well as tonsillitis.

Dosage: It comes in boxes of ten honey pills, with complete instructions on dosage.

Hookworm—see Larva Migrans

Hot Flashes—see Menopause

Hyperacidity—see Acid Reflux

Hypertension

Hypertension, the clinical term for high blood pressure, refers to abnormally high pressure of blood in the main arteries. Whereas blood pressure ordinarily increases as a response to stress and physical activity, a person suffering from hypertension has high blood pressure even in the absence of stress or physical exertion. Hypertension is defined as a blood-pressure reading greater than 140 (systolic) over 90 (diastolic). Even though elderly people normally have blood pressure readings above these values (because blood pressure increases with age), children and adults under fifty years of age should under normal circumstances have lower blood pressure levels.

Hypertension usually causes no symptoms and generally goes undiscovered until it is detected by a physician during a routine physical examination. Tobacco smoking, a high-fat diet, obesity, lack of physical exercise, and stress are considered common causes or at the very least significantly increase the risks of developing hypertension. Possible complications of untreated hypertension include stroke, heart failure, kidney damage, and retinopathy (damage to the retina at the back of the eye). Mild hypertension may respond to weight reduction and a reduction in stress. Discontinuing tobacco smoking, decreasing the amount of alcohol consumed, and the restriction of salt intake can all be helpful.

If these measures bear no effect, Western medicine usually resorts to chemical drug therapy as the only alternative. The drugs that are commonly prescribed unfortunately have undesirable side effects such as an overall decrease in libido in both men and women and varying degrees of impotence in men. These side effects are seen as a necessary evil that must be tolerated because of the grave consequences that can occur when hypertension is left untreated. All of this increases the desirability of using Chinese herbs for treating high blood pressure. They have proven to be effective while totally lacking the negative side effects associated with chemical drugs. In addition, the practice of Chiang Chung Kung (invigorated breathing and Chi Kung exercises) is recommended for reducing stress levels.

The following herbal formulas can be used to lower and regulate blood pressure:

Ling Jiao Gou Teng Tang (Antelope Horn and Uncaria Decoction)

Original Source: *Chong Ding Tong Su Shang Han Lun* (according to *Chinese Herbal Medicine Formulas and Strategies*)

Ingredients:

Quantity (Grams)	Chinese Herbs	English Translation
4.5	Ling Yang Jiao	Antelope Horn
9	Gou Teng	Stems and Thorns of Gambir Vine (Uncaria)
6	Sang Ye	White Mulberry Leaf
9	Ju Hua	Chrysanthemum Flowers
9	Bai Shao	White Peony Root
15	Sheng Di Huang	Chinese Foxglove Root, Raw
12	Chuan Bei Mu	Fritillaria Bulb
15	Zhu Ru	Bamboo Shavings
9	Fu Shen	Tuckahoe Spirit Fungus
2.4	Gan Cao	Licorice Root

Description: This formula is useful for treating essential hypertension with symptoms of dizziness, restlessness, and irritability.

Analysis: Ling Yang Jiao, one of the chief ingredients, benefits the liver and clears heat. Gou Teng is effective for eliminating dizziness or lightheadedness. Sang Ye and Ju Hua also clear heat from the liver. Bai Shao and Sheng Di Huang increase production of body fluids, which assists in quelling the heat. Chuan Bei Mu and Zhu Ru assist in clearing heat. Fu Shen treats irritability and restlessness. Gan Cao harmonizes the actions of the ingredients in this formula.

Dosage and Method of Preparation: Prepare a decoction. Drink four ounces of Ling Jiao Gou Teng Tang tea three times daily, as needed.

Zhen Gan Xi Feng Tang (Sedate the Liver and Extinguish Wind Decoction)

Original Source: *Yi Xue Zhong Zong Can Xi Lu* (according to *Chinese Herbal Medicine Formulas and Strategies*)

Ingredients:

Quantity (Grams)	Chinese Herbs	English Translation
30	Huai Niu Xi	Ox Knee Root
30	Zhi Shi	Green Bitter Orange Fruit
15	Long Gu	Dragon Bones
15	Mu Li	Oyster Shell
15	Gui Ban	Land Tortoise Shell
15	Xuan Shen	Ningpo Figwort Root
15	Tian Men Dong	Tuber of Chinese Asparagus
15	Bai Shao	White Peony Root
6	Yin Chen Hao	Capillaris Herb
6	Chuan Lian Zi	Fruit of Szechuan Pagoda Tree
6	Mai Ya	Barley Sprout
4.5	Gan Cao	Licorice Root

Description: This formula is useful for essential hypertension, renal hypertension (high blood pressure caused by a kidney disorder), and cerebral arteriosclerosis.

Analysis: The chief ingredient, Huai Niu Xi, conducts the circulation of blood downward away from the head, preventing dizziness. Zhi Shi directs the vital energy (Chi) downward. Long Gu and Mu Li both have a sedative effect. Gui Ban, Xuan Shen, Tian Men Dong, and Bai Shao disperse heat by generating body fluids. Yin Chen Hao, Chuan Lian Zi, and Mai Ya work in concert with the chief herb to pacify liver heat and prevent dizziness or lightheadedness. Gan Cao harmonizes the other herbs in this formula and improves taste.

Dosage and Method of Preparation: Prepare a decoction. Drink four ounces of Zhen Gan Xi Feng Tang tea three times daily, as needed.

Du Zhong Pian (Cortex Eucommine Tablets); also known as Compound Cortex Eucommiae

Description: This patent formula decreases cholesterol, lowers blood pressure, reduces hardening of the arteries, and calms the spirit.

Dosage: It comes in bottles of one hundred tablets, with complete instructions on dosage.

Ci Wu Jia Pian (Acanthopanax Senticosus)

Description: This patent formula normalizes blood-pressure levels, lowering high blood pressure and raising low blood pressure.

Dosage: It comes in bottles or boxes containing one hundred tablets, with complete instructions on dosage.

Chiang Ya Wan (Decrease Pressure Pills); also known as Jiang Ya Wan

Description: This patent formula is used to treat hypertension with symptoms of dizziness, headache, tinnitus.

Caution: This formula is prohibited for use during pregnancy.

Dosage: This patent medicine comes in bottles of two hundred pills, with complete instructions on dosage.

Jing Ya Ping Pian (Hypertension Repressing Tablets); also known as Jiang Ya Ping Pian

Description: This patent formula's primary function is to reduce high blood pressure, soften the blood vessels, and decrease cholesterol levels in the blood.

Dosage: This patent medicine comes in boxes with twelve small bottles, twelve tablets per bottle, with complete instructions on dosage.

Hyperthyroidism—see Goiter

Hypoglycemia (see also Diabetes; Pancreas, Disorders of)

Hypoglycemia is an abnormally low level of blood sugar (glucose). In almost all cases, it occurs in sufferers of diabetes mellitus. The principal symptoms include sweating, weakness, hunger, dizziness, trembling, headache, palpitations, and confusion. These usually occur when diabetics take a too-high dose of either insulin or hypoglycemic drugs, miss a meal, fail to eat enough carbohydrates, or exercise too much. On rare occasions, hypoglycemia can result from drinking large amounts of alcohol or from insulinoma, an insulin-producing tumor of the pancreas.

Hypoglycemia and diabetes are both serious conditions; therefore, insulin-dependent diabetics should always carry a sugary snack to take at the first signs of a hypoglycemic attack. The reader should be reminded that the following Chinese herbal formulas are only useful as an adjunct and should not be relied upon in case of an emergency.

Xiao Jian Zhong Tang (Minor Construct the Middle Decoction)

Original Source: *Shang Han Lun* (according to *Chinese Herbal Medicine Formulas and Strategies*)

Ingredients:

Quantity (Grams)	Chinese Herbs	English Translation
30	Yi Tang	Barley Malt Sugar
9	Gui Zhi	Saigon Cinnamon Twig
18	Shao Yao	Peony Root
6	Zhi Gan Cao	Honey-Cooked Licorice Root
9	Sheng Jiang	Fresh Ginger Root
12 pieces	Da Zao	Jujube Fruit

Description: This formula is useful for hypoglycemia, pernicious anemia, weakness, and poor appetite.

Analysis: Yi Tang relieves spasmodic abdominal pain. Gui Zhi benefits the stomach and spleen by dispersing cold. Sheng Jiang and Shao Yao benefit digestion. Da Zao and Zhi Gan Cao move the vital energy (Chi) and harmonize the herbs in this formula.

中草藥

Dosage and Method of Preparation: Prepare a decoction. Drink four ounces of Xiao Jian Zhong Tang tea three times daily, as needed.

Jian Pi Su (Build Spleen Single Ingredient)

combined with

Bu Zhong Yi Qi Wan (Tonify Center to Invigorate Qi Pills); also known as Central Qi Pills, or Bu Zhong Yi Chi Wan

Description: The combined usage of these two patent formulas is especially effective for treating hypoglycemia. Use when there are signs of weakness, poor appetite, and spontaneous sweating.

Dosage: Bu Zhong Yi Qi Wan comes in bottles of two hundred pills, and Jian Pi Su comes in bottles of one hundred tablets, both with complete instructions on dosage.

Ren Shen Feng Wang Jiang (Ginseng Royal Jelly Syrup); also known as Ling Zhi Feng Wang Jiang

Description: This patent formula is a nutritive tonic that promotes appetite, aids in nutritional absorption, and is helpful in treating hypoglycemia.

Dosage: It comes in boxes of ten vials, each 10cc, with complete instructions on dosage.

Impotence—see Erection (Penile), Disorders of

Incontinence, Fecal and Urinary

A person's inability to control bowel or bladder function has several possible causes. These include injury to muscles during childbirth or surgery, general weakness of either the anal or urinary sphincters, paraplegia or paralysis of the legs and lower trunk, and mental handicap or dementia. While the conditions described can be chronic, except in the case of paralysis, incontinence need not be permanent. Indeed, most of us have experienced temporary loss of continence when the need to evacuate the bowel or bladder becomes too great. Of the two types of incontinence, urinary incontinence is more prevalent, especially among the elderly. Uncontrollable, involuntary urination is often due to diseases of the urinary tract and loss of efficiency of the sphincter muscles surrounding the urethra, which decline with age. Other causes are obstruction from an enlarged prostate gland or prolapse of the uterus or vagina. On rare occasions incontinence can be caused by prostate cancer. For reasons that are unknown, urinary incontinence usually affects women more often than men.

Traditional Chinese medicine's treatment includes the use of the following herbal formulas, which are used as an adjunct to internal exercises to strengthen the sphincters and the muscles of the pelvic floor. Practice of these exercises (called "the deer"; see Erection [Penile], Disorders of) is considered critical to resolving problems of fecal and urinary incontinence. Additionally, a little-known but fairly common traditional dietary remedy is eating pig's bladder that has been steamed with hops!

Chin So Ku Ching Wan (Golden Lock [Tea] Pill); also known as Jin Suo Gu Jing Wan, or Golden Lock Consolidate Jing Pills

Description: This patent formula is used to astringe discharges of urine, diarrhea, and semen (nocturnal emissions). A recent report by Jake Fratkin, who is a source for a number of the patent formulas in this book and the author of *Chinese Herbal Patent Formulas,* recommends limiting use of this formula to short periods of time.

Dosage: It comes in bottles of one hundred pills, with complete instructions on dosage.

Du Zhong Bu Tian Su (Eucommia Benefit Heaven Basic Pill)

Description: This patent formula is useful for incontinence of urine or frequent urination.

Dosage: It comes in boxes of twelve vials, eight tablets per vial, with complete instructions on dosage.

Bow Sun Wan (Male Gender Tonify Kidney Pills); also known as Nan Xing Bu Shen Wan

Description: This patent formula enhances kidney function and relieves urinary incontinence or leaking.

Dosage: It comes in boxes of twenty capsules, with complete instructions on dosage.

Indigestion (see also Acid Reflux)

The term indigestion covers a wide variety of symptoms (heartburn, stomachache, nausea, and gas), all of which are usually caused by eating too much, eating too quickly, or eating rich, spicy, or fatty foods. Persistent or recurrent indigestion is associated with peptic ulcers, gallstones, or esophagitis (inflammation of the esophagus). Many of the symptoms of indigestion can be effectively treated with some of the same herbal formulas that are recommended in the section of this book on acid reflux.

Po Chi Pills (Protect and Benefit Pills); also known as Bao Ji Wan, China Po Chi Pills, or Zhong Guo Bao Ji Wan

Description: This patent formula resolves nausea, vomiting with stomach cramps, and abdominal distention.

Dosage: It comes in bottles of one hundred pills, with complete instructions on dosage.

Kang Ning Wan (Curing Pill); also known as Pill Curing

Description: This formula is primarily used for every kind of digestive disturbance with symptoms including nausea, abdominal cramping, vomiting, heartburn, headache, and abdominal bloating.

Dosage: It comes in boxes of ten vials, with complete instructions on dosage.

Note: These doses are suitable for use by children.

Ren Dan/Yang Cheng Brand (Ren Dan Peoples Powder); also known as Benevolence Pills

Description: This patent formula is used for acute and emergency stomach disorders, including abdominal bloating with pain, headache, nausea, vomiting, motion sickness, heartburn, and indigestion.

Dosage: It comes in boxes of twelve vials, with complete instructions on dosage.

Infection

Infection is the establishment in the body of a colony of disease-causing microorganisms such as bacteria, viruses, or fungi. There are two basic types of infection. The first, systemic infection, in which the microorganisms are spread throughout the body, is usually associated with infectious disease (smallpox, diphtheria, tuberculosis). The other kind, localized infection, in which the microorganisms are confined within a particular area, often results from bacteria entering cuts, wounds, or from inadequate dental hygiene. Systemic infection normally exhibits symptoms such as fever, weakness, and aching joints, while localized infection normally causes inflammation, pain, redness, swelling, the formation of pus-filled abscesses, and occasionally a rise in temperature.

Infections are universally treated with antimicrobial agents. In the case of traditional Chinese medicine, this means the use of antibiotic herbs to quell the infection.

Xian Fang Huo Ming Yin (Sublime Formula For Sustaining Life)

Original Source: *Jiao Zhu Fu Ren Liang Fang* (according to *Chinese Herbal Medicine Formulas and Strategies*)

Ingredients:

Quantity (Grams)	Chinese Herbs	English Translation
9	Jin Yin Hua	Honeysuckle Flower
3	Gan Cao	Licorice Root
3	Zhi Bei Mu	Fritillaria Zhebei Bulb
3	Tian Hua Fen	Heavenly Flower Root

12	Dang Gui	Tangkuei
3	Chi Shao	Red Peony Root
3	Ru Xiang	Frankincense Resin
3	Mo Yao	Resin of Myrrh
3	Fang Feng	Guard Against the Wind Root
3	Bai Zhi	Angelica Dahuricae Root
3	Chuan Shan Jia	Pangolin Scales
3	Zao Jiao Ci	Spine Chinese Honeylocust Fruit
9	Chen Pi	Ripe Tangerine Peel

Description: This formula is used for infections. It alleviates pain and resolves sores, carbuncles, and painful skin lesions; it reduces swelling and promotes the discharge of pus.

Analysis: The chief ingredient in this formula, Jin Yin Hua, is widely used in Chinese medicine because of its ability to relieve toxicity (infection), clear pus, and reduce swelling. Chen Pi increases the vital energy (Chi) and reinforces the actions of the other ingredients. Dang Gui, Chi Shao, Ru Xiang, and Mo Yao circulate and strengthen the blood in addition to reducing pain. Fang Feng and Bai Zhi reduce superficial swelling, while Zhe Bei Mu and Tian Hua Fen clear heat (reduce fever). Chuan Shan Jia and Zao Jiao Ci open the meridians and resolve pus, thereby accelerating healing. Gan Cao relieves toxicity and harmonizes the herbs in this formula.

Dosage and Method of Preparation: Prepare a decoction. Drink four ounces of Xian Fang Huo Ming Yin tea three times daily, as needed.

Lien Chiao Pai Tu Pien (Forsythia Defeat Toxin Tablet); also known as Lian Qiao Bai Du Pian

Description: This patent formula is used for acute inflammation and infections (including ulcerated abscesses with pus), for skin itching with rash and redness, or for infection with fever due to local or systemic toxic infection.

Caution: This formula is prohibited for use during pregnancy.

Dosage: It comes in boxes of twelve vials, eight tablets per vial, with complete instructions on dosage.

Hua She Jie Yang Wan (Pit Viper Dispel Itching Pill); also known as Kai Yeung Pills

Description: This patent formula clears up skin rashes and dispels toxins. It is used to relieve fungal infections of the skin with itching, dermatitis (inflammation of the skin), and infection with pus.

Caution: This formula is prohibited for use during pregnancy.

Dosage: It comes in bottles of sixty pills, with complete instructions on dosage.

Chuan Xin Lian-Antiphlogistic Pills (Penetrate Heart, Repeatedly Fight Heat Pills); also known as Chuan Xin Lian Kang Yan Pian

Description: This formula is used to purge heat from the infection. It resolves inflammation, soothes the throat in strep throat infections with swollen glands; it is also used for viral infections that cause fever such as flu, measles, and hepatitis.

Dosage: It comes in bottles of sixty pills, with complete instructions on dosage.

Infertility

Infertility, the inability to conceive or father a child, is a relatively common problem affecting both men and women, with a variety of causes. Common causes for male infertility are a failure to produce enough healthy sperm, sperm that are malformed, or sperm whose life span after ejaculation is too short for them to travel far enough to reach the egg. Other causes are defects in the sperm due to a blockage of the spermatic tubes; damage to the spermatic ducts, usually resulting from a sexually transmitted disease such as gonorrhea; varicose veins in the scrotum; or abnormal development of the testes. Infertility in men may also be caused by failure to deliver the sperm into the vagina due to impotence or other disorders affecting ejaculation such as inhibited or retrograde ejaculation (see also Ejaculation,

Disorders of; Impotence). In rare cases, chromosomal abnormalities or genetic diseases like cystic fibrosis may cause infertility.

Female infertility is usually caused by a failure to ovulate, often occurring for no obvious reason, although sometimes attributed to a hormonal imbalance, stress, or ovarian disorders like tumors or cysts. Another possible cause is blocked fallopian tubes, frequently occurring after pelvic inflammatory disease or disorders of the uterus such as fibroid tumors or endometriosis (see also Endometriosis; Fibroid Tumor; Pelvic Inflammatory Disease). On rare occasions, infertility is caused by a woman's cervical mucus providing a hostile environment to her partner's sperm by producing antibodies that kill or immobilize them.

Quite often when none of these specific causes can be found, traditional Chinese medicine begins treatment by attempting to improve the patient's general state of health. This may include suggestions concerning dietary changes, reducing alcohol and marijuana consumption (both known to lower sperm counts), and instructions in both Taoist sexual practices and relaxation techniques. Otherwise, specific disorders such as those discussed above, if determined as an obstacle to conception, are treated, and the following herbal formulas are prescribed:

Wen Jing Tang (Warm the Menses Decoction)

Original Source: *Jin Gui Yao Lue* (according to *Chinese Herbal Medicine Formulas and Strategies*)

Ingredients:

Quantity (Grams)	Chinese Herbs	English Translation
9	Wu Zhu Yu	Evodia Fruit
6	Gui Zhi	Saigon Cinnamon Twig
9	Dang Gui	Tangkuei
6	Chuan Xiong	Szechuan Lovage Root
6	Shao Yao	Peony Root
9	Mai Men Dong	Lush Winter Wheat Tuber
6	Mu Dan Pi	Tree Peony Root, Bark of
6	Ren Shen	Ginseng

6	Gan Cao	Licorice Root
6	Sheng Jiang	Fresh Ginger Root
6	Ban Xia	Half Summer
6	E Jiao★	Donkey Skin Glue

★See special instructions for preparation below.

Description: This formula is used for infertility due to polycystic ovaries, chronic pelvic inflammatory disease, dysmenorrhea, and functional uterine bleeding.

Analysis: The chief herbs, Wu Zhu Yu and Gui Zhi, warm the uterus, dispel cold, and unblock blood vessels. Dang Gui and Chuan Xiong and, to a lesser degree, Shao Yao enrich and circulate the blood and also regulate the menstrual period. E Jiao and Mai Men Dong focus on moistening dryness and clearing heat. Mu Dan Pi assists the two chief herbs. Ren Shen, Sheng Jiang, Gan Cao, and Ban Xia strengthen the entire body, improve digestion by benefiting the spleen and stomach, and also harmonize the actions of the other herbs in the formula.

Dosage and Method of Preparation: Prepare a decoction. E Jiao should not be cooked with the other herbal ingredients, but added after the formula has been cooked and strained. Stir E Jiao into the decoction and allow the herb to dissolve. It will not be necessary to re-strain the decoction. Drink four ounces of Wen Jing Tang tea three times daily, as needed.

Zan Yu Dan Tang (Special Formula to Aid Fertility Decoction)

Original Source: *Jing Yue Quan Shu* (according to *Chinese Herbal Medicine Formulas and Strategies*)

Ingredients:

Quantity (Grams)	Chinese Herbs	English Translation
9	Fu Zi	Accessory Root of Szechuan Aconite
9	Rou Gui	Saigon Cinnamon Inner Bark
12	Rou Cong Rong	Fleshy Stem of Broomrape

12	Ba Ji Tian	Morinda Root
12	Yin Yang Huo	Licentious Goat Wort Leaf
9	She Chuang Zi	Cnidium Fruit Seed
12	Jiu Zi	Chinese Leek Seed
12	Xian Mao	Golden Eye-Grass Rhizome
12	Shan Zu Yu	Fruit Asiatic Cornelian Cherry
12	Du Zhong	Eucommia Bark
24	Shu Di Huang	Chinese Foxglove Root, Wine-Cooked
18	Dang Gui	Tangkuei
18	Gou Qi Zi	Matrimony Vine Fruit
24	Bai Zhu	Atractylodes Rhizome

Description: This formula is useful for treating impotence, infertility, listlessness, and general fatigue.

Analysis: The chief herbs in this formula are Fu Zi, Rou Gui, Rou Cong Rong, Ba Ji Tian, Yin Yang Huo, She Chuang Zi, Jiu Zi, Xian Mao, Shan Zu Yu, and Du Zhong. Combined, their action for strengthening the kidneys becomes quite powerful. Shu Di Huang, Dang Gui, and Gou Qi Zi are supportive by enriching the blood and replenishing sperm levels. Bai Zhu is added to strengthen the spleen and eliminate dampness.

Dosage and Method of Preparation: Prepare a decoction. Drink four ounces of Zan Yu Dan Tang tea three times daily, as needed.

Fu Ke Zhong Zi Wan (Gynecology Pregnancy Pill); also known as Zhong Zi Wan, or De Sheng Dan

Description: This patent formula invigorates the blood, warms the uterus, resolves amenorrhea, and is useful for infertility and for treating women suffering from miscarriage.

Dosage: It comes in bottles of one hundred pills, with complete instructions on dosage.

Tai Pan Tang Yi Pian (Placenta Sugar Coated Tablets); also known as Sugar-Coated Placenta Tablets

Description: This patent formula consists of pure human placenta extract and is used as a nutritive tonic for blood, Chi, and sperm. It is useful for impotence or deficiency of sperm. It resolves fatigue and weakness and is suitable for both men and women.

Dosage: It comes in bottles of one hundred tablets, with complete instructions on dosage.

Inflammation

Inflammation is redness, swelling, heat, and pain in tissue due to chemical or physical injury or infection. Inflammation is an essential part of the body's response to injury and infection and is usually accompanied by an accumulation of white blood cells, which are attracted by histamine, a protein formed in tissue during allergic reactions. White blood cells help destroy invading microorganisms and are involved in repairing damaged tissue. Treatment of inflammation typically involves assisting normal body processes by using anti-inflammatory agents to help reduce inflammation and resolve swelling and pain. Western medicine typically uses corticosteroid drugs and non-steroidal anti-inflammatory drugs such as aspirin and ibuprofen. Traditional Chinese medicine has basically the same objectives and employs the following antibiotic anti-inflammatory herbal formula:

Niu Huang Jie Du Pian (Cow Gallstone Dispel Toxin Tablet); also known as Niu Huang Chieh Tu Pien, or Bezoar Antidotal Tablets

Description: This patent formula is used to resolve inflamed throat or gums; red, irritated eyes; earaches; toxic swelling; and oral ulcers.

Caution: This formula is prohibited for use during pregnancy.

Dosage: It comes in boxes of ten vials, eight tablets per vial, with complete instructions on dosage.

Inflammatory Bowel Disease—see Colitis; Crohn's Disease; Intestine, Disorders of; Ulcer

Inflammatory bowel disease is a general term for two chronic inflammatory disorders that affect the small and/or large intestines: Crohn's disease and ulcerative colitis. The causes for these conditions are unknown. Refer to the entries listed above for description and treatment information.

Influenza—see Colds and Flu

Insect Bites

We've all experienced puncture wounds in the skin that were inflicted by blood-sucking insects. Common perpetrators of these annoyances include fleas, mosquitoes, lice, midges, gnats, sand fleas, and bed bugs. Some small arachnids (eight-legged animals—such as ticks and mites—that are similar to insects) can also inflict similar injuries. All insect bites provoke what is primarily an allergic reaction to substances in the insect's saliva or feces, which is often deposited at or near the site of the bite and is rubbed in by scratching. Most insect bites cause only temporary pain or itching, but occasionally a victim suffers a severe reaction. Reactions vary from innocuous red pimples, to painful swellings, to a severe rash.

Insects that bite do so to obtain a blood meal, so they normally attack exposed body parts such as the head, hands, arms, or legs. Avoiding tick bites can be particularly important for campers and hikers because of the possibility of contracting Lyme disease. Special precautions should also be taken by residents and travelers in tropical countries because of the possibility of contracting malaria as a result of being bitten by infected mosquitoes (see also Malaria). The use of insect repellents, mosquito nets, and screens over open windows is highly recommended. The following herbal formula treats insect bites after they have occurred:

Jing Wan Hong (Capitol City [Beijing] Many Red Colors); also known as Ching Wan Hung

Description: This patent formula is used to reduce pain, swelling, and rashes. It is useful for sunburn, rash, and insect bites.

Dosage: It comes in tubes, with complete instructions for topical use.

Insomnia

Chronic sleeplessness or insomnia is most often caused by worry or mental hyperactivity. Occasionally, it can be the result of a physical disorder such as sleep apnea (a breathing problem), environmental factors such as noise and light, or lifestyle factors such as too much caffeine in the diet, a lack of exercise during the day, or abuse of drugs (including antianxiety drugs, barbiturates, and amphetamines). Insomnia can also be a symptom of a psychiatric illness; people suffering from anxiety or depression often have difficulty getting to sleep, and schizophrenics are sometimes awakened by "voices" or delusions.

When there is an obvious physical or psychological cause for insomnia, this cause should be treated. Simple lifestyle changes can also resolve the problem. In cases resulting from stress or hyperactivity, meditation and the use of calming herbs have proven very helpful.

Shen Jing Shuai Rou Wan (Nerve Neurasthenia Weakness Pills); also known as Shen Ching Shuai Jao Wan

Description: This patent formula tranquilizes the mind and calms the spirit. It is used for symptoms of fatigue, insomnia, restlessness, and agitation.

Note: Results commonly are experienced only after the formula has been taken for one or two weeks.

Dosage: It comes in bottles of two hundred pills, with complete instructions on dosage.

Suan Zao Ren Tang Pian (Ziziphus Seed Soup Tablets); also known as Tabellae Suanzaoren Tang

Description: This patent formula is used to treat uneasiness, insomnia, and nightmares.

Dosage: It comes in bottles of forty-eight tablets, with complete instructions on dosage.

Intestine, Disorders of

The more serious intestinal disorders include congenital defects, infections and inflammations, parasitic infections, impaired blood supply, ulcers, bowel obstruction, tumors, and cancer.

Congenital defects occur at birth. Babies can be born with intestinal obstructions caused by atresia (congenital closure of the intestine), stenosis (narrowing of the intestine), or volvulus (twisting of the bowels). These conditions are among the most serious intestinal disorders and normally require early corrective surgery.

Infections and inflammations—generally referred to as gastroenteritis—are most often caused by viral or bacterial infection. The diseases associated with gastroenteritis can range from trivial to life threatening, from simple food poisoning to cholera and typhoid fever. Two other important inflammatory diseases of the intestines are ulcerative colitis, which mainly affects the colon, and Crohn's disease, which can affect any part of the digestive tract but usually affects the small intestine (see also Colitis; Crohn's Disease).

Parasitic infection may be caused by single-cell parasites, as in the cases of giardiasis and amebiasis. More commonly, it is caused by intestinal worms such as roundworms, tapeworms, or pinworms (see also Larva Migrans; Roundworms).

Impaired blood supply, or ischemia, is considered life threatening because of the possibility of developing gangrene. Normally, it is the result of partial or complete obstruction of arteries in the abdominal wall from diseases such as atherosclerosis, thrombosis, or embolism. Or blood vessels can be compressed or trapped, which can impede or interrupt blood supply in conditions like volvulus (twisting of the bowels) or a strangulated hernia (protrusion of the intestine through the abdominal wall).

Ulcers of the duodenum (small intestine), called peptic ulcers, occur in typhoid and Crohn's disease and can cause bleeding and perforation (a hole in the intestines). Ulceration of the large intestine can occur in both amebiasis and ulcerative colitis (see also Colitis; Crohn's Disease; Ulcer).

Bowel obstruction from diverticula is a rather common intestinal disorder. Diverticula are small pockets attached to the bowel walls that obstruct the inside of the bowel. These out-pouchings can become infected and inflamed, causing fever, pain in the lower abdominal area, tenderness, and occasionally abscess; this condition is called diverticulitis.

Tumors and cancer in the small intestine are extremely rare, but in the United States, the large intestine is the second most common site of cancerous malignancy after the lungs. Two types of tumors are found in both the large and small intestine: carcinoid tumors and lymphomas. Carcinoid tumors are very slow-growing and usually symptomless; however, they may spread to the liver, leading to carcinoid syndrome. Lymphomas, which damage the walls of the intestine and nearby lymph nodes, cause malabsorption of food.

The high incidence of colon-rectal cancer in Western countries suggests environmental and dietary factors. It is believed by both traditional Chinese and Western medicine that a high-meat, high-fat, low-fiber diet encourages the production and concentration of carcinogens in the intestinal tract. Genetics may also be a factor. Brothers, sisters, and children of people suffering from cancer of the colon are more likely to acquire the disease later in life. Cancer of the colon frequently occurs in association with other intestinal diseases such as ulcerative colitis and familial polyposis, a rare inherited disorder in which numerous—often a thousand or more—polyps are present in the colon or rectum.

Symptoms of tumors or cancer include inexplicable change in bowel movements (either constipation or diarrhea) lasting ten days or more, blood mixed in the feces, and pain or tenderness in the lower abdomen. Sometimes, however, no symptoms are present until the tumor grows so big that it obstructs or ruptures the intestine. (See also Colon-Rectal Cancer.)

The following herbal formulas can be used for treating a wide range of intestinal disorders. However, diagnosis by a physician is strongly recommended due to the grave consequences that can result from misdiagnosis or lack of proper treatment.

Da Huang Mu Dan Tang (Rhubarb and Moutan Decoction)

Original Source: *Jin Gin Yao Lue* (according to *Chinese Herbal Medicine Formulas and Strategies*)

Ingredients:

Quantity (Grams)	Chinese Herbs	English Translation
12	Da Huang	Rhubarb Root
9	Mu Dan Pi (Moutan)	Tree Peony Root, Bark of
15	Tao Ren	Peach Kernel
30	Dong Gua Ren	Wintermelon Seed
12	Mang Xiao★	Mirabilite

★See special instructions for preparation below.

Description: This raw-herb preparation is used for lower abdominal distention, tenderness, and pain, intestinal abscess, and low-grade fever.

Analysis: The chief ingredient, Da Huang, dispels heat and improves the circulation of both blood and vital energy (Chi) in the intestines. Mang Xiao assists the chief herb by softening the stool and reinforcing the promotion of bowel movements. Mu Dan Pi cools the blood and eliminates any masses or blood clots. Tao Ren circulates blood and has a mild laxative effect. Dong Gua Ren expels pus, reduces abscesses, and eliminates heat.

Dosage and Method of Preparation: Prepare a decoction. Do not cook Mang Xiao with the other herbs in the formula. Add it after the decoction has finished cooking and the other herbs have been strained off. At this point gently stir in Mang Xiao until the herb has dissolved. It will not be necessary to re-strain the decoction. Drink four ounces of Da Huang Mu Dan Tang tea three times daily, as needed.

Yi Yi Fu Zi Bai Jiang Tang (Coicis Prepared Aconite and Bai Jian Cao Decoction)

Original Source: *Jin Gui Yao Lue* (according to *Chinese Herbal Medicine Formulas and Strategies*)

Ingredients:

Quantity (Grams)	Chinese Herbs	English Translation
30	Yi Yi Ren	Seeds of Job's Tears
9	Fu Zi	Accessory Root of Szechuan Aconite
18	Bai Jiang Cao	Herba Baijiangcao

Description: This herbal formula expels pus and reduces swelling. It is useful for intestinal abscesses.

Analysis: Yi Yi Ren eliminates inflammation and discharges pus while benefiting the spleen, thus arresting diarrhea. Fu Zi assists by benefiting the spleen and supporting in the control of diarrhea. Bai Jiang Cao, which is anti-inflammatory and also discharges pus and toxins, is specific in its ability to heal intestinal abscesses.

Dosage and Method of Preparation: Prepare a decoction. Drink four ounces of Yi Yi Fu Zi Bai Jiang Tang tea three times daily, as needed.

Wu Mei Tang (Mume Decoction)

Original Source: *Shang Han Lun* (according to *Chinese Herbal Medicine Formulas and Strategies*)

Ingredients:

Quantity (Grams)	Chinese Herbs	English Translation
30	Wu Mei	Dark Plum Fruit
3	Chaun Jiao	Szechuan Pepper Fruit
3	Xi Xin	Chinese Wild Ginger Plant
12	Huang Lian	Golden Thread Root
9	Huang Bai	Amur Cork Tree Bark
9	Gan Jiang	Dried Ginger Root
6	Fu Zi	Accessory Root Szechuan Aconite
6	Gui Zhi	Saigon Cinnamon Twig
9	Ren Shen	Ginseng Root
9	Dang Gui	Tangkuei

Description: This herbal formula eliminates intestinal roundworms.

Analysis: The chief herb, Wu Mei, is very sour tasting, but effective in eliminating roundworms. Chuan Jiao and Xi Xin are both more general in their ability to expel parasites and warm the organs. Huang Bai and Huang Lian assist in attacking parasites. Gan Jiang, Fu Zi, and Gui Zhi all warm the interior to offset the cold, sour nature of the "attacking" herbs. Ren Shen and Dang Gui strengthen the vital energy (Chi) and enrich the blood.

Dosage and Method of Preparation: Prepare a decoction. Drink four ounces of Wu Mei Tang tea three times daily, as needed.

Xiao Jian Zhong Tang (Minor Construct the Middle Decoction)

Original Source: *Shang Han Lun* (according to *Chinese Herbal Medicine Formulas and Strategies*)

Ingredients:

Quantity (Grams)	Chinese Herbs	English Translation
30	Yi Tang	Barley Malt Sugar
9	Gui Zhi	Saigon Cinnamon Twig
18	Shao Yao	Peony Root
6	Zhi Gan Cao	Honey-Cooked Licorice Root
9	Sheng Jiang	Fresh Ginger Root
12 pieces	Da Zao	Jujube Fruit

Description: This raw herb formula reduces pain, eliminates fever, and is useful for treating duodenal ulcers and inflammatory bowel disease.

Analysis: Yi Tang strengthens the stomach and relieves abdominal pain. The other chief ingredient, Gui Zhi, warms the spleen and stomach as well as disperses cold. Shao Yao benefits digestion when it is combined with the previous herb. Zhi Gan Cao assists in reducing abdominal pain while benefiting the stomach and spleen. Sheng Jiang and Da Zao work together to improve digestion and harmonize the actions of the other herbs.

Dosage and Method of Preparation: Prepare a decoction. Drink four ounces of Xiao Jian Zhong Tang tea three times daily, as needed.

Chen Xiang Hua Qi Wan (Aquilariae Move Chi Pills)

Description: This patent formula is useful for gastritis, stomach or duodenal ulcers, and intestinal obstruction.

Dosage: It comes in bottles of one hundred pills, with complete instructions on dosage.

Iron-Deficiency Anemia—see Anemia

Irritable Bladder—see Cystitis; Incontinence; Prostate, Disorders of; Urinary Tract Infection

The most recognizable symptom of irritable bladder syndrome is intermittent, uncontrolled contractions of the muscles in the bladder. These uncontrolled muscle contractions usually cause discomfort and in some cases urinary incontinence. Irritability of the bladder is often due to urinary tract infection, bladder stones, or an enlarged prostate gland. Therefore, treatment for irritable bladder syndrome is directed at resolving the underlying cause. See the entries listed in the heading for more-detailed descriptions of these disorders along with herbal formulas for treating them.

Irritable Bowel Syndrome—see Constipation; Diarrhea; Flatulence; Intestine, Disorders of

Irritable bowel syndrome, also known as spastic colon, is a combination of intermittent abdominal pain and irregular bowel habits. There can be constipation, diarrhea, or alternating incidences of both. Although symptoms subside and even disappear for a period of time, the condition is usually recurrent throughout one's life. Even though it is the most common intestinal disorder, the cause is not fully understood. It occurs as often in China as it does in the West, which more or less excludes the Western diet as the most plausible cause. The condition is twice as common in women as in men.

Symptoms include intermittent cramplike abdominal pain, abdominal distention (often on the left side), transient relief of pain by moving the bowels or passing gas, and a sense of incomplete evacuation of the bowels.

Traditional Chinese medicine recommends colon cleansing with bulk-forming agents such as psyllium seed, along with the use of herbal formulas for relieving the disorder's troublesome symptoms. Unfortunately, there is no known cure for irritable bowel syndrome. Refer to the entries in this chapter on diarrhea, constipation, flatulence, and intestinal disorders for herbal formulas, which treat the accompanying symptoms of irritable bowel syndrome.

Itching (see also specific complaint, e.g., Athlete's Foot; Jock Itch; Rash; etc.)

Itching is a distracting irritation or tickling sensation in the skin that may be generalized (felt all over the skin) or local (confined to one area). Generalized itching can be caused by, among other things, excessive bathing (which removes the skin's natural oils), taking certain drugs, woolen or other textured clothing, and many skin conditions such as rash, chicken pox, hives, eczema, psoriasis, and fungal infections. Additionally, generalized itching can result from diabetes mellitus, renal (kidney) failure, jaundice, certain thyroid disorders, and blood disorders such as leukemia.

Local itching around the anus, called pruritus ani, often occurs in adults with problems such as hemorrhoids, anal fissure, and persistent diarrhea. Worm infestation is the most likely cause for anal itching in children. Other causes for localized itching are pruritus vulvae and candidiasis (both of which affect the external genitalia in women), lice, scabies, and insect bites.

Traditional Chinese medical treatment for itching depends on the underlying cause. The herbal formulas are normally directed at clearing infection, cooling the blood, and resolving hives and rashes with topical ointments.

Xiao Feng Tang (Eliminate Wind Powder from True Lineage)

Original Source: *Wai Ke Zheng Zong* (according to *Chinese Herbal Medicine Formulas and Strategies*)

Ingredients:

Quantity (Grams)	Chinese Herbs	English Translation
3	Jing Jie	Schizonepeta Stem/Bud
3	Fang Feng	Guard Against the Wind Root
3	Niu Bang Zi	Great Burdock Fruit
3	Chan Tui	Cicada Molting
3	Cang Zhu	Atractylodes Cangzhu
3	Ku Shen	Bitter Root
1.5	Mu Tong	Wood with Holes
3	Shi Gao	Gypsum, Mineral
3	Zhi Mu	Anemarrhena Root
3	Sheng Di Huang	Chinese Foxglove Root, Raw
3	Dang Gui	Tangkuei
3	Hei Zhi Ma	Black Sesame Seeds
1.5	Gan Cao	Licorice Root

Description: This herbal formula clears heat (infection from the body), cools the blood, and relieves skin lesions all over the body that are caused by eczema, dermatitis, and psoriasis.

Analysis: Jing Jie, Fang Feng, Niu Bang Zi, and Chan Tui are all chief herbs in this formula; they unblock the pores to allow Cang Zhu, Ku Shen, and Mu Tong to clear heat and eliminate infection. Shi Gao and Zhi Mu assist in clearing heat and prevent rashes from advancing beyond the surface to deeper levels. Sheng Di Huang cools the blood. Dang Gui and Hei Zhi Ma nourish and circulate it. Gan Cao clears heat, relieves toxicity, and harmonizes the actions of the other herbs in the formula.

Dosage and Method of Preparation: Make a decoction. Drink four ounces of Xiao Feng Tang tea three times daily, as needed.

Lien Chiao Pai Tu Pien (Forsythia Defeat Toxin Tablet); also known as Lian Qiao Bai Du Pian

Description: This patent formula clears heat (infection), reduces inflammation, and is useful for treating any kind of skin infection.

Caution: This formula is prohibited for use during pregnancy.

Dosage: It comes in vials containing eight tablets, with complete instructions on dosage.

Xiong Dan Zhi Ling Gao (Fel Ursi Hemorrhoid Effective Ointment); also known as Xiong Dan Zhi Chuang Gao

Description: This patent formula is a salve used to reduce inflammation, stop pain, and resolve itch; it is useful for relief from hemorrhoids and anal fissure.

Dosage: It comes in tubes of four or ten grams, with complete instructions on dosage.

Hua Tuo Gao (Hua Tuo Chinese Physician Ointment)

Description: This patent formula stops itching and is used to treat athlete's foot or fungal infections. It is also effective for treatment of eczema, with redness and scaling crusting the skin.

Dosage: It comes in tubes of four grams, with complete instructions on dosage.

Hua She Jie Yang Wan (Pit Viper Dispel Itching Pill); also known as Kai Yeung Pills

Description: This patent formula stops itching caused by allergic reaction to drugs.

Note: Certain foods are known to interact badly with this formula; do not eat seafood, bamboo shoots, or goose while taking this formula.

Dosage: It comes in bottles of fifty pills, with complete instructions on dosage.

Jaundice (see also Cirrhosis; Gallbladder, Disorders of; Hepatitis; Liver, Disorders of)

A major symptom of many disorders of the liver and biliary system, jaundice is characterized by a yellowing of the skin and the whites of the eyes caused by an accumulation in the blood of the bile pigment bilirubin. There are three major types of jaundice: hemolytic, hepatocellular, and obstructive jaundice. Hemolytic jaundice is caused by a breakdown of red blood cells resulting from the production of excess amounts of bilirubin. Hepatocellular jaundice occurs when bilirubin builds up in the blood and is usually associated with hepatitis, cirrhosis (inflammation of the liver), or liver failure. Obstructive jaundice occurs when bile is prevented from flowing out of the liver because of blockage of the bile ducts, as in disorders such as gallstones and tumors.

The following herbal formulas are all useful for treating disorders associated with jaundice, such as hepatitis, gallstones, cirrhosis, and liver failure:

Li Gan Pian (Benefit Liver Tablets); also known as Liver Strengthening Tablets

Description: This patent formula is used to reduce infection, regulate bile, and to treat jaundice, hepatitis, and gallstones.

Dosage: It comes in bottles of one hundred pills, with complete instructions on dosage.

Ji Gu Cao Wan (Herba Abri Pills); also known as Jigucao Wan

Description: This patent formula nourishes the liver. It was developed specifically for treating chronic hepatitis with jaundice.

Dosage: It comes in bottles of fifty pills, with complete instructions on dosage.

Shi Lin Tong Pian (Stone Dysuria Open Tablets); also known as Te Xiao Pai Shi Wan

Description: This patent formula clears up infection; it is useful for gallstones, hepatitis with jaundice, cirrhosis of the liver with ascites (excess fluids), and edema (excessive accumulation of fluids in the body tissues).

Dosage: It comes in bottles of one hundred tablets, with complete instructions on dosage.

Jock Itch (see also Fungal Infections/Fungal Diseases; Ringworm)

Jock itch, or tinea cruris, is a common infection caused by a group of fungi commonly called ringworm (dermatophytes). Jock itch produces a reddened, itchy area spreading from the genitals outward, usually covering the inside of the thighs. It is more common in males.

Traditional Chinese medicine treats tinea cruris with herbal formulas that contain antifungal ingredients as well as ingredients that eliminate inflammation, cool the blood, and reduce itching. Topical ointments are sometimes used to clear the surface of scaling, flaky skin.

Xiao Feng Tang (Eliminate Wind Powder from True Lineage)

Original Source: *Wai Ke Zheng Zong* (according to *Chinese Herbal Medicine Formulas and Strategies*)

Ingredients:

Quantity (Grams)	Chinese Herbs	English Translation
3	Jing Jie	Schizonepeta Stem/Bud
3	Fang Feng	Guard Against the Wind Root
3	Niu Bang Zi	Great Burdock Fruit

3	Chan Tui	Cicada Molting
3	Cang Zhu	Atractylodes Cangzhu
3	Ku Shen	Bitter Root
1.5	Mu Tong	Wood with Holes
3	Shi Gao	Gypsum, Mineral
3	Zhi Mu	Anemarrhena Root
3	Sheng Di Huang	Chinese Foxglove Root, Raw
3	Dang Gui	Tangkuei
3	Hei Zhi Ma	Black Sesame Seeds
1.5	Gan Cao	Licorice Root

Description: This herbal formula is used to clear heat (infection) and relieve skin lesions from all over the body that are caused by eczema, psoriasis, dermatitis, tinea infection, and diaper rash.

Note: This formula can be used topically or orally.

Analysis: Jing Jie, Fang Feng, Niu Bang Zi, and Chan Tui are all chief herbs in this formula; they unblock the pores and allow Cang Zhu, Ku Shen, and Mu Tong to clear heat and eliminate infection. Shi Gao and Zhi Mu assist in clearing heat and prevent rashes from advancing beyond the surface to deeper levels. Sheng Di Huang cools the blood. Dang Gui and Hei Zhi Ma nourish and circulate it, while Gan Cao clears heat, relieves toxicity, and harmonizes the actions of the other herbs in the formula.

Dosage and Method of Preparation: Make a decoction. For topical application: bathe the affected area with Xiao Feng Tang tea, as needed. For oral application: drink four ounces of Xiao Feng Tang tea three times daily, as needed.

Fu Ling Tu Jin Pi Ding (Complex Tu Jin Bark Tincture); also known as Composita Tujin Liniment

Description: This patent formula reduces inflammation and stops itching. It is used to treat skin infections caused by fungi tinea or sarcoptes scabiei (scabies).

Dosage: It comes in bottles of 15cc, with complete instructions on dosage.

Hua Tuo Gao (Hua Tuo [Chinese Physician's] Ointment)

Description: This formula stops itching and is used to treat dermatitis and eczema (inflammations of the skin) with scaling, oozing sores, and redness.

Dosage: It comes in tubes of four or ten grams, with complete instructions on dosage.

Juvenile Arthritis—see Arthritis

Keratosis Pilaris—see Rash

Keratosis pilaris is a common skin condition in which patches of raised, rough skin appear on the upper arms, thighs, and buttocks.

Kidney, Disorders of: Impaired Blood Supply; Autoimmune Deficiency Disorders; Tumors; Stones; Infection; Cysts; Kidney Failure

Although the kidneys are susceptible to a wide range of disorders, only one healthy kidney is required for good health. Therefore, kidney disease is rarely life threatening, except in situations where both kidneys are affected and the disease has reached an advanced stage. Among the many disorders affecting the kidneys, the most common are hypertension, which can cause kidney damage; nephrotic syndrome, in which fluid collects in the tissue, causing edema; and acute or chronic kidney failure. Other disorders that occur less frequently are congenital abnormalities such as horseshoe kidney, where the two kidneys are joined at the base; cases where both kidneys are on one side of the body; and polycystic disease, where multiple cysts develop on both kidneys.

Some diseases can damage the kidneys or lead to obstruction of

中草藥

the small blood vessels, impairing blood flow. Examples include diabetes mellitus and hemolytic-uremia syndrome, a disease in which the red blood cells are destroyed, leading to kidney damage and ultimately kidney failure. Other fairly common disorders include autoimmune deficiency disorders such as glomerulonephritis, in which the kidneys become inflamed as a result of streptococcal infections, benign kidney tumors, and kidney stones.

Infections and pyelonephritis (inflammation of the kidney; see also Pyelonephritis) are generally associated with obstruction of the urinary tract. Infection resulting from kidney stones, bladder tumors, or, in men, an enlargement of the prostate gland can spread from the bladder to the kidneys. On rare occasions, allergic reactions to certain drugs can cause acute kidney disease or kidney failure, for example the prolonged and excessive use of analgesics (pain medication).

To this long list, traditional Chinese medicine adds sexual overindulgence and alcohol abuse as causes for kidney damage, which is described as kidney emptiness.

The following herbal formulas can be used to treat a variety of kidney disorders:

Xiao Ji Yin Zi (Cephalanoplos Decoction)

Original Source: *Ji Sheng Fang* (according to *Chinese Herbal Medicine Formulas and Strategies*)

Ingredients:

Quantity (Grams)	Chinese Herbs	English Translation
10	Xiao Ji	Small Thistle Plant
10	Ou Jie	Lotus Rhizome, Node
10	Chao Pu Huang	Dry-Fried Cattail Pollen
30	Sheng Di Huang	Chinese Foxglove Root, Raw
10	Hua Shi	Talcum, Mineral
10	Mu Tong	Wood with Holes
10	Dan Zhu Ye	Bland Bamboo Leaves
10	Zhi Zi	Gardenia Fruit
10	Dang Gui	Tangkuei
10	Zhi Gan Cao	Honey-Cooked Licorice Root

Description: This herbal formula is useful for urinary tract infection, kidney stones, renal (kidney) tuberculosis, polycystic kidneys, and renal cysts.

Analysis: Xiao Ji, Ou Jie, Chao Pu Huang, and Sheng Di Huang cool the blood and stop bleeding. Hua Shi clears heat, promotes urination, and stops pain. Mu Tong, Dan Zhu Ye, and Zhi Zi eliminate heat, directing it downward and out of the body through urination. Dang Gui nourishes the blood, and Zhi Gan Cao relieves pain, benefits the spleen and stomach, and harmonizes the actions of the other herbs in the formula.

Dosage and Method of Preparation: Make a decoction. Drink four ounces of Xiao Ji Yin Zi tea three times daily, as needed.

Bei Xie Fen Qing Yin (Dioscorea Hypoglauca Decoction to Separate the Clear)

Original Source: *Dan Xi Xin Fa* (according to *Chinese Herbal Medicine Formulas and Strategies*)

Ingredients:

Quantity (Grams)	Chinese Herbs	English Translation
12	Bei Xie	Fish–Poison Yam Rhizome
9	Yi Zhi Ren	Alpinia Fruit
9	Wu Yao	Lindera Root
9	Shi Chang Pu	Sweet Flag Rhizome

Description: This herbal formula is useful for treating nephrotic syndrome (damage to the filtering units of the kidneys), pyelonephritis (infection of the kidneys), and pelvic inflammatory disease (infection of the internal female reproductive organs).

Analysis: Bei Xie, the chief herb, transforms dampness and turbidity (infection). Yi Zhi Ren warms the kidneys and reduces the frequency of urination. Wu Yao benefits the kidneys and increases vital energy (Chi). Shi Chang Pu resolves infection and eliminates dampness from the urinary bladder.

Dosage and Method of Preparation: Prepare a decoction. Drink four ounces of Bei Xie Fen Qing Yin tea three times daily, as needed.

Shi Lin Tong Pian (Specific Drug Passwan); also known as Te Xiao Pai Shi Wan

Description: This patent formula resolves infection in the kidneys and bladder, cools heat, stops bleeding (blood in the urine), stops pain, and is used for urinary calculi (stones) in kidneys, bladder, and ureters.

Dosage: This patent medicine comes in bottles of 120 pills, with complete instructions on dosage.

Ji Sheng Shen Qi Wan (Kidney Chi Pills/From Formulas to Aid the Living)

Description: This patent formula strengthens the kidneys, promotes urination, and reduces edema (excessive accumulation of fluid in the body tissues).

Dosage: It comes in boxes of one hundred pills, with complete instructions on dosage.

Labyrinthitis—see Ear, Disorders of

Laceration

A laceration is a torn, irregular, or jagged wound (as opposed to an incision), most often treated with antibacterial salves and ointments to prevent infections and hasten healing. It can be treated with the following herbal remedies:

Qi Li San (Seven Unit of Measure Powder)

Description: This patent formula decreases swelling, alleviates pain, and is used for treating injuries including lacerations, open wounds, and bruises.

Dosage: It comes in vial of 1.5 grams, with complete instructions on dosage.

Die Da Wan Hua You (Sports Injury 10,000 Flower Oil); also known as Wan Hua Oil

Description: This patent formula is used to treat cuts and lacerations with bleeding.

Dosage: It comes in bottles containing 15cc, with complete instructions on dosage.

Yu Nan Bai Yao (Yunnan Province White Medicine); also known as Yunnan Paiyao

Description: This patent formula can be taken orally or used topically to stop bleeding from open wounds, lacerations, and bruises.

Dosage: It comes in boxes of sixteen capsules, with complete instructions on usage.

Lactose Intolerance—see Flatulence; Indigestion

The inability to digest lactose (a sugar found in cow's milk) most often results from a deficiency of lactase, an enzyme in the small intestine. Because of the Chinese dietary custom of using soymilk instead of cow's milk, lactose intolerance is a problem seldom encountered in China; therefore, no herbal formula exists specifically for treating this condition. However, a number of formulas exist that are useful for effectively treating the symptoms associated with it, such as gas, bloating, stomach and intestinal cramping. See the entries suggested above.

Larva Migrans (see also Intestine, Disorders of; Ringworm)

Larva migrans refers to infections characterized by the presence of (immature forms of) worms in the body and the symptoms caused by their movement. Visceral larva migrans, more commonly known as toxocariasis, is caused by a type of worm normally found in dogs. Cutaneous larva migrans is caused by a hookworm found in dogs, cats, and other animals. Also known as "creeping eruption," it is contracted by walking barefoot on soil or beaches contaminated with animal feces. The larva penetrate the skin of the feet and move randomly, leaving itchy red lines on the skin that are sometimes accompanied by blistering.

The following herbal formulas can be used for eliminating worms and clearing infection:

Li Zhong An Hui Tang (Regulate the Middle and Calm Roundworm Decoction)

Original Source: *Wan Bing Hui Shen* (according to *Chinese Herbal Medicine Formulas and Strategies*)

Ingredients:

Quantity (Grams)	Chinese Herbs	English Translation
2.1	Ren Shen	Ginseng Root
3	Bai Zhu	Atractylodes Rhizome
3	Fu Ling	Tuckahoe Root
9	Chuan Jiao	Szechuan Pepper Fruit
9	Wu Mei	Dark Plum Fruit
1.5	Gan Jiang	Dried Ginger Root

Description: This raw herbal formula eliminates roundworm or hookworm infections and clears the bowels of infestations.

Analysis: Ren Shen, Bai Zhu, and Fu Ling increase the vital energy (Chi) while focusing or dispelling dampness and strengthening the stomach and spleen. Gan Jiang also benefits the stomach and arrests vomiting. Chuan Jiao alleviates abdominal pain and kills parasites. Wu Mei expels roundworms and stops diarrhea as well as alleviating abdominal pain.

Dosage and Method of Preparation: Prepare a decoction. Drink four ounces of Li Zhong An Hui Tang tea three times daily, as needed.

Lidan Paishi Wan (Benefit Gallbladder Discharge Stone Tablets); also known as Li Dan Tablets, or Li Dan Pai Shi Pian

Description: This patent formula resolves infection, kills worms, and is also useful for ascariasis (roundworm) infection.

Caution: This formula is prohibited for use during pregnancy.

Dosage: It comes in bottles of 120 tablets, with complete instructions on dosage.

Laryngitis (see also Sore Throat)

Laryngitis is inflammation of the larynx (voice box), usually caused by infection, that results in hoarseness or loss of the voice. Laryngitis can be acute, lasting only a few days, or chronic, persisting over a long period of time. Among the possible causes are viral infection due to colds, allergic reaction to drugs or pollen, irritation due to tobacco smoke or air pollutants, damage during surgery, overuse of the voice, or violent coughing. In addition to the hoarseness or loss of voice that is the chief symptom, laryngitis is often accompanied by fever and a general feeling of being sick.

Traditional Chinese medical treatment is directed at resolving inflammation and infection (what is referred to as "heat and poison in the lung"), while soothing the mucus membrane with the following herbal formulas.

Shuang Liao Hou Feng San (Double Ingredient Sore Throat Disease Powder); also known as Superior Sore Throat Powder Spray

Description: This patent formula soothes the throat, stops pain, eliminates infection, and is used to treat tonsillitis and laryngitis.

Dosage: It comes in vials of 1.5 grams, with complete instructions on dosage.

Hou Yan Wan (Laryngitis Pills); also known as Larynx Inflammation Pills

Description: This patent formula is used for sore throat with infection, acute tonsillitis, and laryngitis.

Caution: This formula is prohibited for use during pregnancy.

Dosage: It comes in three vials with ten pills in each, with complete instructions on dosage.

Liu Shen Wan (Six-Spirit Pill); also known as Lu Shen Wan

Description: This patent formula is for acute tonsillitis, sore throat, fever, strep throat, and laryngitis.

Caution: This formula is prohibited for use during pregnancy.

Dosage: It comes in bottles of one hundred pills, with complete instructions on dosage.

Laxatives—see Constipation

Leukemia

Leukemia is any of several types of cancer in which there is a disorganized proliferation of white blood cells in the bone marrow. Leukemia has two basic classifications: acute leukemia, which generally develops very rapidly, and chronic leukemia, which develops more slowly.

Lymphoblastic and myeloblastic are two basic forms of acute leukemia for which there are a number of suspected causes. One theory holds that they are caused by a virus similar to the one that causes AIDS. There has also been speculation that exposure to certain chemicals (such as benzene and some anticancer drugs), atomic radiation, radioactive leaks from nuclear reactors, and certain genetic or inherited factors may play a role. Research has shown that there is an increased incidence of leukemia in people with certain genetic disorders such as Franconi's anemia (a rare type of aplastic anemia), Down's syndrome (a chromosomal abnormality), and other blood disorders, namely, chronic myeloid leukemia and primary polycythemia (an excess of red blood cells). Symptoms include nose bleeding, bleeding gums, bone tenderness, frequent bruising, headache, enlarged lymph nodes (in the neck, armpits, or groin), anemia, and recurrent infections.

Chronic leukemia, which also has two basic forms (lymphocytic and myeloid), is characterized by an uncontrolled proliferation of white blood cells. In both cases the cause is unknown. Although the two bear some similarities, there are distinct differences, most notably in the symptoms and in Western medicine's methods for treating them. In addition to features that are common to acute leukemia, sufferers of lymphocytic leukemia may also have an enlarged liver and spleen, persistent fever, and night sweats. Sufferers of myeloid leukemia, which has two phases, normally experience fatigue, fever, night sweats, weight loss, visual disturbances, abdominal pain, and occasionally priapism (persistent, painful erection of the penis) during the first phase; and symptoms also common to acute leukemia during the second phase.

Western medical treatment for lymphocytic leukemia includes anticancer drugs, sometimes combined with radiation therapy, blood transfusions, and antibiotics. Myeloid leukemia is normally treated with anticancer drugs and bone marrow transplantation. Traditional Chinese medicine attributes the cluster of conditions called leukemia to stagnation of blood and Chi (vital energy); treatment usually consists of herbal therapy, acupuncture and massage.

The severe symptoms and the life-threatening nature of leukemia make it advisable to consider using herbal therapy only as an adjunct to the recommendations of a medical professional.

Bai Hu Tang (White Tiger Decoction)

Original Source: *Shang Han Lun* (according to *Chinese Herbal Medicine Formulas and Strategies*)

Ingredients:

Quantity (Grams)	Chinese Herbs	English Translation
30	Shi Gao	Gypsum, Mineral
9	Zhi Mu	Anemarrhena Root
3	Zhi Gan Cao	Honey-Cooked Licorice Root
15	Geng Mi	Raw Rice

Description: This raw-herb formula is used for symptoms associated with acute leukemia, including fever, profuse sweating, and bleeding nose and gums.

Analysis: The extremely cold nature of Shi Gao, the chief ingredient, makes it very effective for clearing heat (reducing fever). Zhi Mu assists the chief herb by moistening or replenishing fluids, avoiding the dehydration that usually results from high fever. Zhi Gan Cao and Geng Mi benefit the stomach by protecting it and guarding fluid levels from the effects of the extremely cold ingredients, which might otherwise harm the spleen and stomach.

Dosage and Method of Preparation: Prepare a decoction. Do not cook this decoction any longer than it takes the Geng Mi (rice) to become done, then strain off herbs and rice and retain the liquid. Drink four ounces of Bai Hu Tang tea three times daily, as needed.

Sheng Tian Qi Fen (Raw Pseudo Ginseng Powder); also known as Tien Chi Powder Raw

Description: This patent formula will stop bleeding. It is useful for bleeding gums and nosebleed and for relief of all bleeding associated with leukemia. Sheng Tian Qi Fen can be used internally as well as topically.

Caution: This formula is prohibited for use during pregnancy.

Dosage: It comes in boxes of forty grams, with complete instructions on dosage.

Yung Sheng He Ah Chiao (Externally Vigorous Combination Donkey Skin Glue); also known as Yong Sheng He A Jiao

Description: This patent formula is useful for bleeding disorders, including nosebleed and excessive bleeding associated with leukemia, as well as uterine bleeding and excessive menstrual bleeding.

Dosage: It comes in a thirty-gram solid block. Break it in half and dissolve fifteen grams in one liter of boiling water; drink one to two times daily, or as needed.

Leukorrhea (see also Candidiasis; Trichomoniasis; Vaginal Discharge)

It is customary in traditional Chinese medicine to name a disease after certain conditions or circumstances that are associated with it. An example of this is wind and dampness, which are known to be major contributing factors to arthritic suffering. For this reason, Chinese medicine literally refers to arthritis as "wind damp disease." Likewise, infection known to flourish in a moist, warm environment is referred to as "damp heat." Leukorrhea, a vaginal discharge associated with vaginitis (vaginal inflammation or infection), is referred to in Chinese medical language as "vaginal damp heat."

Normal vaginal secretions, which vary considerably among women and occur at different times in the menstrual cycle, tend to be more copious during pregnancy and sexual stimulation. These normal secretions should not be confused with leukorrhea, the abnormal discharge associated with vaginitis, which is profuse, unpleasant smelling, and usually accompanied by vaginal itching.

Two of the most common vaginal infections are candidiasis (generally known as yeast infection, or thrush, and caused by the microscopic organism *Candida albicans*), which causes a thick, white cottage cheese-like discharge; and trichomoniasis or trich (caused by the organism *Trichomonas vaginalis*), which causes a profuse yellow-green discharge. Treatment usually takes the form of antibiotic patent formulas that are taken internally and antibiotic herbal formulas that are used topically as a douche or surface wash.

She Chuang Zi Tang (Cnidium Tea)

Original Source: *Zhong Yi Fang Ji Ling Chuang Shou Ce* (according to *Chinese Herbal Medicine Formulas and Strategies*)

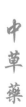

Ingredients:

Quantity (Grams)	Chinese Herbs	English Translation
15	She Chuang Zi	Cnidium Fruit Seed
15	Chuan Jiao	Szechuan Pepper Fruit
15	Ming Fan★	Alum, Mineral
15	Ku Shen	Bitter Root
15	Bai Bu	Stemona Root

★See special instructions for preparation below.

Description: This herbal formula clears up vaginal infection while it dries dampness, kills parasites, and resolves itching. It is useful for trichomoniasis and vaginitis.

Caution: This formula is for external use only; do not drink it.

Analysis: She Chuang Zi, the chief herb, dries dampness, clears infection, and kills parasites. Chuan Jiao assists the chief herb in attacking parasitic infestation. Ming Fan is effective for alleviating itching. Ku Shen clears infection and also stops itching. Bai Bu reinforces the action of the chief herb and is powerful in its ability to kill all forms of bacteria as well as pinworms, head or body lice, and fleas.

Dosage and Method of Preparation: Make a decoction. Ming Fan should not be cooked with the other herbs, but added after the normal cooking procedure, then allowed to steep with the decoction for thirty minutes before straining. Use this formula as a douche or a vaginal wash. Wash with four ounces of room-temperature tea as needed. Douche with eight ounces of room-temperature tea twice daily or as needed.

Yu Dai Wan (Heal Leukorrhea Pill); also known as Yudai Wan

Description: This patent formula clears vaginal infection (damp heat), and astringes discharge with dark color and odor, including symptoms such as lower backache and vaginal itching.

Dosage: It comes in bottles of one hundred pills, with complete instructions on dosage.

中草藥

Chien Chin Chih Tai Wan (Thousand Pieces of Gold Stop Leukorrhea Pill); also known as Qian Jin Zhi Dai Wan

Description: This patent formula clears vaginal infection while it astringes discharge. It is useful for leukorrhea and trichomoniasis with symptoms of lower back pain, fatigue, abdominal distention, and pain.

Dosage: It comes in bottles of 120 pills, with complete instructions on dosage.

Liver, Disorders of: Abscess, Infection, Inflammation, Hepatitis, Cancer, Autoimmune Disorders, Tumors, Failure, Fluke

Traditional Chinese medicine's assertion that the health of the liver is reflected in the eyes appears to be validated by the fact that in most diseases affecting the liver, yellowing or discoloration of the eyes is usually a major symptom.

Heading the list of liver diseases are alcohol-related disorders, which include alcohol-related hepatitis and cirrhosis (see also Cirrhosis; Hepatitis). Enlargement of the liver, jaundice, and yellowing of the skin and eyes are common symptoms of both diseases. Apart from alcohol-induced diseases, the liver can also be affected by congenital defects, which occur at birth. These usually occur as malformations of the bile ducts that obstruct the flow of bile in infants or by the total absence of bile ducts. Both abnormalities cause jaundice (see also Jaundice).

Hepatitis, a general term for inflammation of the liver, is most often caused by viruses such as type A, type B, and type C. All three strains create a condition commonly known as viral hepatitis (see also Hepatitis). Other problems affecting the liver are bacteria spreading through the biliary system, causing liver abscesses; and parasitic diseases such as liver flukes, hydatid disease, and amebiasis.

Additionally, many drugs (namely painkillers such as acetaminophen) when taken in large doses can cause severe liver damage, while some other drugs, taken even in normal doses, have been known to cause an allergic reaction resulting in acute or chronic hepatitis. Poisoning by certain types of mushrooms has also been associated with severe liver damage and in some instances complete liver failure.

Some of the more rare disorders affecting the liver are metabolic disorders in which there is too much iron in the body (hemochromatosis) or too much copper (Wilson's disease). Primary malignant tumors, which originate in the liver, are seldom seen. The liver is, however, a common site of malignant tumors that have spread from cancers of the stomach, pancreas, or large intestine.

Traditional Chinese medicine has been successful in the treatment of liver disorders with the following formulas:

Zhen Wu Tang (True Warrior Decoction)

Original Source: *Shang Han Lun* (according to *Chinese Herbal Medicine Formulas and Strategies*)

Ingredients:

Quantity (Grams)	Chinese Herbs	English Translation
9	Fu Zi	Accessory Root of Szechuan Aconite
6	Bai Zhu	Atractylodes Rhizome
9	Fu Ling	Tuckahoe Root
9	Sheng Jiang	Fresh Ginger Root
9	Bai Shao	White Peony Root

Description: This herbal formula is useful for treating cirrhosis of the liver or other chronic hepatic (liver) disorders.

Analysis: Fu Zi, the chief herb, whose nature is very hot, strengthens the kidneys by warming them. Fu Ling and Bai Zhu drain dampness, thus strengthening the spleen while promoting urination. Sheng Jiang assists in harmonizing the center (spleen and stomach). Bai Shao nourishes the blood.

Dosage and Method of Preparation: Make a decoction. Drink four ounces of Zhen Wu Tang tea three times daily, as needed.

Da Huang Zhe Chong Tang (Rhubarb and Eupolyphaga Decoction)

Original Source: *Jin Gui Yao Lue* (according to *Chinese Herbal Medicine Formulas and Strategies*)

Ingredients:

Quantity (Grams)	Chinese Herbs	English Translation
30	Da Huang	Rhubarb Root
3	Tu Bie Chong	Wingless Cockroach
6	Tao Ren	Peach Kernel
3	Gan Qi	Dried Lacca Sinica
6	Qi Cao	Dried Larva of Scarab
6	Shui Zhi	Leech
6	Meng Chong	Horse Flies
6	Huang Qin	Baical Skullcap Root
6	Xing Ren	Almond Kernel
30	Sheng Di Huang	Chinese Foxglove Root, Raw
12	Bai Shao	White Peony Root
9	Gan Cao	Licorice
9	Chai Hu	Bupleurum Hare's Ear Root

Description: This herbal formula is used to treat chronic hepatitis, alcoholic liver disease, fibrosis of the liver (the abnormal formation of fibrous tissue in the liver), hepatic neoplasm (liver tumors or growths), and cirrhosis of the liver.

Caution: This formula is prohibited for use during pregnancy.

Analysis: Da Huang cools the blood, clears heat, and moves the bowels. Tu Bie Chong circulates the blood and breaks up blood clots and fixed abdominal masses. Tao Ren, Gan Qi, Qi Cao, Shui Zhi, and Meng Chong assist the chief ingredients by circulating blood, unblocking the meridians, and reducing abdominal masses. Huang Qin and Xing Ren benefit the liver by reducing heat and moistening, which offsets the dryness created by liver heat. Sheng Di Huang and Bai Shao cool and nourish the blood. Gan Cao harmonizes the herbs. Chai Hu, which is not normally part of the formula, is added because of the tremendous benefits it provides by strengthening the liver, relieving surface heat, and clearing heat.

Dosage and Method of Preparation: Make a decoction. Drink four ounces of Da Huang Zhe Chong Tang tea three times daily, as needed.

Ji Gu Cao Wan (Herba Abri Pills); also known as Jigucao Wan

Description: This patent formula clears liver heat (infection), clears the bile ducts, decreases inflammation in the liver, stops pain, and is used to treat acute and chronic hepatitis with or without jaundice.

Dosage: It comes in bottles of fifty pills, with complete instructions on dosage.

Lung, Disorders of—see Asthma; Bronchitis; Pleurisy; Pneumonia; Tuberculosis

Lymph Nodes, Enlarged

Lymph nodes (located in the neck, armpits, and groin) play an important role in fighting infection. More commonly known as lymph glands, in addition to producing antibodies, they also form large cells called macrophages that engulf bacteria and other foreign particles. Microphages form a barrier to prevent the spread of infection by filtering out bacteria before it can enter the bloodstream.

When lymph nodes become enlarged, they are said to be overloaded, which is usually a clear indication of local infection. Sore throat, tonsillitis, and laryngitis are common examples of infections causing enlarged lymph nodes in the neck, while inflammation, cysts, and abscesses of the breasts are causes for enlargement of those in the armpits. Infections of the urethra and prostate glands as well as certain sexually transmitted diseases are some of the possible causes for enlarged lymph nodes in the groin.

Pu Ji Xiao Du Yin Tang (Universal Benefit Decoction to Eliminate Toxin)

Original Source: *Wei Sheng Bao Jian* (according to *Chinese Herbal Medicine Formulas and Strategies*)

Ingredients:

Quantity (Grams)	Chinese Herbs	English Translation
15	Jiu Chao Huang Qin	Wine-Fried Baical Skullcap Root
15	Jiu Chao Huang Lian	Wine-Fried Coptis Root
3	Niu Bang Zi	Great Burdock Fruit
3	Lian Qiao	Forsythia Root
3	Bo He	Peppermint
1.5	Jiang Can	Dead Body of Sick Silkworm
6	Xuan Shen	Ningpo Figwort Root
3	Ma Bo	Puffball Fruit
3	Ban Lan Gen	Woad Root
6	Jie Geng	Balloon Flower Root
6	Gan Cao	Licorice Root
6	Chen Pi	Ripe Tangerine Peel
6	Chai Hu	Bupleurum Hare's Ear Root
1.5	Sheng Ma	Black Cohosh Rhizome

Description: This herbal formula clears heat from the lymph nodes and resolves infection; it is useful for acute tonsillitis and lymphadenitis.

Analysis: Jiu Chao Huang Qin and Jiu Chao Huang Lian are used together to clear toxic heat (infection) from the upper part of the body. Niu Bang Zi, Lian Qiao, Bo He, and Jiang Can disperse cold and infection in the face and head. Xuan Shen, Ma Bo, Ban Lan Gen, Jie Geng, and Gan Cao clear heat and infection in the throat and relieve toxic fire. Chen Pi regulates the flow of vital energy (Chi) and blood-dispersing pathogenic influences. Chai Hu and Sheng Ma guide the other ingredients to the head and upper body.

Dosage and Method of Preparation: Make a decoction. Drink four ounces of Pu Ji Xiao Du Yin Tang tea three times daily, as needed.

Xi Huang Wan (West Gallstone Pills)

Description: This patent formula is used to reduce swelling associated with lymphadenitis; it is useful for treating abscesses, carbuncles, inflammations, and a wide variety of infections.

Caution: This formula is prohibited for use during pregnancy.

Dosage: It comes in vials of eight pills per vial, with complete instructions on dosage.

Malaria

Malaria is a potentially fatal parasitic disease that is spread by the bite of a mosquito. The parasites responsible for malaria are single-cell organisms called plasmodia that infect the bloodstream, causing symptoms that include shaking, chills, fever with sweating, and severe headache. General malaise, nausea, and vomiting may also occur.

Malaria is prevalent throughout the tropics and kills as many as one million infants and children every year in tropical regions such as Africa. The chance of contracting the disease in the United States is very small. The period between the mosquito bite and the appearance of symptoms is usually a week or two, but it can be as long as a year if the person has taken antimalarial drugs, which suppress rather than cure the disease. Both Western and traditional Chinese medicine offer effective treatment for malaria, but neither has a vaccine or herbal remedy that can be taken in advance to prevent it. The Western drug of choice for treating malaria is quinine. The following Chinese herbal formulas have also proven effective:

Da Chai Hu Tang (Major Bupleurum Decoction)

Original Source: *Shang Han Lun* (according to *Chinese Herbal Medicine Formulas and Strategies*)

Ingredients:

Quantity (Grams)	Chinese Herbs	English Translation
24	Chai Hu	Bupleurum Hare's Ear Root
9	Huang Qin	Baical Skullcap Root
9	Zhi Shi	Green Bitter Orange Fruit
6	Da Huang	Rhubarb Root
9	Bai Shao	White Peony Root
24	Ban Xia	Half Summer
15	Sheng Jiang	Fresh Ginger Root
12 pieces	Da Zao	Jujube Fruit

Description: This herbal formula is used to treat alternating fever and chills, nausea, and vomiting. It is useful for malaria, especially with predominant fever.

Analysis: The chief herb, Chai Hu, is combined with Huang Qin, which strengthens its ability to clear heat from the liver and gallbladder. Zhi Shi benefits the vital energy (Chi) and reduces the feeling of fullness in the chest and abdomen. Da Huang assists in draining heat by moving the bowels in addition to facilitating the flow of bile. Bai Shao enriches the blood and benefits the stomach. Ban Xia calms the stomach and with Sheng Jiang stops vomiting. Da Zao assists in the release of pathogenic influence.

Dosage and Method of Preparation: Prepare a decoction. Drink four ounces of Da Chai Hu Tang tea three times daily, as needed.

Da Yuan Yin (Reach the Membrane Source Decoction)

Original Source: *Wen Yi Lun* (according to *Chinese Herbal Medicine Formulas and Strategies*)

Ingredients:

Quantity (Grams)	Chinese Herbs	English Translation
1.5	Cao Guo	Grass Fruit
3	Huo Po	Magnolia Bark
6	Bing Lang	Betel Nut
3	Huang Qin	Baical Skullcap Root
3	Zhi Mu	Anemarrhena Root
3	Bai Shao	White Peony Root
1.5	Gan Cao	Licorice Root

Description: This herbal formula is used to treat alternating fever and chills with headache, nausea, and vomiting, as is seen in malaria.

Analysis: There are three chief ingredients in this formula: Cao Guo, which transforms turbidity (infection) and stops vomiting; Huo Po, which also transforms turbidity and benefits the vital energy (Chi); and Bing Lang, which disperses dampness and drives out pathogenic influences. Huang Qin clears heat (fever) and dries dampness (resolves sweating) while strengthening the stomach and gallbladder. Zhi Mu also clears heat and balances fluids to prevent dehydration. Bai Shao nourishes the blood, and Gan Cao harmonizes the actions of the other herbs in the formula.

Dosage and Method of Preparation: Prepare a decoction. Drink four ounces of Da Yuan Yin tea three times daily, as needed.

Measles

Traditional Chinese medicine cites viral infection causing heat in the blood, stomach, and lungs as the principal cause for measles. Not coincidentally, rubella (as it is clinically known) is characterized by two prominent symptoms: rash and high fever.

Measles is highly infectious and mainly affects children, although it can occur at any age. Normally, once infected with the disease, the recipient is immune for life. The incubation period for measles is nine to eleven days before symptoms appear. Common symptoms are fever, runny nose, sore eyes, and a cough. After three to four days, a red rash appears, usually starting on the head and neck and spreading downward to cover the entire body. Complications include ear and chest infections and, on rare occasions, encephalitis (infection of the brain).

Note: Pregnant women who have never had measles or been immunized against the disease should take extra precautions to avoid becoming infected. Measles during pregnancy results in death of the fetus in 20 percent of all cases.

Immunization is, of course, the preferred course of action for preventing the disease; if, however, you become infected with measles, the following herbal formula should prove helpful in relieving symptoms and speeding up a cure:

Sheng Ma Ge Gen Tang (Cimicifuga and Kudzu Decoction)

Original Source: *Xiao Er Yao Zheng Zhi Jue* (according to *Chinese Herbal Medicine Formulas and Strategies*)

Ingredients:

Quantity (Grams)	Chinese Herbs	English Translation
6	Zi Cao	Groomwell Root
6	Sheng Ma	Black Cohosh (Cimicifuga) Rhizome
9	Ge Gen	Kudzu Root
3	Zhi Gan Cao	Honey-Cooked Licorice Root
9	Chi Shao	Red Peony Root

Description: This herbal formula is useful for measles; it brings rashes to the surface and disperses them, quells fever and chills, and abates coughing, red eyes, and thirst.

Analysis: The chief herbs, Zi Cao and Sheng Ma, effectively treat rashes. Ge Gen supports this action by opening the pores and replenishing fluid levels to offset dehydration caused by heat (fever). Chi Shao and Zhi Gan Cao harmonize the herbs in the formula, preventing their harsh nature from injuring the Chi and Yin, and consequently causing nausea and thirst.

Dosage and Method of Preparation: Prepare a decoction. Drink four ounces of Sheng Ma Ge Gen Tang tea three times daily, as needed.

An Kung Niu Huang Wan (Peaceful Palace Ox Gallstone Pill); also known as An Gong Niu Huang Wan

Description: This patent formula quells fever and calms shaking (chills); it is efficacious for measles with high fever in children or adults.

Caution: This formula is prohibited for use during pregnancy.

Dosage: It comes in a box of one pill, with complete instructions on dosage.

Memory Loss

There are two basic types of memory loss. The first and more serious type, amnesia, is brought on by shock, hysteria, alcohol or drug use, and on rare occasions by brain tumors, syphilis, or epilepsy. With amnesia, the storage and recall of information in long-term memory is impaired. Amnesia can also occur in some forms of psychiatric illness in which there is no apparent disease or physical damage. The second type of memory loss, senile dementia (forgetfulness), mainly affects elderly people.

As logic might dictate, traditional Chinese medicine's method for treating memory loss is largely determined by the cause. Some of the possible causes of amnesia are head injuries, including concussion resulting in temporary memory loss; degenerative disorders such as Alzheimer's disease, causing a gradual yet permanent loss of memory; infections such as encephalitis, which can cause either temporary or permanent loss of memory; and brain tumors, strokes, and subarachnoid hemorrhage, which normally cause irreversible brain damage resulting in the permanent loss of memory. When amnesia is caused by damage or disease in areas of the brain concerned with memory function—except in cases where there is irreversible brain damage—memory loss is often temporary and can be restored by treating the underlying cause (such as mental fatigue, aging, or menopause).

The following herbal formulas can be used for treating these causes of memory loss or forgetfulness:

Bu Nao Wan (Supplement Brain Pills); also known as Cerebral Tonic Pills

Description: This patent formula is useful to abate restlessness and mental agitation and to improve concentration and poor memory.

Dosage: It comes in bottles of three hundred pills, with complete instructions on dosage.

Jian Nao Wan (Healthy Brain Pills)

Description: This patent formula is useful for mental agitation, lack of concentration, forgetfulness, and mental fatigue.

Dosage: It comes in bottles of three hundred pills, with complete instructions on dosage.

Note: Limit the use of this formula to two weeks.

Meningitis

Traditional Chinese medicine treats meningitis (inflammation of the membrane covering the brain and spinal cord) with a decoction made from various species of bamboo (Zhu Ye) and calcium sulfate (Shi Gao). Although the rationale behind such treatment is based on sound medical principles, in order to avoid what could be a fatal outcome, immediate medical attention should be sought if any of the following symptoms are experienced: fever with severe headache accompanied by nausea, vomiting, an aversion to light, or a stiff neck.

There are two basic forms of meningitis, viral and bacterial. Viral meningitis usually is not serious, clears up in two to three weeks, and has no aftereffects. Bacterial meningitis, the more serious of the two, is a medical emergency that can result in permanent brain damage. Nearly 70 percent of meningitis sufferers are children under age five.

Western treatment for bacterial meningitis usually involves administering large doses of intravenous antibiotics. The following Chinese herbal formulas can be useful for treating mild cases of viral meningitis:

Yin Qiao Tang (Honeysuckle and Forsythia Decoction)

Original Source: *Wen Bing Tiao Bian* (according to *Chinese Herbal Medicine Formulas and Strategies*)

Ingredients:

Quantity (Grams)	Chinese Herbs	English Translation
15	Jin Yin Hua	Honeysuckle Flower
15	Lian Qiao	Forsythia Fruit
6	Jie Geng	Balloon Flower Root
12	Niu Bang Zi	Great Burdock Fruit
6	Bo He★	Peppermint
6	Dan Dou Chi	Prepared Black Bean
9	Jing Jie	Schizonepeta Stem/Bud
6	Dan Zhu Ye	Bland Bamboo Leaves
30	Xian Lu Gen	Reed Root
6	Gan Cao	Licorice Root

★See special instructions for preparation on the next page.

Description: This herbal formula is used for viral meningitis, fever, headache, nausea, and encephalitis.

Analysis: The chief herbs, Jin Yin Hua and Lian Qiao, clear heat and relieve toxicity. Jie Geng and Niu Bang Zi benefit the throat and lungs by spreading the vital energy (Chi). Bo He and Dan Dou Chi assist the chief herbs in clearing heat. Jing Jie nourishes the fluids, preventing dryness. Dan Zhu Ye, Xian Lu Gen, and Gan Cao all generate fluids and eliminate thirst.

Dosage and Method of Preparation: Prepare a decoction. Bo He (Peppermint) should not be cooked as long as the other herbs. Instead, add it to the simmering herbal decoction when five minutes of cooking time remains. Overcooking this herb will reduce its effectiveness. Drink four ounces of Yin Qiao Tang tea three times daily, as needed.

Zi Xue Dan (Purple Snow Crystals); also known as Tzu Hsueh Tan

Description: This patent formula eliminates inflammation and infection, fever, epidemic encephalitis, and viral meningitis.

Caution: This formula is prohibited for use during pregnancy.

Dosage: It comes in vials containing .8 grams, with complete instructions on dosage.

Wan Shi Niu Huang Qing Xin Wan (Cow Gallstone Clear Heat Heart Syndrome Pills); also known as Niu Huang Qin Xin Wan, or Bezoar Sedative Pills

Description: This patent formula is used for high-grade fever, encephalitis, inflammation, infection, infantile convulsions, and viral meningitis.

Caution: This formula is prohibited for use during pregnancy.

Dosage: It comes in ten honey pills, with complete instructions on dosage.

Menopause

Menopause, also known as climacteric, is quite simply the cessation of menstruation. Usually occurring in women between ages forty-five and fifty-five, menopause is associated with complaints that include hot flashes, night sweats, vaginal dryness, dry skin, and brittle bones. These physical symptoms are said to be caused by a reduction in the production of estrogen, a hormone produced by the ovaries. There are also psychological symptoms, but it is not clear whether they are caused by a lack of estrogen or are a reaction to the physical symptoms and the sleep disturbances that are created by night sweats. The most common psychological symptoms are depression, poor memory, lack of concentration, anxiety, mood swings, and a loss of interest in sex. Additionally, a rise in blood pressure is not uncommon.

According to traditional Chinese medicine, menopause is caused by a decrease in estrogen production, blood deficiency, and an imbalance between the kidneys and the liver; it can be effectively treated with herbal therapy as an alternative to hormone replacement therapy (Premarin, etc.), which has become Western medicine's standard method of treatment.

Xiao Yao Tang (Rambling Decoction)

Original Source: *Tai Ping Hui Min He Ji Ju Fang* (according to *Chinese Herbal Medicine Formulas and Strategies*)

Ingredients:

Quantity (Grams)	Chinese Herbs	English Translation
9	Chai Hu	Bupleurum Hare's Ear Root
9	Dang Gui	Tangkuei
9	Bai Shao	White Peony Root
9	Bai Zhu	Atractylodes Rhizome
9	Fu Ling	Tuckahoe Root
6	Zhi Gan Cao	Honey-Cooked Licorice Root

Description: This herbal formula is used for treating menopause with symptoms of vertigo, fatigue, dry mouth, low-grade fever, alternating fever and chills, mood swings, insomnia, and hot flashes.

Analysis: Chai Hu is assisted by Dang Gui and Bai Shao in treating the liver and nourishing the blood to improve its function. Bai Zhu and Fu Ling benefit the spleen while moderating spasmodic abdominal pain. Zhi Gan Cao harmonizes the herbs in the formula. Although the symptoms of menopause seem not to be addressed in the analysis of this formula, many of them are attributed to an imbalance of the liver, which is treated by the chief herbs.

Dosage and Method of Preparation: Prepare a decoction. Drink four ounces of Xiao Yao Tang tea three times daily, as needed.

Zhi Bai Di Huang Wan (Anemarrhenae Phellodendri Rhemannia Pills); also known as Eight Flavor Tea, Chih Pai Di Huang Wan, or Chih Pai Pa Wei Wan

Description: This patent formula reduces low-grade fever, eliminates night sweats, and is useful for treating hot flashes associated with menopause.

Dosage: It comes in bottles of two hundred pills, with complete instructions on dosage.

Da Bu Yin Wan (Super Supplement Yin Pill)

Description: This patent formula is useful for treating hot flashes, night sweats, insomnia, and dizziness associated with menopause.

Dosage: This patent medicine comes in bottles of two hundred pills, with complete instructions on dosage.

Tian Wang Bu Xin Wan (Heavenly Spirit Benefit Heart Pills); also known as Emperor's Tea, Tien Wang Pu Hsin Tan, or Tien Wang Bu Xin Wan

Description: This patent formula is used for menopausal symptoms such as restlessness, insomnia, poor memory, short attention span, and poor concentration.

Dosage: It comes in bottles of two hundred pills, with complete instructions on dosage.

Deng Xin Wan (Stabilize Heart Pills); also known as Ding Xin Wan

Description: This patent formula is used for menopausal syndrome with symptoms of palpitations, insomnia, poor memory, dizziness, restlessness, hot flashes, and dry mouth.

Dosage: It comes in bottles of one hundred pills, with complete instructions on dosage.

He Che Da Zao Wan (Placenta Great Creation Pill); also known as Placenta Compound Restorative Pills, Ho Cheh Ta Tsao Wan, or Restorative Pills

Description: This patent formula is used for treating menopausal disorders such as fatigue, fever with thirst, night sweating, hot flashes, and restlessness insomnia.

Dosage: It comes in bottles of one hundred pills, with complete instructions on dosage.

Menorrhagia (see also Vaginal Bleeding)

Traditional Chinese medicine describes a normal menstrual cycle as one that lasts from three to five days, with an average blood loss of approximately two fluid ounces (sixty milliliters). Anything in excess of that is considered menorrhagia, the clinical term for excessive loss of blood during menstruation. Although excessive menstrual bleeding normally results from an imbalance of the hormones estrogen and progesterone or a physical disorder such as polyps, fibroid tumors, pelvic infections or the use of an IUD, in some women no physical cause can be found. (See also Endometriosis; Ovarian Cyst; Pelvic Inflammatory Disease.)

Western treatment for menorrhagia includes prescribing hormone supplements (usually birth control pills or Premarin) when hormone imbalance is suspected, performing a D and C (dilation and curettage), or in severe cases a hysterectomy (surgical removal of the uterus).

The Chinese herbal formulas given below can be considered for regulating the period and arresting excessive bleeding. Sufferers of menorrhagia may also want to consider using blood tonics to improve blood quality, since menorrhagia is a leading cause of pernicious anemia. (See also Anemia; Tonics [in Chapter 2].)

Qing Re Zhi Beng Tang (Clear Heat and Stop Excessive Uterine Bleeding Decoction)

Original Source: *Zhong Yi Fu Ke Zhi Liao Xue* (according to *Chinese Herbal Medicine Formulas and Strategies*)

Ingredients:

Quantity (Grams)	Chinese Herbs	English Translation
9	Zhi Zi	Gardenia Fruit
15	Chao Huang Qin	Stir-Fried Baical Skullcap Root
9	Huang Bai	Amur Cork Tree Bark
24	Sheng Di Huang	Chinese Foxglove Root, Raw
9	Mu Dan Pi	Tree Peony Root, Bark of
24	Di Yu	Burnet-Bloodwort Root
30	Ce Bai Ye Tan	Leafy Twig of Arborvitae
30	Chun Gen Bai Pi	Ailanthus Bark
15	Duan Gui Ban	Land Tortoise Shell, Calcined
30	Bai Shao	White Peony Root

Description: This herbal formula is used for menorrhagia. It stops excessive bleeding and clears heat.

Analysis: Zhi Zi, Huang Bai, and Chao Huang Qin collectively clear heat from the liver. Sheng Di Huang and Mu Dan Pi cool the blood and improve its functioning. Di Yu, Ce Bai Ye Tan, and Chun Gen Bai Pi all address the main complaint and powerfully stop bleeding. Duan Gui Ban and Bai Shao nourish the blood and also benefit the liver.

Dosage and Method of Preparation: Prepare a decoction. Drink four ounces of Qing Re Zhi Beng Tang tea three times daily, as needed.

Bu Xue Tiao Jing Pian (Nourish Blood Adjust Period Tablet); also known as Bu Tiao Tablets—A Blood Tonic for Menstrual Disorders

Description: This patent formula nourishes the blood, inhibits bleeding, warms the uterus, and is useful for irregular bleeding and excessive uterine bleeding.

Dosage: This patent medicine comes in bottles of one hundred tablets, with complete instructions on dosage.

Kwei Be Wan (Restore Spleen Pill); also known as Gui Pi Wan, or Angelicae Longana Tea

Description: This patent formula is a classical prescription to nurture blood and is useful for abnormal uterine bleeding and heavy menstrual periods.

Dosage: It comes in bottles of two hundred pills, with complete instructions on dosage.

Menstruation, Disorders of, Painful—see Amenorrhea; Dysmenorrhea; Menorrhagia

Middle Ear Infection—see Ear, Disorders of; Otitis Media

Migraine—see Headache; Pain

Migraines are severe headaches lasting from several hours to several days, sometimes accompanied by visual disturbances, nausea, and/or projectile vomiting. There are two basic types of migraines: "common" and "classical." In common migraine headaches, the pain develops slowly, often increasing to throbbing, severe pain that is made worse by the slightest movement or noise. In classical migraine headaches (which are comparatively rare), the headache is preceded by a slowly expanding area of blindness surrounded by a sparkling edge that increases to involve up to one-half of the field of vision of each eye. This state normally lasts for approximately twenty minutes and is often followed by a severe, one-sided headache accompanied by nausea, vomiting, and sensitivity to light.

中草藥

There is no single cause for migraine headaches; a number of factors exist that singly or in combination can bring on an attack. These factors may be stress related, such as anger, anxiety, worry, excitement, depression, shock, overexertion, or changes of climate. Attacks can also be triggered by certain foods, such as chocolate, cheese and other dairy products, red wine, and citrus fruits. Somewhat less commonly, migraines have been brought on by bright light, glare, loud noise, intense or penetrating odors, and menstruation.

Chinese herbal formulas used for treating migraine headaches can be found in this chapter's entries for headache and pain.

Miscarriage

Miscarriage, clinically known as spontaneous abortion, occurs in 10 to 30 percent of all pregnancies. Most miscarriages occur in the first ten weeks of pregnancy. Symptoms include cramping and/or bleeding. Light bleeding during the early months of pregnancy occurs in approximately 50 percent of all pregnancies, and many of these pregnancies continue uneventfully to term. Heavy bleeding with cramping, on the other hand, is generally more serious since it may signal impending miscarriage.

Wide ranges of problems exist that can cause miscarriage. Many miscarriages occur because of developmental defects or abnormalities in the fetus. Less common causes are genetic defects such as cervical incompetence (the inability of the cervix to hold the pregnancy), a septate (subdivided) uterus, large fibroid tumors, and severe maternal infection or illness or exposure to toxins.

A woman who miscarries three or more times consecutively is called a habitual aborter. Habitual abortion can be caused by genetic or hormonal abnormalities, chronic infection, autoimmune deficiency disease, or uterine abnormalities.

It is a good idea to investigate any cramping or spotting that occurs after the first trimester. When immediate medical attention is given, a significant number of possible miscarriages can be treated, and in many cases miscarriage is avoided. The following Chinese herbal formulas can be useful for preventing a threatened abortion or in the aftermath of unpreventable abortion:

Bao Tai Zi Sheng Tang (Protect the Fetus and Aid Life Decoction)

Original Source: *Xian Xing Zhai Yi Xue Guang Bi Ji* (according to *Chinese Herbal Medicine Formulas and Strategies*)

Ingredients:

Quantity (Grams)	Chinese Herbs	English Translation
10	Ren Shen	Ginseng
10	Bai Zhu	Atractylodes Rhizome
4.5	Fu Ling	Tuckahoe Root
1.5	Zhi Gan Cao	Honey-Cooked Licorice Root
4.5	Shan Yao	Peony Root
4.5	Bai Bian Dou	Hyacinth Bean
4.5	Lian Zi	Lotus Seeds
4.5	Yi Yi Ren	Seeds of Job's Tears
1.2	Bai Dou Kou	White Cardamon Fruit
1.5	Huo Xiang	Patchouli
1.2	Ze Xie	Water Plantain Rhizome
3	Mai Ya	Barley Sprout
1.5	Jie Geng	Balloon Flower Root
6	Chen Pi	Ripe Tangerine Peel
6	Shan Zha	Hawthorne Fruit
.9	Huang Lian	Golden Thread Root
4.5	Qian Shi	Euralye Seed

Description: This herbal formula "nourishes the fetus" and is used for threatened miscarriage, as well as for morning sickness.

Analysis: Ren Shen increases the vital energy (Chi). Bai Zhu and Fu Ling resolve dampness and improve the appetite by strengthening the stomach and spleen. Shan Yao assists in this function. Bai Bian Dou, Yi Yi Ren, Lian Zi, Bai Dou Kou, and Huo Xiang all benefit the center, reducing nausea and arresting both vomiting and diarrhea. Ze Xie is diuretic; it reduces edema by promoting urination. Mai Ya, Chen Pi, and Shan Zha improve digestion. Jie Geng clears excess heat. Qian Shi stabilizes the kidneys. Huang Lian clears heat and stops uterine bleeding. Zhi Gan Cao harmonizes all of the other herbs in the formula.

Dosage and Method of Preparation: Prepare a decoction. Drink four ounces of Bao Tai Zi Sheng Tang tea three times daily, during the first trimester of pregnancy.

E Jiao Ai Tang (Ass-Hide Gelatin and Mugwort Decoction)

Original Source: *Jin Gui Yao Lue* (according to *Chinese Herbal Medicine Formulas and Strategies*)

Ingredients:

Quantity (Grams)	Chinese Herbs	English Translation
6	E Jiao	Donkey Skin Glue (Ass Hide)
9	Ai Ye	Mugwort Leaf
18	Sheng Di Huang	Chinese Foxglove Root, Raw
9	Dang Gui	Tangkuei
6	Chuan Xiong	Szechuan Lovage Root
12	Shao Yao	Peony Root
6	Gan Cao	Licorice Root

Description: This herbal formula nourishes the blood, stops bleeding, nourishes the fetus, and is useful for threatened miscarriage and uterine bleeding.

Analysis: E Jiao, the chief ingredient, nourishes the blood and stops uterine bleeding. Ai Ye warms the womb, pacifies the fetus, and stops uterine bleeding. Sheng Di Huang cools the blood. Dang Gui nourishes it and relieves pain. Chuan Xiong circulates the blood. Shao Yao assists in nourishing the blood and stopping the pain. Gan Cao harmonizes the other herbs in the formula.

Dosage and Method of Preparation: Make a decoction. Drink four ounces of E Jiao Ai Tang tea three times daily, as needed.

An Tai Wan (Soothe Embryo Pills); also known as Bao Tia Wan, Shi San Tai Bao Wan, or Bao Chan Wu Yu Wan

Description: This patent medicine relaxes the muscles and calms the fetus; it is used to help prevent miscarriage or premature delivery by stopping bleeding from the uterus.

Dosage: It comes in bottles of one hundred pills, with complete instructions on dosage.

Bu Zhong Yi Qi Wan (Tonify Center to Invigorate Qi Pills); also known as Central Qi Pills, or Bu Zhong Yi Chi Wan

Description: This patent formula is useful for uterine bleeding as seen in habitual miscarriage.

Dosage: It comes in bottles of one hundred pills, with complete instructions on dosage.

Morning Sickness (see also Nausea; Pregnancy)

The nausea and vomiting experienced by pregnant women result from increased hormone production. Although these symptoms can occur at any time, they are most often experienced in the morning upon waking.

Normally only lasting for the first trimester of pregnancy, in rare cases morning sickness can become severe and prolonged, causing the risk of dehydration, nutritional deficiency, and weight loss. In such cases medical attention should be sought to replace lost fluids and rule out any serious underlying disorders.

Traditional Chinese medicine offers centuries-old dietary advice that is simple but effective: avoid all cold foods and consume only warm foods, along with infused ginger tea to alleviate nausea and vomiting. The following herbal formulas should also prove useful:

Sheng Jiang Tang (Raw Ginger Tea)

Ingredient:

Quantity (Grams)	Chinese Herb	English Translation
9	Sheng Jiang	Fresh Ginger Root

Description: An infusion of this herb settles the stomach and relieves nausea and vomiting.

Analysis: Sheng Jiang is used alone to warm the stomach and relieve vomiting.

中草藥

Dosage and Method of Preparation: Prepare an infusion by placing sliced fresh ginger root (Sheng Jiang) in a coffee cup; fill the cup with boiling water, cover the cup, and allow the tea to steep for fifteen minutes. Strain off herb, and drink the tea. Drink eight ounces of Sheng Jiang Tang tea, as needed.

Kang Ning Wan (Curing Pill); also known as Pill Curing

Description: This patent medicine helps with the symptoms of morning sickness, including nausea and vomiting. It is safe in pregnancy and for children.

Dosage: It comes in boxes containing ten vials per box, with complete instructions on dosage.

Shen Ling Bai Zhu Pian (Codonopsis Poria Atractylodes Formula); also known as Shenling Baizhupian

Description: This patent formula is used during pregnancy for morning sickness; it alleviates nausea and vomiting. Excellent for children as well.

Dosage: It comes in bottles of 150 pills, with complete instructions on dosage.

Mosquito Bites—see Insect Bites; Malaria

Motion Sickness (see also Headache; Nausea; Stomachache)

Motion sickness is brought on by road, sea, or air travel. In its mild form it causes a feeling of uneasiness, headache, and slight abdominal discomfort. Severe cases include symptoms of distress, sweating, lightheadedness, nausea, and vomiting.

Recommendations for avoiding motion sickness are to avoid eating a large meal before traveling (a full stomach will only exacerbate the condition) and to get as much fresh air as possible by opening windows during the trip (good ventilation is an important preventive measure). The following herbal formulas should be taken in advance of travel (one-half to one full hour before departure time) or during the trip if an attack occurs:

Ren Dan Yang Cheng Brand (Ren Dan People's Powder); also known as Benevolence Pills

Description: This patent formula is useful for treating motion sickness with dizziness, vomiting, and nausea.

Dosage: It comes in a package containing 320 small silver pills, with complete instructions on dosage.

Kang Ning Wan (Curing Pill); also known as Pill Curing

Description: This patent medicine relieves headache, abates nausea, stops vomiting, and is effective for preventing motion sickness.

Dosage: It comes in boxes containing ten vials per box, with complete instructions on dosage.

Mumps

Mumps is a viral illness causing inflammation and swelling of the parotid (salivary) glands that usually occurs during childhood. Although serious complications are uncommon, mumps can be very uncomfortable when contracted by teenage boys and grown men. Unlike in juvenile sufferers, who experience swollen parotid glands, mumps in teenage or adult males causes inflammation and swelling in one or both testes.

Mumps, which are highly infectious, are spread in airborne droplets. Normally a two- or three-week period passes between infection and the appearance of symptoms. Typical symptoms are fever, headache, difficulty swallowing, and swollen salivary glands. An occasional complication is meningitis; even more rarely, mumps can lead to sterility in older males.

Normally, a vaccination is administered to young children in their second year; once vaccinated or infected, a person is immune from the disease for life. Traditional Chinese medicine uses the following herbal formulas to treat the symptoms of mumps:

Gan Lu Xiao Du Dan (Sweet Dew Special Formula to Eliminate Toxin)

Original Source: *Wen Re Jing Wei* (according to *Chinese Herbal Medicine Formulas and Strategies*)

Ingredients:

Quantity (Grams)	Chinese Herbs	English Translation
15	Lian Qiao	Forsythia Fruit
15	Huang Qin	Baical Skullcap Root
9	Bo He	Peppermint
12	She Gan	Arrow Shaft Rhizome
9	Chuan Bei Mu	Fritillaria Bulb
21	Hua Shi	Talcum, Mineral
12	Mu Tong	Wood with Holes
30	Yin Chen Hao	Capillaris Herb
12	Huo Xiang	Patchouli
6	Shi Chang Pu	Sweet Flag Rhizome
12	Bai Dou Kou	White Cardamon Fruit

Description: This herbal formula is used to treat symptoms of mumps, including fever, sore throat, swollen glands, and inflammation of tonsils.

Analysis: This formula contains eleven herbs, which are divided into three groups. The first group, Lian Qiao, Huang Qin, and Bo He, clears heat from the upper body, thus reducing fever; She Gan and Chuan Bei Mu drain heat from the lungs, resolving phlegm and benefiting the throat. The second group, Hua Shi, Mu Tong, and Yin Chen Hao, releases the heat from the lower body. The last group, Huo Xiang, Shi Chang Pu, and Bai Dou Kou, benefits the spleen and eliminates infection.

Dosage and Method of Preparation: Prepare a decoction. Drink four ounces of Gan Lu Xiao Du Dan tea three times daily, as needed.

Hou Yan Wan (Larynx Inflammation Pills); also known as Laryngitis Pills

Description: This patent formula resolves inflammation, reduces fever, relieves sore throat, and is useful for treatment of mumps and tonsillitis.

Dosage: It comes in a box of three vials, ten pills per vial, with complete instructions on dosage.

Liu Shen Wan (Six-Spirit Pill); also known as Lu Shen Wan

Description: This patent formula is used for mumps, fever, infections, sore throat, and acute tonsillitis.

Dosage: It comes in bottles of ten, thirty, or one hundred pills, with complete instructions on dosage.

Myocardial Infarction

The heart is considered by both Western and traditional Chinese medicine to be the chief organ in the body. All other bodily systems depend on it for delivery of the most precious vital fluid: blood. When it fails to function, death is usually immediate. Myocardial infarction, the clinical term for heart attack, is the single most common cause of death in developed countries. Each year in the United States alone, approximately one million people suffer from heart attacks that all too often are fatal.

The characteristic symptoms of heart attack are sudden pain in the center of the chest, shortness of breath, restlessness, cold clammy skin, nausea or vomiting, pain or numbness radiating down the left arm, or a sudden loss of consciousness. Men are more likely to suffer heart attacks than women; smokers are more likely than nonsmokers; and the children of someone who died of a heart attack are more likely also to die from one. Other risk factors include increased age, unhealthy diet, stress, obesity, and disorders such as hypertension (high blood pressure), diabetes, and hyperlipidemia (excessive fat in the blood).

Note: If someone is suspected of having a heart attack, a physician or ambulance should be summoned immediately! Most people who die of a myocardial infarction do so within the first few hours of the attack, due to what is called ventricular fibrillation, which is an arrhythmia (irregular heartbeat) that seriously interferes with the heart's pumping action.

I wish to emphasize that no matter your personal preference for so-called alternative or conventional Western medicine, one of the best preventive health practices you can engage in is to learn how to administer CPR (cardiopulmonary resuscitation).

The following Chinese herbal formulas are offered only as a possible adjunct to typical Western medical treatment for myocardial infarction:

Shen Fu Tang (Ginseng and Prepared Aconite Decoction)

Original Source: *Jiao Zhu Fu Ren Liang Fang* (according to *Chinese Herbal Medicine Formulas and Strategies*)

Ingredients:

Quantity (Grams)	Chinese Herbs	English Translation
12	Ren Shen	Ginseng
9	Fu Zi	Accessory Root of Szechuan Aconite
9	Long Gu	Dragons Bones
9	Mu Li	Oyster Shell
9	Bai Shao	White Peony Root
6	Zhi Gan Cao	Honey-Cooked Licorice Root

Description: This herbal formula is useful in aiding recovery from cardiac failure, myocardial infarction, or cardiogenic shock, with symptoms of cold extremities, sweating, and shortness of breath.

Analysis: This is normally a two-herb formula that has been augmented with four additional herbs. Ren Shen, one of the two main ingredients, tonifies or strengthens the vital energy (Chi) and is useful for treating shallow respiration, shortness of breath, and cold limbs. Fu Zi, the second main ingredient, is recommended for cold extremities and for an imperceptible pulse with severe sweating. Long Gu aids palpitations and sweating. Mu Li also treats palpitations. Bai Shao nourishes the blood and relieves pain. Zhi Gan Cao harmonizes the herbs in the formula.

中
草
藥

Dosage and Method of Preparation: Prepare a decoction. Drink four ounces of Shen Fu Tang tea three times daily, as needed.

Kuan Hsin Su Ho Wan (Cardiovascular Styrax Pills); also known as Guan Xin Su Ho Capsules, or Guan Xin Su He Wan

Description: This patent formula is a recent treatment for blood stagnation in the heart; it is useful for prevention of as well as following acute myocardial infarction.

Caution: This formula is prohibited for use during pregnancy.

Dosage: It comes in bottles of thirty pills, with complete instructions on dosage.

Nasal Congestion (see also Allergies; Colds and Flu; Sinusitis)

Nasal congestion is partial blockage of the nasal passage caused by inflammation of the mucus membrane, usually brought on by infection that has developed as the result of a cold or an allergic reaction. Traditional Chinese medicine generally frowns on Western medicine's use of nasal sprays for treating nasal congestion, considering them of doubtful value. Instead, treatment is directed at resolving the underlying cause—either a cold or mucus—and eliminating infection.

Xiao Qing Long Tang (Minor Blue Green Dragon Decoction)

Original Source: *Shang Han Lun* (according to *Chinese Herbal Medicine Formulas and Strategies*)

Ingredients:

Quantity (Grams)	Chinese Herbs	English Translation
9	Ma Huang★	Yellow Hemp
9	Gui Zhi	Saigon Cinnamon Twig
9	Sheng Jiang	Fresh Ginger Root
9	Xi Xin	Chinese Wild Ginger Plant

9	Wu Wei Zi	Schizandra Fruit
9	Chi Shao	Red Peony Root
9	Ban Xia	Half Summer
9	Zhi Gan Cao	Honey-Cooked Licorice Root
9	Fang Feng	Guard Against the Wind Root
9	Jing Jie	Schizonepeta Stem/Bud

*Persons with high blood pressure should not use Ma Huang; instead substitute 9 grams of Bai Qian (White Before Rhizome).

Description: This herbal formula provides relief from pronounced nasal congestion and nasal headache.

Analysis: Ma Huang and Gui Zhi open the pores and cause sweating; they also relieve wheezing and benefit the lungs. Sheng Jiang and Xi Xin warm the interior and prevent chills while transforming congestive fluids. Wu Wei Zi and Chi Shao are added to benefit the lungs and nourish the blood. Ban Xia calms the stomach; Fang Feng and Jing Jie relieve head and body ache and guard against chills. Zhi Gan Cao harmonizes the herbs in this formula.

Dosage and Method of Preparation: Prepare a decoction. Drink four ounces of Xiao Qing Long Tang tea three times daily, as needed.

Cang Er Zi Tang (Xanthium Decoction)

Original Source: *Ji Sheng Fang* (according to *Chinese Herbal Medicine Formulas and Strategies*)

Ingredients:

Quantity (Grams)	Chinese Herbs	English Translation
9	Cang Er Zi	Xanthium Fruit
9	Bai Zhi	Angelica Dahuricae Root
6	Bo He*	Peppermint
9	Jin Yin Hua	Honeysuckle Flower
6	Xin Yi Hua	Magnolia Flower

*See special instructions for preparation below.

Description: This herbal formula relieves frontal headache, nasal discharge, nasal obstruction, and dizziness.

Analysis: Cang Er Zi, the chief herb, and Xin Yi Hua unblock nasal passages and arrest nasal discharge. Bai Zhi resolves dampness, while Bo He clears the eyes and head. Jin Yin Hua treats infection.

Dosage and Method of Preparation: Make a decoction. Bo He should not be added to the decoction until the last five minutes of cooking time. Overcooking Bo He will reduce its effectiveness. Drink four ounces of Cang Er Zi Tang tea three times daily, as needed.

Chuan Xiong Cha Tiao Wan (Ligusticum Tea Adjust Pills); also known as Chuan Qiong Cha Tiao Wan

Description: This patent formula is useful for headache due to nasal congestion, sinusitis, and rhinitis.

Note: This formula should be taken with strong green tea to enhance its effects.

Dosage: It comes in bottles of two hundred pills, with complete instructions on dosage.

Bi Yuan Wan (Nasal Sinusitis Pills)

Description: This patent formula opens nasal passages, relieves stuffy nose, and is useful for removing nasal polyps and blood stasis (clogged blood in the nasal passages).

Dosage: It comes in bottles of one hundred pills, with complete instructions on dosage.

Nasal Obstruction—see Nasal Congestion

Nasal obstruction on one or both sides of the nasal passage that interferes with breathing is usually caused by inflammation, severe deviation of the septum, polyps, hematoma (blood clots), or in rare instances a malignant tumor. In children, enlargement of the adenoids is a common cause for nasal obstruction. Many of the herbal formulas helpful for nasal congestion can be used for nasal obstruction, unless the case involves a deviated septum. In such cases surgery is usually required.

Nausea (see also Morning Sickness; Motion Sickness)

Nausea is the sensation of needing to vomit. Although nausea may occur independently of vomiting and vice versa, they usually happen concurrently and result from the same cause. Traditionally, Chinese herbal formulas for treating nausea include herbs that address the underlying cause as well as herbs for resolving the nausea and vomiting that are merely symptoms. An example is food poisoning, whose treatment principle is directed at eliminating the bacterial infection that is the underlying cause; in addition, a secondary effort in the remedy aims to resolve the accompanying symptoms of nausea and diarrhea.

General nausea remedies follow:

Ji Zhong Shui (Benefit Many Problems Liquid); also known as Liu Shen Shui, or Chi Chung Shui

Description: This patent formula harmonizes the center (settles the stomach). It is an emergency remedy for the stomach that is recommended for travelers to treat a variety of acute stomach aliments characterized by cramping, nausea, vomiting, and diarrhea.

Caution: This formula is prohibited for use during pregnancy.

Dosage: It comes in boxes of twelve vials, compete with instructions on dosage.

Ping Wei Pian (Peaceful Stomach Tablets); also known as Tabellae Ping Wei

Description: This patent formula benefits the stomach (eliminates stomachaches); it soothes gastric imbalance, dyspepsia, abdominal cramping, nausea, vomiting, and diarrhea.

Dosage: It comes in bottles of forty-eight tablets, with complete instructions on dosage.

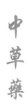

Shen Chu Cha (Fermented Leaven Tea); also known as Shen Qu Cha

Description: This patent formula harmonizes the center (settles the stomach) and calms stomach heat. It contains fourteen herbs for resolving digestive problems with symptoms including belching, nausea, bloating, vomiting, constipation, or diarrhea.

Dosage: It comes in a box of eighteen small blocks, with complete instructions on dosage.

Huo Hsiang Cheng Chi Pian (Pogostemon Normalize Chi Pills); also known as Huo Xiang Zheng Qi Pian, or Lophanthus Antifebrile Pills

Description: This patent formula is valuable for resolving nausea with vomiting, diarrhea, and stomach flu with headache; it is traditionally used for cholera.

Dosage: It comes in bottles of one hundred pills, with complete instructions on dosage.

Po Chi Pills (Protect and Benefit Pills); also known as Bao Ji Wan, Zhong Guo Bao Ji Wan, or China Po Chi Pills

Description: This patent formula is useful for a variety of stomach complaints, such as stomach flu, indigestion, motion sickness, alcohol hangover characterized by nausea, vomiting, diarrhea, stomach cramps.

Dosage: It comes in boxes of ten vials, with complete instructions on dosage.

Nicotine Addiction—see Addiction to Nicotine

Nosebleed

Anosebleed is a loss of blood from the mucus membrane that lines the nose. The occurrence is fairly common in childhood, less frequent in healthy young adults, but becomes increasingly more common and more serious in old age. The most common causes are a blow to the nose, fragile blood vessels, colds, or other sinus infections. A recurring bloody nose is usually a sign of hypertension (high blood pressure), a bleeding disorder such as leukemia or hemophilia, or a tumor of the nose or sinuses.

Most nosebleeds can be controlled by simple first aid measures and/or the use of Chinese herbs that are famous for their ability to stop bleeding. Both are listed below. If a bloody nose persists for more than thirty minutes, seek immediate medical help.

Zi Su Ye (Perilla Leaf)

The patient should lean forward with mouth open; stuff the bleeding nostril with the Chinese herb Zi Su Ye, a large leafy herb whose raw form will instantly check bleeding. Insert as much of the leaf as the nostril will hold; after the leaf has been inserted, pinch and hold the nose for ten to fifteen minutes. Instruct the patient to breathe through the mouth until the bleeding stops.

If Zi Su Ye is not available, use gauze; it is less effective but will get the job done.

Analysis: Zi Su Ye is mainly used to correct digestive disturbances; it is also effective in stopping nosebleeds.

Yu Nan Bai Yao (Yunnan Providence White Medicine); also known as Yunnan Paiyao

Description: This patent formula is used to stop bleeding. To arrest a nosebleed, break open two capsules, pour the loose powder onto a cotton swab, and apply directly to the wound. Alternatively, the powder can be inhaled or snuffed into the bleeding nostril. Immediately, apply direct pressure (pinch the nose and hold the pressure) for ten to fifteen minutes.

Caution: This formula is prohibited for use by pregnant women.

Dosage: It comes in boxes of sixteen capsules, with complete instructions on dosage.

Obesity

Aperson is considered obese when he or she weighs 20 percent or more than the maximum desirable weight for his or her height and build. Obesity occurs when the net energy intake exceeds the net energy expenditure—in other words, when more calories are taken in then are being used to fuel the body. It is not always the case that obese people eat more than thin people eat. A person's energy requirements are determined by his or her basal metabolic rate (the amount of energy needed to maintain vital body functions at rest) and level of physical activity. Obese people may have an extremely low basal metabolic rate, or they may require fewer calories because they are less physically active.

Research has shown that children of obese parents are ten times more likely to be obese than children of parents with normal weight—which supports the theory that genetic factors play a role in the development of obesity. In only a minority of cases, hormonal imbalances are associated with obesity.

Possible complications of obesity include hypertension, stroke, coronary heart disease, and adult-onset diabetes. Obesity in men is associated with an increased risk of cancers of the colon, rectum, and prostate; obesity in women shows a progressive increase in the risk of cancers of the breast, uterus, and cervix.

Osteoarthritis is aggravated by obesity. Extra weight on the hips, knees, and back places undue strain on the joints. Although weight loss does not reverse the disease, it does help relieve stress and pain.

An obese person should assume a diet that provides five hundred to one thousand fewer calories per day than his or her energy requirements. The energy deficit is met by using some of the excess stored body fat. Such a reduction will typically yield an average weight loss of one to two pounds per week. Regular exercise (especially aerobic exercise) increases weight loss by burning even more calories and by increasing the metabolic rate.

Anyone who follows a basic Chinese diet, which is based on five thousand years of culinary experience, suffers few problems with obesity. Recent scientific research in Western dietetics has confirmed what the Chinese have known for thousands of years: the basic Chinese diet provides adequate nutrition while minimizing the intake of fat, which is a major contributor to obesity. The Chinese diet contains practically no dairy products (including no cheese, butter, and cream) and is based on caloric proportions as follows: 10 percent of calories from meat and fish, 30 percent from vegetables and fruits, 40 percent from grains and cereals, and 20 percent from miscellaneous seasonings (honey, etc.).

Losing weight requires a willingness to make lifestyle changes that include regular exercise and dietary modifications. The following Chinese herbal formulas can also be useful in your effort:

Fang Feng Tong Sheng Tang (Ledebouriella Powder That Sagely Unblocks)

Original Source: *Huang Di Su Wen Xuan Ming Lun Fang* (according to *Chinese Herbal Medicine Formulas and Strategies*)
Ingredients:

Quantity (Grams)	Chinese Herbs	English Translation
1.5	Fang Feng	Guard Against the Wind Root
1.5	Ma Huang★	Yellow Hemp Root
1.5	Jiu Da Huang	Wine-Fried Rhubarb Rhizome
1.5	Mang Xiao	Mirabilite
1.5	Jing Jie	Schizonepeta Stem/Bud
1.5	Bo He★★	Peppermint
1.5	Zhi Zi	Gardenia Fruit
9	Hua Shi	Talcum, Mineral
3	Shi Gao	Gypsum, Mineral
3	Jie Geng	Balloon Flower Root
1.5	Chuan Xiong	Szechuan Lovage Root
1.5	Dang Gui	Tangkuei
1.5	Bai Shao	White Peony Root
1.5	Bai Zhi	Angelica Dahuricae Root
6	Gan Cao	Licorice Root

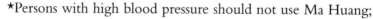
★Persons with high blood pressure should not use Ma Huang;

instead substitute 1.5 grams of Bai Qian (White Before Rhizome).

★★See special instructions for preparation below.

Description: This traditional herbal formula induces sweating and reduces edema and water accumulation in the body. It also gently purges the body, keeping the bowels open so that food is quickly metabolized and purged. This formula can be used long-term while fighting obesity.

Analysis: Fang Feng and Ma Huang open the pores and cause sweating to relieve water retention. Jiu Da Huang and Mang Xiao promote bowel movement, while Jing Jie, Bo He, Zhi Zi, and Hua Shi drain heat through the urine. Shi Gao and Jie Geng are included in the formula to clear heat from the organs. Chuan Xiong, Dang Gui, and Bai Shao all nourish the blood. Bai Zhi benefits the spleen, which improves digestion and metabolism of food. Gan Cao protects the stomach (because of the large number of herbs in this formula).

Dosage and Method of Preparation: Prepare a decoction. Bo He should not be added to the decoction until the last five minutes of cooking time. Overcooking Bo He will reduce its effectiveness. Drink four ounces of Fang Feng Tong Sheng Tang three times daily, as needed.

Bao Jian Mei Jian Fei Cha (Bojenmi Chinese Tea)

Description: This patent formula reduces fat, expels excess water, maximizes nutrient absorption, and is useful for weight reduction.

Dosage: It comes in cans of one hundred grams of tea or boxes of tea bags, with complete instructions on dosage.

Astra 18-Diet Fuel

Description: This patent formula is a traditional remedy for obesity and eating disorders.

Note: Combine use of this formula with #274 Astra Diet Tea (below).

Dosage: It comes in bottles of sixty or ninety tablets of 500 mg each, with complete instructions on dosage.

274 Astra Diet Tea

Description: This patent formula regulates the functions of the stomach, suppresses appetite, and invigorates energy levels.

Note: Combine use of this formula with Astra 18-Diet Fuel.

Dosage: It comes in boxes of sixteen tea bags, with complete instructions on dosage.

Osteoarthritis—see Arthritis

Otitis Media (see also Ear, Disorders of)

Otitis media, or inner-ear infection, is inflammation of the cavity between the eardrum and the inner ear. It normally occurs as a result of an upper respiratory tract infection (such as a cold) that extends upward into the Eustachian tube, the passage connecting the back of the nose to the middle ear. The tube may become blocked by the inflammation or by enlarged adenoids, which are often associated with infections of the nose and throat. As a result, fluid and pus produced by the inflammation and by bacterial infection fail to drain through the tube and thus accumulate in the middle ear. Children are particularly susceptible to otitis media, probably because of the short length of their Eustachian tubes. Approximately one in six children suffer from the acute form in the first year of life, and about one in ten between ages two and eight. Acute otitis media is marked by sudden severe earache, a feeling of fullness in the ear, deafness, tinnitus (ringing in the ear), and fever.

In chronic otitis media, pus constantly exudes from a perforation in the eardrum; some degree of deafness also results. Complications include otitis externia (inflammation of the outer ear) and damage to the bones in the middle ear, which can cause total deafness; in rare cases the infection spreads inward from the ear, causing mastoiditis or a brain abscess.

Traditional Chinese medicine uses antibiotic herbs to eliminate pus and infection and anti-inflammatory herbs to resolve inflammation and the resulting fever.

Pu Ji Xiao Du Yin (Universal Benefit Decoction to Eliminate Toxin)

Original Source: *Wei Sheng Bao Jian* (according to *Chinese Herbal Medicine Formulas and Strategies*)

Ingredients:

Quantity (Grams)	Chinese Herbs	English Translation
15	Jiu Chao Huang Qin	Wine-Fried Baical Skullcap Root
15	Jiu Chao Huang Lian	Wine-Fried Coptis Root
3	Niu Bang Zi	Great Burdock Fruit
3	Lian Qiao	Forsythia Fruit
3	Bo He★	Peppermint
3	Jiang Can	Dead Body of Sick Silkworm
6	Xuan Shen	Ningpo Figwort
3	Ma Bo	Puffball Fruit
3	Ban Lan Gen	Woad Root
6	Jie Geng	Balloon Flower Root
6	Gan Cao	Licorice Root
6	Chen Pi	Ripe Tangerine Peel
6	Chai Hu	Bupleurum Hare's Ear Root
1.5	Sheng Ma	Black Cohosh Rhizome

★See special instructions for preparation below.

Description: This herbal formula is used to eliminate infection and swelling in the ear; it reduces fever and is used for infection of the ear, throat, and sinuses.

Analysis: Jiu Chao Huang Qin and Jiu Chao Huang Lian are used together to clear toxic heat (infection) from the upper part of the body. Niu Bang Zi, Lian Qiao, Bo He, and Jiang Can disperse cold and infection in the face and head. Xuan Shen, Ma Bo, Ban Lan Gen, Jie Geng, and Gan Cao clear heat and infection in the throat and relieve toxic fire. Chen Pi regulates the flow of vital energy (Chi) and blood–dispersing pathogenic influences. Chai Hu and Sheng Ma guide the other ingredients to the head and upper body.

Dosage and Method of Preparation: Prepare a decoction. Bo He should not be added to the decoction until the last five minutes of cooking time. Overcooking Bo He will reduce its effectiveness. Drink four ounces of Pu Ji Xiao Du Yin tea three times daily, or as needed.

Niu Huang Jie Du Pian (Cow Gallstone Dispel Toxin); also known as Niu Huang Chieh Tu Pien, or Bezoar Antipyretic Pills

Description: This patent formula is useful for ear infections with fever and inflammation with or without pus; it is useful for otitis media, tonsillitis, and sinusitis.

Dosage: It comes in bottles of twenty tablets, with complete instructions on dosage.

Shuang Liao Hou Feng San (Double Ingredient Sore Throat Disease Powder); also known as Superior Sore Throat Powder Spray

Description: This patent formula reduces fever, clears infection, and eliminates pus. It is useful for ear, throat, and sinus infections.

Dosage: It comes in 2.2-gram bottles of powder spray. Wash infected area with hydrogen peroxide and spray as directed.

Ovarian Cyst

Ovarian cysts are abnormal fluid-filled swellings (sacs) on the ovary. Approximately 95 percent of ovarian cysts are benign and often disappear without treatment. There are three types of ovarian cysts. The most common, follicular cysts, result when the egg-producing follicle of the ovary enlarges and fills with fluid. Dermoid cysts are cysts containing embryonic elements of all three germ layers including hair and teeth. Malignant cysts are more commonly referred to as ovarian cancer. Some ovarian cysts cause no symptoms; others can cause abdominal discomfort, pain during intercourse, or menstrual irregularities including amenorrhea (lack of menstruation), menorrhagia (heavy periods), or dysmenorrhea (painful periods). See also the specific entries for these conditions.

Traditional Chinese medical treatment is directed at moving the stagnation (fluid in the sacs) and resolving the cyst. Herbal diuretics (herbs that cause urination) as well as herbs for moving the bowels are also an important part of treatment. This is because of the anatomical proximity of the bowels and bladder to the ovaries; when bowels and bladder remain full, they press against the cyst, increasing the lower abdominal pain and discomfort.

The following two formulas are well known for resolving and/or removing ovarian cysts:

Gui Zhi Fu Ling Tang (Cinnamon Twig and Poria Decoction)

Original Source: *Jin Gui Yao Lue* (according to *Chinese Herbal Medicine Formulas and Strategies*)

Ingredients:

Quantity (Grams)	Chinese Herbs	English Translation
12	Gui Zhi	Saigon Cinnamon Twig
12	Fu Ling	Tuckahoe (Poria) Root
15	Chi Shao Yao	Red Peony Root
12	Mu Dan Pi	Tree Peony Root, Bark of
12	Tao Ren	Peach Kernel

Description: This herbal formula is useful for ovarian cysts. It invigorates the blood, moves stagnation of the blood, reduces fixed lower abdominal masses, and is also used for uterine fibroids.

Caution: This formula is prohibited for use during pregnancy.

Analysis: Gui Zhi and Fu Ling, the chief herbs, unblock the blood vessels and eliminate clotting and cysts by improving circulation. Chi Shao Yao, Mu Dan Pi, and Tao Ren promote blood circulation and reduce fixed abdominal masses.

Dosage and Method of Preparation: Make a decoction. Drink four ounces of Gui Zhi Fu Ling Tang tea three times daily, as needed.

Tao He Cheng Qi Tang (Peach Pit Decoction to Order the Chi)

Original Source: *Shuan Han Lun* (according to *Chinese Herbal Medicine Formulas and Strategies*)

Ingredients:

Quantity (Grams)	Chinese Herbs	English Translation
15	Tao Ren	Peach Kernel
12	Da Huang	Rhubarb Root

6	Gui Zhi	Saigon Cinnamon Twig
6	Mang Xiao★	Mirabilite
9	Hong Hua	Safflower Flowers
12	Chi Shao Yao	Red Peony Root
9	Dang Gui	Tangkuei
6	Zhi Gan Cao	Honey-Cooked Licorice Root

★See special instructions for preparation below.

Description: This herbal formula is used to move blood stasis; it resolves lower abdominal masses and eliminates lower abdominal pain while it lubricates and moves the bowels. It is useful for more difficult ovarian cysts and fibroid tumors. This formula can be used for long periods of time.

Analysis: Tao Ren, Hong Hua, and Chi Shao Yao dissolve blood clots and eliminate pathogenic heat. Gui Zhi unblocks blood vessels, which improves circulation. Dang Gui nourishes blood. Da Huang and Mang Xiao promote bowel movement, which reduces pain. Zhi Gan Cao harmonizes the other herbs in the formula and improves the taste.

Dosage and Method of Preparation: Make a decoction. Do not cook the Mang Xiao with the other herbs in this formula. Add it after the decoction has finished cooking and the other herbs have been strained off. At this point, gently stir in Mang Xiao until it is dissolved. It is not necessary to re-strain the decoction. Drink four ounces of Tao He Cheng Qi Tang tea twice daily, as needed.

Overweight—see Obesity

Pain

Among the many functions of the nervous system, one of the most important is the transmission of the sensation of pain. Pain acts as the body's alarm system, proclaiming malfunction or damage caused by trauma or the presence of disease. Although unpleasant, pain operates to our advantage; without it, we would have no knowledge of harmful conditions, which would go untreated and grow progressively worse.

Many adjectives are used to describe different types of pain. Common descriptive terms include throbbing, penetrating, gnawing, aching, burning, gripping, sharp, and shooting. These descriptions are extremely important because the extent to which a patient is able to accurately describe his or her pain can be a valuable clue to a doctor in making a diagnosis. Of course, it is not unreasonable for a person to seek some form of relief from pain, but it is imperative that pain not be treated without attempting to diagnose or determine the underlying cause.

Chinese medicine uses the following formula for relief of pain caused by a variety of ailments; for more specific relief, refer to the entry that deals with the particular underlying ailment:

Yan Hu Suo Zhi Tong Pian (Yan Hu Extract, Stop Pain Tablets); also known as Corydalis Yanhusus-Analgesic Tablets, or Yan Hu Su Zhi Tong Pian

Description: This patent formula can be used for a wide variety of pain, including stomachache, headache, toothache, and joint inflammation. This formula can be combined with other herbal formulas.

Dosage: It comes in bottles of twenty-four pills, with complete instructions on dosage.

Pancreas, Disorders of: Infection, Tumor (see also Diabetes; Hypoglycemia)

The pancreas is located in back of the abdomen near the spleen (with which it is paired in traditional Chinese medicine). The pancreas has two important functions. The first is the secretion of digestive enzymes that break down carbohydrates, fats, proteins, and acids; the second is secretion of the hormones insulin and glucagon, which regulate the level of glucose (sugar) in the blood.

Disorders of the pancreas include acute pancreatitis, which is an infection often caused by the mumps virus or occasionally by the Coxsackie virus. Pancreatitis can be a contributing factor in the development of diabetes. Trauma or injury to the pancreas, most often caused by a blow to the abdomen, can also cause acute pancreatitis. Other causes of pancreatic infection are excessive alcohol intake and the overuse of certain drugs, including sulfur, estrogen, thiazide, and corticosteroid.

Although not a frequent cause of pancreatitis, gallstones occasionally block the exit of the pancreatic duct, leading to inflammation of the pancreas. Tumors or pancreatic cancer, although very uncommon compared to the number of cases of pancreatitis, is nevertheless one of the most common cancers in the United States. Characterized by symptoms such as upper abdominal pain, loss of appetite, nausea, weight loss, vomiting, and fatigue, it is difficult to diagnose and in many cases has spread extensively by the time it is detected.

Traditional Chinese medicine uses the following herbal formulas to treat the pancreas:

Da Chai Hu Tang (Major Bupleurum Decoction)

Original Source: *Shang Han Lun* (according to *Chinese Herbal Medicine Formulas and Strategies*)

Ingredients:

Quantity (Grams)	Chinese Herbs	English Translation
24	Chai Hu	Bupleurum Hare's Ear Root
9	Huang Qin	Baical Skullcap Root
9	Zhi Shi	Green Bitter Orange Fruit
6	Da Huang	Rhubarb Root
9	Bai Shao	White Peony Root
24	Ban Xia	Half Summer
15	Sheng Jiang	Fresh Ginger Root
12 pieces	Da Zao	Jujube Fruit

Description: This herbal formula is used for pain in the upper abdomen, nausea, vomiting, diarrhea, and is useful for treating pancreatitis.

Analysis: When the chief ingredient, Chai Hu, is combined with Huang Qin, its ability to clear heat from the liver and gallbladder is strengthened. Zhi Shi moves the vital energy (Chi), and Da Huang moves the bowels, which indirectly stimulates the flow of bile. Bai Shao nourishes the blood and reduces abdominal spasms. Ban Xia calms the stomach. Sheng Jiang and Da Zao also benefit the stomach by improving digestion.

Dosage and Method of Preparation: Make a decoction. Drink four ounces of Da Chai Hu Tang tea three times daily, as needed.

Qing Yi Tang (Clear the Pancreas Decoction)

Original Source: *Zhong Xi Yi Jie He Zhi Liao Ji Fu Zheng* (according to *Chinese Herbal Medicine Formulas and Strategies*)

Ingredients:

Quantity (Grams)	Chinese Herbs	English Translation
15	Chai Hu	Bupleurum Hare's Ear Root
9	Huang Qin	Baical Skullcap Root
9	Huang Lian	Golden Thread Root
15	Bai Shao	White Peony Root
9	Yan Hu Sou	Corydalis Rhizome
15	Da Huang	Rhubarb Root
9	Mu Xiang★	Costus Root
9	Mang Xiao★	Mirabilite

★See special instructions for preparation below.

Description: This is one of the best-known formulas in traditional Chinese medicine for treating acute and chronic pancreatitis. This herbal formula clears inflammation from the pancreas, reduces fever, and alleviates pain.

Analysis: Chai Hu benefits the liver, clears heat, reduces pain, and eliminates vomiting. Huang Qin and Huang Lian disperse heat and resolve turbidity (infection) while arresting diarrhea. Bai Shao and Yan Hu Sou are used together for treating pain. Mu Xiang promotes the movement of vital energy (Chi) and improves the function of the stomach and the spleen, thus benefiting digestion. Da Huang and Mang Xiao promote bowel movement.

Dosage and Method of Preparation: Make a decoction. (1) Add Mu Xiang to the rest of the herbs during the last ten minutes of cooking time. (2) Do not cook Mang Xiao with the other herbs in this formula. Add this herb after the decoction has finished cooking and the other herbs have been strained off. At this point gently stir in Mang Xiao until the herb has dissolved. It will not be necessary to re-strain the decoction. Drink four ounces of Qing Yi Tang tea three times daily, as needed.

Paralysis

Paralysis is a condition of loss of movement in a body part with accompanying loss of sensation. Paralysis may be temporary or permanent. Perhaps one of the most complex conditions in all of medicine, paralysis results from strokes or diseases of the nervous system where there is impairment of motor or sensory nerves. Traditional Chinese medicine's approach to treatment normally involves acupuncture, herbal therapy, massage, electrostimulation, and remedial exercises. These therapies usually produce a return of some sensation, but unfortunately they are rarely completely curative.

Paralysis of one half of the body is called hemiplegia; paralysis of all four limbs and the trunk is called quadriplegia; paralysis of only the legs and sometimes part of the trunk is called paraplegia. Paralysis may be flaccid, giving the limbs a floppy appearance, or spastic, causing the affected parts of the body to be rigid.

Although one of the most common causes of paralysis is stroke, it can be caused by any brain disorder in which the portion of the brain that controls movement is damaged. Such causes include a brain tumor, brain abscess, brain hemorrhage, cerebral palsy, or encephalitis (brain infection). Other causes include spinal cord disorders, such as damage caused by trauma (fractures), or diseases affecting nerves in the spinal cord, for example, multiple sclerosis, poliomyelitis, myelitis, Friedreich's ataxia, meningitis, or motor neuron disease. Muscle disorders, most commonly muscular dystrophy, are also culprits. Temporary paralysis can also occur in myasthenia gravis.

For paralyzed people confined to a bed or wheelchair, nursing care is essential to avoid complications such as bed sores, deep vein thrombosis, urinary tract infections, constipation, and limb deformities. The following Chinese herbal formulas can also be useful:

Bu Yang Huan Wu Tang (Tonify the Yang to Restore Five [Tenths] Decoction)

Original Source: *Yi Lin Gai Cuo* (according to *Chinese Herbal Medicine Formulas and Strategies*)

Ingredients:

Quantity (Grams)	Chinese Herbs	English Translation
6	Shi Gao	Gypsum Mineral
120	Huang Qi	Milk-Vetch Root
6	Dang Gui Wei	Tangkuei Root
3	Chuan Xiong	Szechuan Lovage Root
4.5	Chi Shao	Red Peony Root
3	Tao Ren	Peach Kernel
3	Hong Hua	Safflower Flowers
3	Di Long	Earthworm
6	Dai Zhe Shi	Red Stone from Dai County

Description: This herbal formula is used for treatment of paralysis. It is useful for hemiplegia, paralysis, and atrophy of the lower limbs, facial paralysis, slurred speech, and incontinence.

Caution: This formula is prohibited for use during pregnancy.

Analysis: The chief herb, Huang Qi, powerfully tonifies the vital energy (Chi). Dang Gui Wei, Chuan Xiong, and Chi Shao together nourish and circulate the blood. Tao Ren and Hong Hua assist in blood circulation by unblocking the channels. Di Long unblocks the meridians, allowing efficient circulation of both blood and Chi to the lower extremities. Shi Gao and Dai Zhe Shi are required to balance the formula because of the high dose of the chief herb.

Dosage and Method of Preparation: Make a decoction. Drink four ounces of Bu Yang Huan Wu Tang tea three times daily, as needed.

Comment: This formula should be taken throughout physical therapy treatments until the patient has fully recovered—for at least six months.

Tian Ma Wan (Gastrodiae Pills)

Description: This patent formula promotes blood circulation, relaxes muscles and tendons, relieves numbness of limbs, and treats hemiplegia. It is useful for treating post-stroke paralysis of face, arm, and legs. It is especially effective for treating Bell's palsy.

Dosage: It comes in bottles of one hundred pills, with complete instructions on dosage.

Ren Shen Zai Zao Wan (Ginseng Restorative Pills); also known as Tsai Tsao Wan

Description: This patent formula contains fifty-eight herbs that promote blood circulation; it is useful for treating post-stroke paralysis, facial paralysis, limb paralysis (spastic or flaccid), and impaired speech and articulation. It is also used to prevent strokes in patients who have had transient ischemic attacks.

Caution: This formula is prohibited for use during pregnancy.

Dosage: It comes in bottles of fifty pills, with complete instructions on dosage.

Comment: This formula must be taken for at least six months during physical therapy and until the patient is fully recovered.

Parkinson's Disease

Parkinson's disease is a brain disorder that causes muscle tremors, stiffness, and weakness. Most noticeable of these symptoms are the tremors that characterize the disease. Traditional Chinese medicine attributes Parkinson's to deficiency of the liver and kidney Chi along with a blood disorder that leads to a lack of nourishment of the brain. Western medicine recognizes the brain damage to the basal ganglia (nerve cell clusters in the brain) but considers the causes of unknown origin.

Although Parkinson's disease is degenerative and incurable, it is treatable; best treatment results occur in the early stages of the disease. Western medicine's course of treatment includes the drugs levodopa, bromocriptine, and amantadine. By contrast, traditional Chinese medicine uses acupuncture, remedial exercises, electro-acupuncture, and herbal therapy. The following herbal formulas have provided some benefits in managing the symptoms of Parkinson's disease in its early stages:

E Jiao Ji Zi Huang Tang (Ass-Hide Gelatin and Egg Yolk Decoction)

Original Source: *Chong Ding Tong Su Shang Han Lun* (according to *Chinese Herbal Medicine Formulas and Strategies*)

Ingredients:

Quantity (Grams)	Chinese Herbs	English Translation
6	E Jiao	Donkey Skin Glue (Ass-Hide)
2 whole yolks	Ji Zi Huang★	Chicken Egg Yolk
12	Sheng Di Huang	Chinese Foxglove Root, Raw
9	Bai Shao	White Peony Root
1.8	Zhi Gan Cao	Honey-Cooked Licorice Root
6	Gou Ten	Stem and Thorns of Gambir Vine
15	Shi Jue Ming	Abalone Shell
12	Mu Li	Oyster Shell
12	Fu Shen	Tuckahoe Spirit Fungus
9	Luo Shi Teng	Star Jasmine Stem

★See special instructions for preparation below.

Description: This herbal formula provides relief from rigid extremities, muscle spasms, and uncontrollable twitching.

Analysis: The chief ingredients in this formula, E Jiao and Ji Zi Huang, nourish the blood, adjust body fluids, and reduce spasms. Sheng Di Huang, Bai Shao, and Zhi Gan Cao benefit the liver and assist in reducing tremors. Gou Ten, Shi Jue Ming, and Mu Li have a sedative effect that helps to calms spasms. Fu Shen is calming and also benefits the liver. Luo Shi Teng focuses the actions of the other herbs in the formula.

Dosage and Method of Preparation: Prepare a decoction. Do not add the Ji Zi Huang (two egg yolks) until the decoction has been completely cooked, strained, and cooled. Then add the egg yolks and blend well. Drink four ounces of E Jiao Ji Zi Huang Tang tea three times daily, or as needed.

Jian Bu Hu Qian Wan (Walk Vigorously [Like] a Tiger Stealthily Pills); also known as Chen Pu Hu Chien Wan

Description: This patent formula is used for treatment of weak limbs, debility in walking, limbs that are flaccid and weak, and muscle atrophy.

中草藥

Dosage: It comes in bottles of two hundred pills, with complete instructions on dosage.

Ren Shen Zai Zao Wan (Ginseng Restorative Pills); also known as Tsai Tsao Wan

Description: This patent formula is useful for treating hemiplegia, speech disturbances, contractive or flaccid muscle tone in the extremities (legs, feet, hands, and arms), as well as numbness and tingling in the limbs.

Caution: This formula is prohibited for use during pregnancy.

Dosage: It comes in boxes of ten wax pills, with complete instructions on dosage.

Pelvic Inflammatory Disease

Pelvic inflammatory disease (P.I.D.) is an infection of the internal female reproductive organs that often occurs after a sexually transmitted disease such as gonorrhea or chlamydial infection. It may also occur after miscarriage, abortion, or childbirth. IUD users have a higher incidence than women using other forms of birth control. P.I.D. is one of the most common causes of pelvic pain in women. Symptoms include pain and tenderness in the pelvic region, fever, and an unpleasant-smelling vaginal discharge (see also Vaginal Discharge). The pain occurs most often following menstruation and may be worse during intercourse. Sufferers may also experience malaise, vomiting, and backache. Pelvic inflammatory disease may cause infertility or an increased risk of ectopic pregnancy, primarily from scarring of the fallopian tubes that prevents the egg from reaching the uterus.

Western treatment normally involves the use of antibiotic drugs and analgesics. Traditional Chinese medicine similarly prescribes herbal formulas containing antibiotic herbs that are decocted and taken in tea form. Sometimes, it is possible to eliminate the infection by using an herbal douche. In severe cases, the simultaneous use of both oral decoction and douche is usually recommended to bring about a quicker cure.

Long Dan Xie Gan Tang (Gentiana Longdancao Decoction to Drain the Liver)

Original Source: *Yi Fang Ji Jie* (according to *Chinese Herbal Medicine Formulas and Strategies*)

Ingredients:

Quantity (Grams)	Chinese Herbs	English Translation
9	Long Dan Cao	Chinese Gentina Root
12	Huang Qin	Baical Skullcap Root
12	Zhi Zi	Gardenia Fruit
6	Mu Tong	Wood with Holes
15	Che Qian Zi	Plantago Seed
12	Ze Xie	Water Plantain Rhizome
9	Chai Hu	Bupleurum Hare's Ear Root
15	Sheng Di Huang	Chinese Foxglove Root, Raw
12	Dang Gui	Tangkuei
6	Gan Cao	Licorice

Description: This herbal formula is used to clear pelvic infection, eliminate foul vaginal discharge, and reduce pain.

Analysis: Long Dan Cao, the chief herb, is powerful in its ability to clear heat and eliminate infection from the lower body. Huang Qin and Zhi Zi assist the chief herb. Chai Hu disperses heat in the liver and gallbladder. Mu Tong, Che Qian Zi, and Ze Xie remove the heat by promoting urination. Sheng Di Huang and Dang Gui nourish the blood, and Gan Cao harmonizes the herbs in this formula.

Dosage and Method of Preparation: Prepare a decoction. Drink four ounces of Long Dan Xie Gan Tang tea three times daily as needed. In severe cases, combine oral use of this formula with the following vaginal douche:

Vaginal Douche

Ingredients:

Quantity (Grams)	Chinese Herbs	English Translation
9	Chuan Lian Zi	Fruit of Szechuan Pagoda Tree

12	Gou Qi Gen	Matrimony Vine Root
9	Huang Bai	Amur Cork Tree Bark
12	Ku Shen	Bitter Root
9	She Chuang Zi	Cnidium Fruit Seed
9	Ku Fan★	Alum, Mineral Salt

★See special instructions for preparation below.

Description: This vaginal douche is for all types of vaginal infections with discharge, foul odor, itching, irritation, lower abdominal discomfort, and discomfort when urinating.

Caution: This formula is for external use only as a douche; do not drink this formula.

Analysis: Chuan Lian Zi, Gou Qi Gen, Huang Bai, Ku Shen, and She Chuang Zi are all combined to create a powerful infection-eliminating action. Ku Fan eliminates the discharge with its astringent action.

Dosage and Method of Preparation: Make a decoction. Ku Fan should not be cooked with the other herbs but added after the normal cooking procedure, then allowed to steep with the decoction for thirty minutes before straining. Douche with eight ounces of this decocted tea at room temperature twice daily, as needed.

Peptic Ulcer—see Ulcer

Pernicious Anemia—see Anemia

Pertussis

Pertussis, commonly known as whooping cough, is an infectious disease that mainly affects infants and young children. Pertussis is caused by the bacterium *Bordetella pertussis,* which is spread in airborne droplets coughed out by the infected person.

In developed countries most infants are vaccinated against pertussis in their first year, but not all children are suitable for vaccination, so epidemics of the illness still occur. Symptoms begin with a mild cough, sneezing, nasal discharge, fever, and sore eyes—during the noninfectious period. After a few days, the cough becomes more persistent and severe. Sometimes, the cough can cause vomiting. Infants sustain a risk of apnea (cessation of breathing) or an inability to catch the breath due to spastic coughing. Pertussis can last for up to ten weeks and can develop complications such as pneumonia, nosebleeds, and recurrent vomiting, which can cause dehydration and malnutrition.

Once a person is infected, antibiotic drugs are usually of little use. An infected child should be kept warm, avoiding drafts or smoke that can trigger coughing. He or she should be given small, frequent meals and plenty of fluids.

Note: An infant or child who turns blue, who regurgitates or coughs up blood, or who repeatedly vomits after coughing should be seen by a physician.

The following Chinese herbal remedies can aid in treating pertussis:

Sang Xing Tang (Mulberry Leaf and Almond Kernel Decoction)

Original Source: *Wen Bing Tiao Bian* (according to *Chinese Herbal Medicine Formulas and Strategies*)

Ingredients:

Quantity (Grams)	Chinese Herbs	English Translation
3	Sang Ye	White Mulberry Leaf
3	Zhi Zi	Gardenia Fruit
3	Dan Dou Chi	Prepared Black Bean
4.5	Xing Ren	Almond Kernel
3	Zhe Bei Mu	Fritillaria Zhebei Bulb
6	Sha Shen	Root of Silvertop Beech Tree
3	Li Pi	Pear Peel

Description: This herbal formula reduces fever, nourishes the lungs, stops cough, and is useful for whooping cough.

Analysis: Sang Ye moistens and benefits the throat. Zhi Zi and Dan Dou Chi reduce fever and cause mild sweating to relieve heat. Xing Ren and Zhe Bei Mu moisten and eliminate the "dry" coughing. Together, Sha Shen and Li Pi have a cooling and moistening effect.

Dosage and Method of Preparation: Make a decoction. Drink four ounces of Sang Xing Tang tea three times daily, or as needed.

Lo Han Kuo Infusion (Momordica Fruit Instant Medicine); also known as Luo Han Guo Chong Ji

Description: This patent formula is used to treat stubborn cough, such as that associated with whooping cough or tuberculosis. This formula stops cough, nourishes the lungs, and clears lung heat (infection).

Dosage: This patent medicine comes in packages containing twelve small boxes, with complete instructions on dosage.

Pharyngitis—see Sore Throat

Pink Eye—see Conjunctivitis

Pinworms—see Roundworms

Pleurisy

Pleurisy is characterized by sharp chest pain that results from inflammation of the membrane lining the lungs. It is usually caused by a viral infection such as pleurodynia or pneumonia. Other possible causes include pulmonary embolism and lung cancer. Both Western and traditional Chinese medical treatment are directed at clearing the infection (except in the case of lung cancer) that is the underlying cause.

Hsiao Yao Wan (Bupleurum Sedative Pills); also known as Xiao Yao Wan

Description: This patent formula is useful for pleurisy. It nourishes the blood, counters fatigue, and reduces pain.

Dosage: It comes in bottles of two hundred pills, with complete instructions on dosage.

PMS—see Premenstrual Syndrome

Pneumonia

Chinese medicine refers to pneumonia as "heat and stagnation of fluid in the lungs." This is an apt description of two of the disease's most prominent symptoms: high fever and mucus congestion. Western medicine's more detailed explanation cites viruses and bacteria as the most common causes. Although rarely, pneumonia can also be caused by other classes of organisms, such as fungi, yeast, or protozoa. These types usually occur only in people with immunodeficiency disorders. Pneumocystic pneumonia, for example, is caused by a protozoan commonly occurring in people with AIDS.

There are two main types of pneumonia: lobar pneumonia and bronchopneumonia. In lobar pneumonia, one lobe of one lung is affected. In bronchopneumonia, inflammation starts in the bronchi and bronchioles (airways) and then spreads to affect patches of tissue in either one or both lungs. Symptoms typically include fever, chills, shortness of breath, pain, and a cough, producing phlegm that is occasionally streaked with blood. Potential complications are pleural effusion (fluid around the lungs), empyema (pus in the pleural cavity), and lung abscess.

Several useful herbal formulas follow for treating both types of pneumonia.

Ma Xing Shi Gan Tang (Ephedra, Almond Kernel, Gypsum, and Licorice Decoction)

Original Source: *Shang Han Lun* (according to *Chinese Herbal Medicine Formulas and Strategies*)

Ingredients:

Quantity (Grams)	Chinese Herbs	English Translation
12	Ma Huang*	Yellow Hemp Root (Ephedra)
48	Shi Gao	Gypsum
18	Xing Ren	Almond Kernel
6	Zhi Gan Cao	Honey-Cooked Licorice Root

*Persons with high blood pressure should not use Ma Huang; instead, substitute 12 grams of Bai Qian (White Before Rhizome).

Description: This herbal formula reduces fever, eliminates coughing with labored breathing; it is useful for bronchitis, pertussis, lobar pneumonia, and bronchial pneumonia.

Analysis: Ma Huang, the chief ingredient, circulates vital energy (Chi), benefits the lungs, and reduces wheezing. Shi Gao is used to drain heat from the lungs while its cool nature controls the sweating created by the chief herb. Xing Ren moistens and stops coughing. Zhi Gan Cao assists in this action and also improves the taste of the formula.

Dosage and Method of Preparation: Prepare a decoction. Drink four ounces of Ma Xing Shi Gan Tang tea three times daily, as needed.

Wei Jing Tang (Reed Decoction)

Original Source: *Qian Jin Yao Fang* (according to *Chinese Herbal Medicine Formulas and Strategies*)

Ingredients:

Quantity (Grams)	Chinese Herbs	English Translation
30	Lu Gen	Reed Rhizome Root
30	Yi Yi Ren	Seeds of Job's Tears
24	Dong Gua Ren	Wintermelon Seeds
9	Tao Ren	Peach Kernel

Description: This herbal formula is used to clear heat (infection) from lungs; it transforms phlegm, resolves blood stasis, discharges pus, and is useful for pneumonia, asthma, pertussis, and bronchitis.

Analysis: Lu Gen, the main ingredient, clears heat and is especially effective for treating lung abscesses. Dong Gua Ren resolves phlegm, reduces heat, and eliminates pus. Yi Yi Ren disperses heat and pus as well as opening the bowels, providing an outlet. Tao Ren improves circulation and lubricates the intestines, creating a mild laxative effect.

Dosage and Method of Preparation: Prepare a decoction. Drink four ounces of Wei Jing Tang tea three times daily, as needed.

Ching Fei Yi Huo Pien (Clear Lungs Restrain Fire Tablets); also known as Qing Fei Yi Huo Pian

Description: This patent formula clears lung heat, treats cough, stops bleeding, increases fluids; it is useful for pneumonia, pulmonary abscess, bronchitis.

Caution: This formula is prohibited for use during pregnancy.

Dosage: It comes in tubes of eight tablets, with complete instructions on dosage.

Chuan Xin Lian-Antiphlogistic Pills (Penetrate Heart, Repeatedly Fight Heat Pills); also known as Chuan Xin Lian Kang Yan Pian

Description: This patent formula clears heat and reduces inflammation; it is used for treating pneumonia, tuberculosis, pulmonary abscess, and other infections associated with lung heat.

Dosage: It comes in bottles of sixty pills, with complete instructions on dosage.

Poisoning

It is strongly recommended that anyone who has ingested poison contact the poison control center immediately.

For an herbal formula to treat nonchemical food poisoning, see Food Poisoning.

Poison Ivy, Poison Oak, Poison Sumac—see Rash

Postnatal Care

The postnatal period, considered to begin with delivery and to last for approximately six weeks, presents a number of conditions that are a normal result of childbirth. The list of maladies experienced after giving birth can include hemorrhoids, postpartum hemorrhaging, depression, and the most common complaint, weakness and fatigue. The following Chinese herbal formulas can be used for strengthening the body and restoring energy levels as well as addressing many of the residual problems often encountered after childbirth:

Wu Ji Bai Feng Wan (Black Chicken White Phoenix Pill/Condensed); also known as Wu Chi Pai Feng Wan, or Wu Ji Bai Feng Wan Nong Suo

Description: This patent formula is useful for postpartum weakness, bleeding, fatigue, low back pain, and pain or weakness in the legs.

Dosage: It comes in boxes containing ten wax, egg-shaped capsules encasing the herbs, or bottles of 120 pills, with complete instructions on dosage.

Tai Pan Tang Yi Pian (Placenta Sugar-Coated Tablets); also known as Sugar-Coated Placenta Tablets

Description: This patent formula is used to treat general debility, fatigue, and weakness following long-term illness or childbirth.

Dosage: It comes in bottles of one hundred pills, with complete instructions on dosage.

Ren Shen Feng Wang Jiang (Ginseng Royal Jelly Syrup); also known as Ling Zhi Feng Wang Jiang

Description: This nutritive tonic is beneficial following illness or childbirth. It promotes appetite, restores strength, and counters fatigue.

Dosage: It comes in vials of 10cc each, with complete instructions on dosage.

Dang Gui Gin Gao (Angelica Dang Gui Syrup); also known as Tankwe Gin for Tea

Description: This general women's tonic is recommended for improving blood quality, improving vitality, and increasing strength following childbirth, illness, or surgery.

Dosage: It comes in bottles of 100cc or 200cc, with complete instructions on dosage.

Ba Zhen Wan (Eight Treasure Tea Pills); also known as Nu Ke Ba Zhen Wan

Description: This patent formula is an excellent women's general tonic, useful for fatigue, postpartum hemorrhaging, and weakness after childbirth and to correct anemia.

Dosage: It comes in bottles of two hundred pills, with complete instructions on dosage.

Bei Jing Feng Wang Jing (Peking Royal Jelly)

Description: This patent medicine tonifies Chi (increases energy), benefits digestion, nourishes the blood, and is used as a nutritional support and general tonic following childbirth, illness, surgery, or trauma.

Dosage: It comes in vials of 10cc each, with complete instructions on dosage.

Pregnancy (see also Morning Sickness)

Pregnancy, the period from conception to birth, typically lasts forty weeks and has certain common features of discomfort such as nausea, backache, and constipation. Many of the symptoms that are a normal part of pregnancy are treatable. What follows is a list of Chinese herbal formulas that can be used to manage and eliminate some of the discomfort of pregnancy. These formulas should not be considered a substitute for prenatal care or for coaching by a trained midwife, but they can be safely used throughout pregnancy without concern for harming the mother or the fetus.

Ba Zhen Wan (Eight Treasure Tea Pills); also known as Nu Ke Ba Zhen Wan

Description: This patent formula is an excellent general women's tonic to tonify the Chi (improve energy) and nourish the blood (correct anemia).

Dosage: It comes in bottles of two hundred pills, with complete instructions on dosage.

Dang Gui Gin Gao (Angelica Dang Gui Syrup); also known as Tankwe Gin for Tea

Description: This patent formula is recommended as a general tonic for women exhibiting signs of blood deficiency and fatigue.

Dosage: It comes in bottles of 100cc or 200cc, with complete instructions on dosage.

Kang Ning Wan (Curing Pill); also known as Pill Curing

Description: This patent formula is used to settle the stomach and to relieve nausea, morning sickness, and vomiting.

Dosage: It comes in boxes of ten vials, with complete instructions on dosage.

Huo Hsiang Cheng Chi Pien (Pogostemon Normalize Chi Pills); also known as Huo Xiang Zheng Qi Pian, or Lophanthus Antifebrile Pills

Description: This patent formula is used for relief of nausea, headache, morning sickness, and vomiting.

Dosage: It comes in bottles of one hundred sugar-coated pills, with complete instructions on dosage.

Hsiang Sha Yang Wei Pien (Saussurea Amomum Nourish Stomach Tablet); also known as Xiang Sha Yang Wei Pian

Description: This patent formula is used for nausea, vomiting, and morning sickness.

Dosage: It comes in bottles of twenty or sixty pills, with complete instructions on dosage.

Bu Zhong Yi Qi Wan (Tonify Center to Invigorate Qi Pills); also known as Central Qi Pills, or Bu Zhong Yi Chi Wan

Description: This patent formula is useful for hemorrhoids, varicose veins, uterine bleeding, and habitual miscarriage.

Dosage: It comes in bottles of one hundred pills, with complete instructions on dosage.

An Tai Wan (Soothe Embryo Pills); also known as Bao Tai Wan, Shi San Tai Bao Wan, or Bao Chan Wu Yu Wan

Description: This patent formula is used to relieve back and leg pain or to treat uterine bleeding; it also helps to prevent miscarriages.

Dosage: It comes in bottles of one hundred pills, with complete instructions on dosage.

Premature Ejaculation—see Ejaculation, Disorders of

Premenstrual Syndrome

Premenstrual syndrome, more commonly referred to as PMS, is the combination of physical and emotional symptoms that begin at ovulation and continue until the onset of menstruation. Many theories exist concerning the causes of PMS. The theories range from hormonal imbalances (estrogen and progesterone levels) to vitamin and mineral deficiencies. None of these suggested causes has been conclusively confirmed.

The most frequent emotional symptoms are irritability, tension, depression, and fatigue. Physical symptoms include breast tenderness, fluid retention, headache, backache, and lower abdominal pain and congestion. Traditional Chinese medicine suspects that most often the emotional symptoms can be attributed to anticipation of the pain and discomfort that is all too often associated with the menstrual period. Herbal treatment is directed at correcting menstrual irregularities by harmonizing the blood (resolving blood clots), eliminating pain, and regulating the length of the cycle (maximum three to five days). The following Chinese herbal formulas have proven to be extremely effective for treating premenstrual syndrome:

Wu Ji Bai Feng Wan (Black Chicken White Phoenix Pills/Condensed); also known as Wu Chi Pai Feng Wan, or Wu Ji Bai Feng Wan Nong Suo

Description: This patent formula is used to regulate menstruation; it reduces postpartum weakness, stops pain, corrects fluid retention, stops headaches, stops lower abdominal cramping and backaches.

Dosage: It comes in 10 honey pills or bottles of 120 pills, with complete instructions on dosage.

Bu Xue Tiao Jing Pian (Nourish Blood Adjust Period Pills); also known as Bu Tiao Tablets

Description: This patent formula is useful for treating symptoms of PMS such as menstrual cramps, headache, irritability, backache, and fatigue.

Dosage: It comes in bottles of one hundred tablets, with complete instructions on dosage.

Ba Zhen Wan (Eight Treasure Tea Pills); also known as Nu Ke Ba Zhen Wan

Description: This patent formula is an excellent general tonic for women; it is useful for symptoms of PMS as well as improving anemia, eliminating menstrual cramps, regulating menses, and eliminating headaches and backaches.

Dosage: It comes in bottles of two hundred pills, with complete instructions on dosage.

Prostate, Disorders of: Cancer, Enlarged Prostate, Prostatitis

Prostate cancer is the second most frequently occurring cancer in men after cancer of the lung. Although it can occur in middle age, more often it affects the elderly. Symptoms of this disease are enlargement of the prostate gland (which causes difficulty starting urination), impaired urinary flow, and increased frequency of urination. In the advanced stages prostate cancer usually causes pelvic pain that is a result of cancer spreading to the bones. While the precise causes are unknown, hormonal imbalances (testosterone levels) and diets high in fat are suspected of contributing. Western medicine claims to have a relatively high success rate treating prostate cancer when it is discovered in its early stages. Traditional Chinese medicine makes no claims but does offer herbal formulas for treating it. Therefore, it should be understood that the use of these herbal formulas should be adjunctive to Western treatment.

Prostate Cancer Formula

An excellent book on Chinese medicines used to fight cancer is *Anticancer Medicinal Herbs,* by Chang Minyi. According to this book, the following single-herb formula has been used to treat prostate cancer:

Ingredient:

Quantity (Grams)	Chinese Herb	English Translation
10	Lao Guan Cao	Erodium Plant

Description: This formula is for the treatment of cancer of the prostate gland.

Analysis: Lao Guan Cao eliminates fever, relieves toxins, and activates the circulation of blood and vital energy (Chi) to the perineal region.

Dosage and Method of Preparation: Make a decoction. Combine ten grams of herb with 200 ml of water; cook as instructed. Drink eight ounces of this formula three times daily, as needed.

Prostate enlargement, also called benign prostatic hypertrophy, is simply an increase in size of the prostate gland, for which there is no known cause. Usually affecting men over fifty, symptoms gradually develop as the enlarging prostate presses on the urethra, obstructing the flow of urine. Normally, sufferers experience difficulty starting urination, and once started, the stream or flow is weak. Overdevelopment of the bladder muscle (in order to force the urine through the obstructed urethra) can cause swelling in the lower abdomen. There may be incontinence due to overflow of small quantities of urine, or the bladder may become overactive, resulting in frequent urination. Severe abdominal pain and the ability to pass only a few drops of urine indicate acute urinary retention and require immediate treatment.

Chinese herbal therapy has been fairly successful in treating prostate enlargement, yet it is important to undergo a digital rectal examination to confirm the diagnosis since there has been some speculation concerning a relationship between this condition and prostate cancer.

Prostatitis is inflammation of the prostate gland. It is usually caused by bacterial infection that has spread from the urethra. The infection may or may not be sexually transmitted. Presence of a urinary catheter increases the risk of prostatitis. Anyone with frequently recurring prostate infections would be well advised to investigate the cause.

Two Chinese herbs noted for their ability to effectively treat this condition are Che Qian Zi (Plantago Seeds) and Ze Xie (Water Plantain). Complete formulas are given below. Their use is preferable to the standard Western medical treatment of antibiotic drugs requiring long-term use, which can be undesirable because of compromised immunity and with which there is a high rate of recurrence.

Xiao Ji Yin Zi (Cephalanoplos Decoction)

Original Source: *Ji Sheng Fang* (according to *Chinese Herbal Medicine Formulas and Strategies*)

Ingredients:

Quantity (Grams)	Chinese Herbs	English Translation
3.5	Xiao Ji	Small Thistle Plant
3.5	Ou Jie	Lotus Rhizome, Node
3.5	Chao Pu Huang	Dry-Fried Cattail Pollen
30	Sheng Di Huang	Chinese Foxglove Root, Raw
3.5	Hua Shi	Talcum, Mineral
3.5	Mu Tong	Wood with Holes
3.5	Dan Zhu Ye	Bland Bamboo Leaves
3.5	Zhi Zi	Gardenia Fruit
3.5	Dang Gui	Tangkuei
3.5	Zhi Gan Cao	Honey-Cooked Licorice Root

Description: This herbal formula is useful for prostate enlargement with painful and frequent urination and abdominal distention.

Analysis: Xiao Ji, Ou Jie, Chao Pu Huang, and Sheng Di Huang, combined, cool the blood and stop bleeding. Hua Shi clears heat and promotes urination while addressing painful urinary dysfunc-

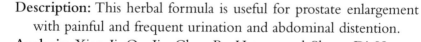

tion. Mu Tong, Dan Zhu Ye, and Zhi Zi eliminate fever and heat in the lower body, directing it out of the body. Dang Gui nourishes the blood, and Zhi Gan Cao relieves pain and settles the stomach.

Dosage and Method of Preparation: Prepare a decoction. Drink four ounces of Xiao Ji Yin Zi tea three times daily, or as needed.

Ba Zheng Tang (Eight Herb Powder for Rectification)

Original Source: *Tai Ping Hui Min He Ji Ju Fang* (according to *Chinese Herbal Medicine Formulas and Strategies*)

Ingredients:

Quantity (Grams)	Chinese Herbs	English Translation
6	Mu Tong	Wood with Holes
30	Hua Shi	Talcum, Mineral
15	Che Qian Zi	Plantago Seed
12	Qu Mai	Fringed Pink Flower Plant
12	Bian Xu	Knotweed Plant
9	Zhi Zi	Gardenia Fruit
9	Zhi Da Huang	Treated Rhubarb Root
6	Deng Xin Cao	Rush Pith
9	Gan Cao	Licorice Root

Description: This herbal formula clears heat (infection), promotes urination, relieves pain, and is useful for prostatitis.

Analysis: The chief ingredient, Mu Tong, clears heat and resolves infection. Hua Shi, Che Qian Zi, Qu Mai, and Bian Xu clear infection by promoting urination. Zhi Zi clears heat and also promotes urination. Zhi Da Huang moves the bowels. Deng Xin Cao directs the action of the other herbs downward, and Gan Cao harmonizes them.

Dosage and Method of Preparation: Make a decoction. Drink four ounces of Ba Zheng Tang tea three times daily, as needed.

Qian Lie Xian Wan (Prostate Gland Pills)

Description: This patent formula reduces inflammation and clears pus, infection, and swelling or enlargement of prostate.

Dosage: It comes in bottles of ninety pills, with complete instructions on dosage.

Jie Jie Wan (Dispel [Prostate] Swelling Pills); also known as Kai Kit Pill

Description: This patent formula is useful for chronic and difficult cases of enlarged prostate; it promotes urination, resolves pain, and is recommended for conditions where swelling is pronounced, with pain in the groin.

Dosage: It comes in bottles of fifty-four pills, with complete instructions on dosage.

Psoriasis

Psoriasis is a skin disease characterized by red scaly patches. Its most common sites are the knees, elbows, scalp, and trunk. Although the exact causes of psoriasis are unknown, it is known to run in families. The classic symptoms of psoriasis are skin eruptions, often accompanied by painful swelling. There are three basic types of the disorder. Discoid (meaning disklike), or plaque psoriasis, the most common form, exhibits red scaly patches; occasionally, the nails become pitted, thickened, or separated from the nail bed. Guttate psoriasis, which occurs most frequently in children, usually begins with a sore throat and develops red patches that quickly spread over a wide area. Pustular psoriasis is characterized by small pustules that may either cover the entire body or be confined to isolated locations such as the palms or soles of the feet.

Traditional Chinese medicine's basic approach for treating psoriasis through the use of blood cleansers contrasts strikingly to Western medicine's use of ultraviolet lamps and emollient creams, coal tar ointments, corticosteroids, and anticancer drugs such as methotrexate.

Xiao Feng Tang (Eliminate Wind Powder from True Lineage)

Original Source: *Wai Ke Zheng Zong* (according to *Chinese Herbal Medicine Formulas and Strategies*)

Ingredients:

Quantity (Grams)	Chinese Herbs	English Translation
3	Jing Jie	Schizonepeta Stem/Bud
3	Fang Feng	Guard Against the Wind Root
3	Niu Bang Zi	Great Burdock Root
3	Chan Tui	Cicada Molting
3	Cang Zhu	Atractylodes Cangzhu
3	Ku Shen	Bitter Root
1.5	Mu Tong	Wood with Holes
3	Shi Gao	Gypsum, Mineral
3	Zhi Mu	Anemarrhena Root
3	Sheng Di Huang	Chinese Foxglove Root, Raw
3	Dang Gui	Tangkuei
3	Hei Zhi Ma	Black Sesame Seeds
1.5	Gan Cao	Licorice Root

Description: This herbal formula is useful for treating itching red skin and lesions with pus. It reduces fever, cools the blood, clears infection, resolves rashes; it is used for various conditions of dermatitis, including psoriasis.

Analysis: The chief herbs in this formula, Jing Jie, Fang Feng, Niu Bang Zi, and Chan Tui unblock the pores, allowing surface heat to be vented. Cang Zhu, Ku Shen, and Mu Tong promote urination and drain infection through the urine. Zhi Mu and Shi Gao reduce fever. Sheng Di Huang and Dang Gui cool and nourish the blood. Hei Zhi Ma nourishes the blood and moistens. Gan Cao clears heat, relieves toxicity, and harmonizes the actions of the other herbs in the formula as well as improving the taste.

Dosage and Method of Preparation: Prepare a decoction. Xiao Feng Tang tea can be used two ways: (1) apply the room-temperature tea to the affected areas of skin to provide relief from swelling and inflammation; (2) drink four ounces of the tea three times daily, as needed.

Lien Chiao Pai Tu Pien (Forsythia Defeat Toxin Tablets); also known as Lian Qiao Bai Du Pian

Description: This patent formula is useful for treating psoriasis, skin eruptions, boils, carbuncles, and similar skin conditions. It clears heat (infection), reduces inflammation, discharges pus, and eliminates swelling.

Caution: This formula is prohibited for use during pregnancy.

Dosage: It comes in vials containing eight tablets each, with complete instructions on dosage.

Pyelonephritis (see also Kidney, Disorders of)

Pyelonephritis, or inflammation of the kidneys, is usually caused by a bacterial infection. More commonly called kidney infection, pyelonephritis may be acute, taking the form of a sudden attack, or chronic, in which repeated attacks may cause scarring of the kidneys. Acute pyelonephritis, which is more common in women and more likely to occur in pregnancy, usually results from cystitis (bladder infection) and spreads to the kidneys. Typical symptoms include high fever, chills, and back pain. Chronic pyelonephritis often starts in childhood, resulting from congenital abnormality, and is usually caused by the reflux of urine from the bladder back into one of the ureters. Persistent infection leading to inflammation and scarring over a period of years can cause permanent kidney damage. Possible complications of chronic pyelonephritis include hypertension, and renal (kidney) failure. Herbal formulas for treating kidney infections include ingredients for clearing infection, reducing fever, and eliminating pain.

Wu Wei Xiao Du Yin (Five Ingredient Decoction to Eliminate Toxin)

Original Source: *Yi Zong Jin Jian* (according to *Chinese Herbal Medicine Formulas and Strategies*)

Ingredients:

Quantity (Grams)	Chinese Herbs	English Translation
9	Jin Yin Hua	Honeysuckle Flower

3.6	Pu Gong Ying	Dandelion Herb
3.6	Zi Hua Di Ding	Yedeon's Violet Root
3.6	Ye Ju Hua	Wild Chrysanthemum Flower
3.6	Zi Bei Tian Kuei	Begonia

Description: This herbal formula is used for treating kidney infections, urinary tract infections, and appendicitis. It clears heat (infection), resolves swelling, and eliminates inflammations.

Analysis: The chief herb, Jin Yin Hua, clears heat and infection and reduces swelling. Pu Gong Ying, Zi Hua Di Ding, Ye Ju Hua, and Zhi Bei Tian Kuei all clear heat and cool the blood and are useful for treating poisonous lesions.

Dosage and Method of Preparation: Prepare a decoction. Drink four ounces of Wu Wei Xiao Du Yin tea three times daily, as needed.

Lung Tan Xie Gan Wan (Gentiana Purge Liver Pills); also known as Long Dan Xie Gan Wan

Description: This patent formula is used to reduce fever, pain, and infection. It is useful for pyelonephritis, cystitis, and urethritis.

Dosage: It comes in bottles of one hundred pills, with complete instructions on dosage.

Quinsy—see Tonsillitis

Rash (see also Fever; Itching; or specific complaint, e.g., Athlete's Foot; Psoriasis; etc.)

A rash is an inflammation of the skin that can be accompanied by red spots, fever, and itching. Rashes are usually caused by eczema, psoriasis or keratosis, vitamin deficiency (as with scurvy), an allergic reaction to something recently eaten, contact with certain plants (poison ivy, oak, or sumac), or a reaction to a particular drug (for example, barbiturates or antibiotics). Rashes are also the main indication of many childhood infectious diseases such as chicken pox, scarlet fever, ringworm, and Rocky Mountain spotted fever. A rash may be localized (affecting a small area of the skin) or generalized (covering the entire body). Traditional Chinese medicine uses herbal teas, ointments, pills, and salves for treating rashes. In difficult cases, or as a means of speeding recovery, it is often suggested that the ingestion of herbal teas and the applications of topical solutions be done simultaneously.

Xiao Feng Tang (Eliminate Wind Powder from True Lineage)

Original Source: *Wai Ke Zheng Zong* (according to *Chinese Herbal Medicine Formulas and Strategies*)

Ingredients:

Quantity (Grams)	Chinese Herbs	English Translation
3	Jing Jie	Schizonepeta Stem/Bud
3	Fang Feng	Guard Against the Wind Root
3	Niu Bang Zi	Great Burdock Fruit
3	Chan Tui	Cicada Molting
3	Cang Zhu	Atractylodes Cangzhu
3	Ku Shen	Bitter Root
1.5	Mu Tong	Wood with Holes
3	Shi Gao	Gypsum, Mineral
3	Zhi Mu	Anemarrhena Root
3	Sheng Di Huang	Chinese Foxglove Root, Raw
3	Dang Gui	Tangkuei
3	Hei Zhi Ma	Black Sesame Seeds
1.5	Gan Cao	Licorice Root

Description: This herbal formula is used to clear infection from the body; it cools the blood and relieves the skin of lesions caused by rash, eczema, dermatitis, and psoriasis. This formula can be used topically (as a soothing bath for the skin) or taken internally as a decoction.

Analysis: Jing Jie, Fang Feng, Niu Bang Zi, and Chan Tui are all chief herbs in this formula; they unblock the pores to allow Cang Zhu,

Ku Shen, and Mu Tong to clear heat and eliminate infection. Shi Gao and Zhi Mu assist in clearing heat and prevent rashes from advancing beyond the surface to deeper levels. Sheng Di Huang cools the blood. Dang Gui and Hei Zhi Ma nourish and circulate it. Gan Cao clears heat and relieves toxicity as well as harmonizes the actions of the other herbs in the formula.

Dosage and Method of Preparation: Make a decoction. Drink four ounces of Xiao Feng Tang tea three times daily, as needed, or bathe the body in room-temperature tea, as needed.

Jing Wan Hong (Capitol City [Beijing] Many Red Colors); also known as Ching Wan Hung

Description: This patent formula is used to stop pain, decrease inflammation, control infection, promote regeneration of damaged skin tissue, and provide relief from rashes and painful skin eruptions.

Dosage: It comes in tubes of thirty grams or five hundred grams, with complete instructions on dosage.

Lien Chiao Pai Tu Pien (Forsythia Defeat Toxin Tablet); also known as Lian Qiao Bai Du Pian

Description: This patent formula is used for inflammation- and infection-causing abscesses, rashes with itching and redness, and carbuncles.

Caution: This formula is prohibited for use during pregnancy.

Dosage: It comes in packages of twelve vials, eight tablets per vial, with complete instructions on dosage.

Cai Feng Zhen Zhu An Chuang Wan (Margarite Acne Pill); also known as Colorful Phoenix Precious Pearl Hide Skin Boil Pill

Description: This patent formula clears heat (infection) while it relieves itching and redness; it is useful for hives, rashes, and acne.

Dosage: It comes in bottles of thirty-six pills, with complete instructions on dosage.

Rectum, Disorders of: Bleeding, Prolapse (see also Intestine, Disorders of; Colon-Rectal Cancer)

Rectal bleeding is most commonly caused by hemorrhoids, but it can also result from several disorders of the rectum, colon, or intestines. Possible causes of rectal bleeding include anal fissures, anal fistula, proctitis, rectal prolapse, diverticular disease, and cancers of the intestines, rectum, or colon. Because of the possibility of serious underlying causes, all incidences of rectal bleeding should be investigated immediately.

There are several different types of bleeding; these often offer telltale signs for determining its origin: for example, hemorrhoids normally produce bright-red blood on the toilet paper or on the surface of the feces (see also Hemorrhoids); diverticulitis causes dark-red feces; bleeding high in the digestive tract produces blackish feces.

Several Chinese herbal formulas can be useful in treating many of the disorders mentioned. It bears repeating that their use should only be considered after a thorough examination and diagnosis has been made by a qualified physician.

Rectal prolapse occurs when the lining of the anus protrudes outside of the rectum as a result of straining. Traditional Chinese medicine holds that this condition results from central Chi deficiency (general weakness of the organs of the digestive system). Common causes of a prolapsed rectum include difficulty defecating, pushing and straining during childbirth, and lifting heavy objects. Often associated with prolapsed hemorrhoids, rectal prolapse causes discomfort, mucus discharge, and bleeding from the rectum (see also Hemorrhoids). In infants and younger people, prolapse is usually temporary and can often be corrected by adopting a high-fiber diet. In elderly people, it tends to be more severe and often permanent due to weakening of the anal sphincter (muscle) and the surrounding tissue that supports the perineum (the area between the scrotum and anus in men or between the vulva and anus in women). Along with herbal therapy, traditional Chinese medicine normally recommends remedial exercises to strengthen the surrounding tissue and muscles (these exercises are called "the deer"; see Erection [Penile], Disorders of, for a description of how to perform them).

Huai Hua Tang (Sophora Japonica Flower Decoction)

Original Source: *Pu Ji Ben Shi Fang* (according to *Chinese Herbal Medicine Formulas and Strategies*)

Ingredients:

Quantity (Grams)	Chinese Herbs	English Translation
30	Huai Hua	Sophora Flower of Pagoda Tree
15	Ce Bai Ye Tan	Leafy Twig of Arborvitae
9	Jing Jie Sui	Schizonepeta Spike
9	Zhi Ke	Bitter Orange Fruit Ripe

Description: This herbal formula cools the intestines, stops bleeding, reduces pain, and promotes healing.

Analysis: Huai Hua, the chief herb, cools the blood, clears infection from the intestines, and also stops bleeding. Jing Jie Sui and Ce Bai Ye Tan assist the chief herb by clearing heat and cooling the blood as well as arresting bleeding. Zhi Ke relaxes the intestines and modifies the actions of the herbs that stop bleeding to prevent an impairment of circulation.

Dosage and Method of Preparation: Make a decoction. Drink four ounces of Huai Hua Tang tea three times daily, as needed.

Xiong Dan Zhi Ling Gao (Fel Ursi Hemorrhoid Effective Ointment); also known as Xiong Dan Zhi Chuang Gao

Description: This patent formula stops pain and bleeding; it clears heat (infection), reduces inflammation, and eliminates burning and itching.

Dosage: It comes in tubes of four or ten grams, with complete instructions on dosage.

Huai Jiao Wan (Fructus Sophorae Japonicae Pill); also known as Fructus Sophorae

Description: This patent formula clears heat (infection) in the intestines, stops bleeding, heals hemorrhoids, and reduces pain.

Dosage: It comes in bottles of one hundred pills, with complete instructions on dosage.

Zhen Ren Yang Zang Tang (True Man's Decoction to Nourish the Organs)

Original Source: *Tai Ping Hui Min He Ji Ju Fang* (according to *Chinese Herbal Medicine Formulas and Strategies*)

Ingredients:

Quantity (Grams)	Chinese Herbs	English Translation
6	Ren Shen	Ginseng
12	Bai Zhu	Atractylodes Rhizome
5	Rou Gui	Saigon Cinnamon Inner Bark
15	Wei Rou Dou Kou	Dry-Fried Nutmeg Seeds
15	He Zi	Myrobalan Fruit
20	Zi Ying Su Ke	Honey-Fried Opium Poppy Husk
15	Bai Shao	White Peony Root
12	Dang Gui	Tangkuei
9	Mu Xiang	Costus Root
9	Zhi Gan Cao	Honey-Cooked Licorice Root

Description: This herbal formula is used to tonify deficient organs (intestines), restrain leakage from the intestines, stop diarrhea, stop bleeding, and reduce pain.

Analysis: Ren Shen and Bai Zhu combined are very effective for strengthening the stomach and spleen. Rou Gui and Wei Rou Dou Kou dispel cold and benefit the kidneys and spleen. He Zi and Zi Ying Su Ke are both effective for arresting diarrhea. Bai Shao and Dang Gui enrich the blood to offset the anemia that is often a result of chronic diarrhea. Mu Xiang supports digestion and relieves abdominal pain. Zhi Gan Cao harmonizes the other herbs in this formula and improves taste.

Dosage and Method of Preparation: Prepare a decoction. Drink four ounces of Zhen Ren Yang Zang Tang tea three times daily, as needed.

Hua Zhi Ling Wan (Fargelin for Piles); also known as Qiang Li Hua Zhi Ling

Description: This patent formula clears heat (from intestines), stops pain and bleeding, and is useful for internal or external hemorrhoids and prolapsed anus.

Dosage: It comes in bottles of thirty-six pills, with complete instructions on dosage. For difficult cases, the normal dosage of three to four pills three times daily should be doubled.

Bu Zhong Yi Qi Wan (Tonify Center to Invigorate Qi Pills); also known as Central Qi Pills, or Bu Zhong Yi Chi Wan

Description: This patent formula is useful for treating prolapsed anus, and it strengthens the organs of the digestive system (intestines, stomach, and spleen).

Dosage: It comes in bottles of one hundred pills, with complete instructions on dosage.

Red Eye—see Conjunctivitis

Respiratory Tract Infection—see Bronchitis; Laryngitis; Pneumonia; Sinusitis; Tonsillitis

Respiratory tract infection is an infection of the breathing passages caused by viruses or bacteria. Infection can occur in the upper respiratory tract (nose, throat, sinuses, and larynx) or the lower one (trachea, bronchi, and lungs). Common respiratory infections include those referenced in the heading. See those specific entries for herbal treatments.

Rheumatism—see Arthritis

A popular term for stiffness in the muscles and joints, rheumatism, like arthritis, is referred to in traditional Chinese medicine as wind damp disease. It can be treated with the herbal formulas recommended for arthritis.

Rheumatoid Arthritis—see Arthritis

Rhinitis—see Allergies; Nasal Congestion

Ringing in the Ears—see Tinnitus

Ringworm (see also Athlete's Foot; Fungal Infections/Fungal Diseases; Jock Itch)

Ringworm is a fungal skin infection whose ring-shaped scaly patches inspire its name. Although the fungal infection can appear on any part of the body, the feet, groin, scalp, and trunk are particularly vulnerable. Because of the relationship between ringworm and athlete's foot (tinea pedia), the herbal formulas used for treating one are usually effective for treating the other.

Hua She Jie Yang Wan (Pit Viper Dispel Itching Pills); also known as Kai Yeung Pills

Description: This patent formula counteracts itching, resolves fungal infections, and is useful for various skin diseases such as ringworm, eczema, pruritus, and dermatitis.

Caution: This formula is prohibited for use during pregnancy.

Dosage: It comes in bottles of sixty pills, with complete instructions on dosage.

Fu Ling Tu Jin Pi Ding (Complex Tu Jin Bark Tincture); also known as Composita Tujin Ointment, or Fu Fang Tu Jin Pi Ding

Description: This patent formula is useful for treating skin infections caused by fungus, tinea, or scabies.

Note: This formula is for external use only.

Dosage: It comes in bottles of 15cc, with complete instructions on dosage.

Roundworms (see also Intestine, Disorders of; Larva Migrans)

Roundworms, also known as nematodes, are a variety of parasitic worms that inhabit the human intestine. Unless there is serious infestation, their presence usually goes undetected due to a lack of symptoms. Normally, their presence becomes apparent when the roundworm larvae pass through various parts of the body. The most common types of roundworm include the pinworm, which mainly affects children, and trichinosis, which affects adults and is often contracted from ingesting undercooked pork.

Traditional Chinese medicine uses the following formulas to treat roundworm:

Wu Mei Tang (Mume Decoction)

Original Source: *Shang Han Lun* (according to *Chinese Herbal Medicine Formulas and Strategies*)

Ingredients:

Quantity (Grams)	Chinese Herbs	English Translation
30	Wu Mei	Dark Plum Fruit
3	Chuan Jiao	Szechuan Pepper Fruit
3	Xi Xin	Chinese Wild Ginger Plant
12	Huang Lian	Golden Thread Root
9	Huang Bai	Amur Cork Tree Bark

9	Gan Jiang	Dried Ginger Root
6	Fu Zi	Accessory Root Szechuan Aconite
6	Gui Zhi	Saigon Cinnamon Twig
9	Ren Shen	Ginseng
9	Dang Gui	Tangkuei

Description: This herbal formula warms the intestines and eliminates roundworms.

Analysis: The chief herb, Wu Mei, is very sour tasting, but effective in eliminating roundworms. Chuan Jiao and Xi Xin are both more general in their ability to expel parasites and warm the organs. Huang Bai and Huang Lian assist in attacking parasites. Gan Jiang, Fu Zi, and Gui Zhi all warm the interior to offset the cold, sour nature of the "attacking" herbs. Ren Shen and Dang Gui strengthen the vital energy (Chi) and enrich the blood.

Dosage and Method of Preparation: Prepare a decoction. Drink four ounces of Wu Mei Tang tea three times daily, as needed.

Lidan Paishi Wan (Benefit Gallbladder Discharge Stone Tablets); also known as Li Dan Pai Shi Pian, or Li Dan Tablets

Description: This patent formula clears infection, kills worms, reduces inflammation, and is useful for roundworm infestation.

Caution: This formula is prohibited for use during pregnancy.

Dosage: It comes in bottles of 120 tablets, with complete instructions on dosage.

Rubella—see Measles

Scarlet Fever

A few centuries ago scarlet fever was considered life threatening; today it is far less common and is not considered nearly as dangerous. An infectious disease that mainly affects children, its initial symptoms include sore throat, fever, and rash. The rash, which normally appears three to five days after the sore throat and fever, begins as a mass of tiny red spots on the neck and upper trunk. The symptom that defines the disease is a white coating with red spots that develops on the tongue, which after a few days peels away to reveal a bright red or scarlet appearance. Soon afterward, the fever subsides, and the rash fades. Although uncommon, if the infection is left untreated, the patient runs a risk of contracting rheumatic fever or inflammation of the kidneys.

Western medical treatment typically relies on an antibiotic such as penicillin or erythromycin. Chinese herbal formulas are also concerned with resolving infection as well as eliminating fever and reducing pain.

Sheng Ma Ge Gen Tang (Cimicifuga and Kudzu Decoction)

Original Source: *Xiao Er Yao Zheng Zhi Jue* (according to *Chinese Herbal Medicine Formulas and Strategies*)

Ingredients:

Quantity (Grams)	Chinese Herbs	English Translation
6	Sheng Ma	Black Cohosh Rhizome (Cimicifuga)
9	Ge Gen	Kudzu Root
3	Zhi Gan Cao	Honey-Cooked Licorice Root
9	Chi Shao	Red Peony Root
9	Jie Geng	Balloon Flower Root
6	Xuan Shen	Ningpo Figwort Root
6	Ma Bo	Puffball Fruit

Description: This herbal formula is used to heal sore throat and reduce swelling; it resolves rashes, reduces fever, stops pain, and is used for scarlet fever and measles.

Analysis: Sheng Ma clears the stomach and effectively reduces rashes. Ge Gen assists by opening the pores of the skin; it also expels heat. Zhi Gan Cao relieves toxicity. Chi Shao moves blood and clears infection. Jie Geng, Xuan Shen, and Ma Bo combine to relieve itching and to clear heat, inflammation, and infection.

Dosage and Method of Preparation: Prepare a decoction. Drink four ounces of Sheng Ma Ge Gen Tang tea three times daily, as needed.

Qing Yin Wan (Clear Voice Pills)

Description: This patent formula is used to nourish fluids (prevent dehydration) and to clear heat (infection) in the throat and lungs; it is useful for painful and swollen throat such as that accompanying scarlet fever, tonsillitis, and Vincent's angina.

Dosage: It comes in boxes of ten honey pills, with complete instructions on dosage.

Liu Shen Wan (Six Spirit Pills); also known as Lu Shen Wan

Description: This patent formula eliminates infection, decreases inflammation, reduces fever, stops pain, and is useful for treating scarlet fever, Vincent's angina, and strep throat.

Caution: This formula is prohibited for use during pregnancy.

Dosage: It comes in bottles of thirty or one hundred pills, with complete instructions on dosage.

Shuang Liao Hou Feng San (Double Ingredient Sore Throat Disease Powder); also known as Superior Sore Throat Powder Spray

Description: This patent formula is a throat spray useful for treating oral infections such as scarlet fever, tonsillitis, pharyngitis, and others.

Note: This formula is to be used only as a spray and is not to be ingested.

Dosage: It comes in a vial containing powder, with complete instructions on dosage.

Seizure (see also Epilepsy)

Generally speaking, seizures result from irregular electrical brain activity that can be caused by a variety of neurological problems. Possible causes include head injury, infection, cerebrovascular accident (stroke), brain tumor, metabolic disturbances, or alcohol or drug withdrawal. When seizures are recurrent, they are called epilepsy. Both Western and Chinese medicine's approach to treatment depends on the cause for the seizure. Herbal formulas can be useful for the specific condition for which they are recommended (refer to Description under each formula).

Zhi Bao Dan (Greatest Treasure Special Decoction)

Original Source: *Tai Ping Hui Min He Ji Ju Fang* (according to *Chinese Herbal Medicine Formulas and Strategies*)

Ingredients:

Quantity (Grams)	Chinese Herbs	English Translation
30	Xi Jiao	Rhinoceros Horn
15	Niu Huang	Cow/Water Buffalo Gallbladder Calculae
30	Dai Mao	Hawksbill Turtle Shell
.3	Bing Pian	Resin of Borneol Camphor
.3	She Xiang	Musk Deer Gland Secretions
45	An Xi Xiang	Benzoin Resin
30	Zha Sha	Cinnabar
30	Hu Po	Amber
30	Xiong Huang	Realgar

Description: This herbal formula is useful for delirium, convulsions, spasms, and seizures such as those associated with encephalitis, meningitis, and epilepsy.

Caution: This formula is prohibited for use during pregnancy.

Analysis: Xi Jiao clears heat and cools the blood. Niu Huang clears heat; it also relieves toxicity and opens the orifices. Dai Mo benefits the liver and is an important ingredient in this formula because of its ability to stop spasms and convulsions. Bing Pian, She Xiang, and An Xi Xiang open the orifices and eliminate internal obstruction. Zha Sha and Hu Po have a sedative effect and Xiong Huang relieves toxicity.

Dosage and Method of Preparation: Grind the herbs into a fine powder. Dissolve three grams of powdered Zhi Bao Dan into eight ounces of warm water, mix well, and drink, as needed.

She Dan Chen Pi San (Snake Gallbladder Tangerine Peel Powder); also known as San She Tan Chen Pi Mo

Description: This patent formula is useful for treating epilepsy, with grand mal or petit mal seizures. This herbal medicine may be taken with other seizure medications such as phenobarbital or Dilantin.

Dosage: It comes in vials containing .6 gram of powder, with complete instructions on dosage.

Septicemia

More commonly known as blood poisoning, septicemia occurs when bacteria rapidly multiply in the blood. Normally, it results from bacteria escaping an infection elsewhere in the body, such as from an abscess, a urinary tract or intestinal infection, pneumonia, or meningitis. People whose resistance is lowered by an immunodeficiency disorder or from taking immunosuppressant drugs are at a greater risk of suffering from septicemia. It causes a person to become suddenly ill, with accompanying chills, high fever, rapid breathing, headache, and clouded consciousness. If anyone exhibits these symptoms, emergency treatment should be sought. If the condition remains unchecked, in most cases the patient passes into a state of septic shock, a life-threatening condition. Traditional Chinese medicine's use of antibiotic herbs and blood cleansers should only be considered when the infection is minor and the fever is low-grade.

Qing Ying Tang (Clear the Nutritive Level Decoction)

Original Source: *Wen Bing Tiao Bian* (according to *Chinese Herbal Medicine Formulas and Strategies*)

Ingredients:

Quantity (Grams)	Chinese Herbs	English Translation
9	Xuan Shen	Ningpo Figwort Root
15	Sheng Di Huang	Chinese Foxglove Root, Raw
9	Mai Men Dong	Lush Winter Wheat Tuber

9	Jin Yin Hua	Honeysuckle Flower
6	Lian Qiao	Forsythia Fruit
4.5	Huang Lian	Golden Thread Root
3	Dan Zhu Ye	Bland Bamboo Leaves
6	Dan Shen	Salvia Root
9	Xi Jiao★	Rhinoceros Horn

★See special instructions for preparation below.

Description: This herbal formula is used to relieve fever, clear infection, and replenish fluids; it is useful for septicemia, meningitis, and encephalitis.

Analysis: Xi Jiao clears heat and has a calming effect. Mai Men Dong and Xuan Shen clear heat and nourish the body fluids. Sheng Di Huang cools the blood. Jin Yin Hua, Lian Qiao, Huang Lian, and Dan Zhu Ye also clear heat in addition to eliminating infection. Dan Shen cools the blood and prevents blood stasis (poor circulation).

Dosage and Method of Preparation: Prepare a decoction. Xi Jiao (Rhinoceros Horn) should be ground into a fine powder and added to the strained, prepared decoction when you are ready to drink the recommended dosage; do not cook this herb with the rest of the ingredients. Drink four ounces of Qing Ying Tang tea (mixed with nine grams of powdered Xi Jiao) three times daily, as needed.

An Kung Niu Huang Wan (Peaceful Palace Ox Gallstone Pills); also known as An Gong Niu Huang Wan

Description: This patent formula is useful for treating diseases with high-grade fever, when the body fluids have been damaged from disorders such as encephalitis, bacillary dysentery, and other serious infections, including septicemia.

Caution: This formula is prohibited for use during pregnancy.

Dosage: It comes in boxes of ten honey pills, with complete instructions on dosage.

Shingles—see Herpes Zoster

Sickle-Cell Anemia

Sickle-cell anemia is a blood disease in which the red blood cells are abnormal, causing a chronic, severe form of anemia. These red blood cells contain a type of hemoglobin known as hemoglobin S; when hemoglobin S crystallizes, it distorts the red cells into a sickle shape. This disease, which is inherited, primarily affects people of African descent, although individuals of Mediterranean and Southeast Asian origin can also be affected. Sickle-cell anemia occurs in people who have inherited hemoglobin S from both parents. If it is inherited from only one parent, the person has what is known as sickle-cell trait and usually does not suffer from the symptoms characteristic of sickle-cell anemia. The symptoms, which include fatigue, headaches, shortness of breath, pallor, and jaundice, usually first appear at approximately six months of age. A sickle-cell crisis can be brought on by a variety of conditions or circumstances, including infection, cold weather, and dehydration. Or, it may occur for no apparent reason. During a crisis, the sufferer may experience pain (especially in the bones), blood in the urine, seizures, and, on rare occasions, a stroke or unconsciousness. Sufferers also sustain an increased risk of contracting pneumococcal pneumonia.

Sickle-cell anemia is treatable but is as yet incurable. When a crisis occurs, it can be life threatening and should be considered a medical emergency requiring immediate treatment. Traditional Chinese medicine uses the following formula to treat sickle-cell anemia:

Xiao Ji Yin Zi (Cephalanoplos Decoction)

Original Source: *Ji Sheng Fang* (according to *Chinese Herbal Medicine Formulas and Strategies*)

Ingredients:

Quantity (Grams)	Chinese Herbs	English Translation
15	Xiao Ji	Small Thistle Plant
15	Ou Jie	Lotus Rhizome, Node
15	Chao Pu Huang	Dry-Fried Cattail Pollen
120	Sheng Di Huang	Chinese Foxglove Root, Raw
15	Hua Shi	Talcum, Mineral

15	Mu Tong	Wood with Holes
15	Dan Zhu Ye	Bland Bamboo Leaves
15	Zhi Zi	Gardenia Fruit
15	Dang Gui	Tangkuei
15	Zhi Gan Cao	Honey-Cooked Licorice Root

Description: This herbal formula is useful for treating sickle-cell anemia, with symptoms of blood in the urine and burning pain. The formula nurtures the yin to resolve dehydration, while it nourishes the blood to resolve anemia.

Analysis: Xiao Ji, Ou Jie, Chao Pu Huang, and Sheng Di Huang cool the blood and stop bleeding. Hua Shi clears heat, promotes urination, and stops pain. Mu Tong, Dan Zhu Ye, and Zhi Zi eliminate heat, directing it downward and out of the body through urination. Dang Gui nourishes the blood, and Zhi Gan Cao relieves pain, benefits the spleen and stomach, and harmonizes the actions of the other herbs in the formula.

Dosage and Method of Preparation: Prepare a decoction. Drink four ounces of Xiao Ji Yin Zi tea three times daily, as needed.

Sinusitis

Inflammation of the sinuses, or sinusitis as it is clinically known, is most often caused by infection spreading to the sinuses from the nose. The infection typically starts as a viral infection such as the common cold. Less commonly, sinuses can become inflamed or infected as a result of an allergic reaction (e.g., hay fever), an abscess in an upper tooth, or a severe facial injury. Stuffy nose, throbbing pain, fever, pus in the affected sinuses, and copious nasal discharge are all common symptoms.

Traditional Chinese medicine offers several flower remedies useful for treating sinus infections from any of these causes.

Cang Er Zi Tang (Xanthium Decoction)

Original Source: *Ji Sheng Fang* (according to *Chinese Herbal Medicine Formulas and Strategies*)

Ingredients:

Quantity (Grams)	Chinese Herbs	English Translation
9	Cang Er Zi	Xanthium Fruit
6	Xin Yin Hua	Magnolia Flower
9	Bai Zhi	Angelica Dahuricae Root
6	Bo He★	Peppermint

★See special instructions for preparation below.

Description: This herbal formula alleviates pain in the sinus region, unlocks the nose, and resolves infection.

Analysis: The chief herb, Cang Er Zi, along with Xin Yin Hua, unblocks the nasal passages and arrests nasal discharge. Bai Zhi resolves dampness, while Bo He clears the eyes and head. Xin Yin Hua treats infection.

Dosage and Method of Preparation: Prepare a decoction. Bo He should not be added to the decoction until the last five minutes of cooking time. Overcooking Bo He will reduce its effectiveness. Drink four ounces of Cang Er Zi Tang tea three times daily, as needed.

Pe Min Kan Wan (Nose Allergy Pill); also known as Bi Min Gan Wan

Description: This patent formula stops headaches and eliminates inflammation; it is useful for symptoms such as runny nose, stuffy nose and sneezing associated with common cold, flu, and allergies.

Dosage: It comes in bottles of fifty pills, with complete instructions on dosage.

Bi Yan Pian (Nose Inflammation Pill)

Description: This patent formula reduces fever, resolves inflammation and infection, and is useful for sinusitis symptoms including sneezing, itchy eyes, facial congestion, and sinus pain caused by allergies or the common cold.

Dosage: It comes in bottles of one hundred tablets, with complete instructions on dosage.

Chuan Xiong Cha Tiao Wan (Ligusticum Tea Adjust Pill); also known as Chuan Qiong Cha Tiao Wan

Description: This patent formula stops sinus pain and eliminates headaches associated with nasal congestion and sinusitis.

Note: The effects of this formula are enhanced when taken with strong green tea.

Dosage: It comes in bottles of two hundred pills, with complete instructions on dosage.

Bi Tong Tablet (Nose Open Tablet); also known as Tablet Bi-Tong

Description: This patent formula resolves phlegm, stops pain associated with allergies, and treats common cold with accompanying symptoms of sneezing, watery eyes, and facial congestion.

Dosage: It comes in bottles of one hundred pills, with complete instructions on dosage.

Sore Throat (see also Laryngitis; Tonsillitis)

In most cases, inflammation of the throat (especially that which causes discomfort from swallowing) is usually the first symptom of the common cold. Occasionally, a sore throat is symptomatic of a number of commonly occurring disorders such as pharyngitis, tonsillitis, laryngitis, or infectious mononucleosis, as well as many common childhood viral illnesses such as chicken pox, measles, or mumps (see also Chicken Pox; Measles; Mumps). In rare instances, it is brought on by the more serious streptococcal infection (causing strep throat), which if left untreated can cause acute glomerulonephritis (inflammation in the kidneys), rheumatic fever, or scarlet fever. The following Chinese herbal formulas are useful for treating simple inflammation of the throat as well as viral infections that cause sore throat:

Qiang Lan Tang (Notopterygium and Isatis Root Decoction)

Original Source: *Fang Ji Xue* (according to *Chinese Herbal Medicine Formulas and Strategies*)

Ingredients:

Quantity (Grams)	Chinese Herbs	English Translation
12	Qiang Huo	Notopterygium Rhizome
30	Ban Lan Gen	Woad Root (Isatis Root)
9	Ma Bo	Puffball Fruit
9	Shan Dou Gen	Mountain Bean Root
9	Xuan Shen	Ningpo Figwort Root

Description: This herbal formula is used for fever and sore, swollen throat with or without swollen lymph glands. It is useful for relief of severe sore throat discomfort.

Analysis: Qiang Huo, the chief herb, relieves painful sore throat, while its assistant, Ban Lan Gen, reduces fever and clears infection. Ma Bo, Shan Dou Gen, and Xuan Shen are all anti-inflammatory; they eliminate infection and benefit the mucus membrane in the throat.

Dosage and Method of Preparation: Prepare a decoction. Drink four ounces of Qiang Lan Tang tea three times daily, as needed.

Hou Yan Wan (Laryngitis Pills); also known as Larynx Inflammation Pills

Description: This patent formula is applicable for sore throat with hoarseness or laryngitis or for tonsillitis or mumps. If strep infection is involved, combine use of this formula with the next formula, Chuan Xin Lian-Antiphlogistic Pills.

Caution: This formula is prohibited for use during pregnancy.

Dosage: It comes in boxes of three vials, ten pills per vial, with complete instructions on dosage.

Chuang Xin Lian-Antiphlogistic Pills (Penetrate Heart, Repeatedly Fighting Heat Pills); also known as Chuang Xin Lian Kang Yan Pian

Description: This patent formula is used for acute throat inflammation with swollen glands and fever, including strep throat and measles.

Dosage: It comes in bottles of sixty pills, with complete instructions on dosage.

Qing Yin Wan (Clear Voice Pills)

Description: This patent formula is useful for treating hoarseness, swollen and painful throat, tonsillitis, and scarlet fever.

Dosage: It comes in boxes of ten honey pills, with complete instructions on dosage.

Ling Yang Shang Feng Ling (Antelope Horn Injured by Wind Efficacious Remedy)

Description: This formula resolves inflammation of the throat and soothes and moistens the mucus membrane (tissue lining the throat).

Dosage: It comes in bottles of sixty tablets, with complete instructions on dosage.

Sprain

A sprain is the tearing or stretching of a ligament, causing painful swelling of the joint. It is a relatively common injury most often incurred during sports or athletic activities. Treatment normally consists of applying an ice pack to reduce swelling, wrapping the injury with a compression bandage, and resting the affected joint. In extremely severe cases involving torn ligaments, surgical repair may be necessary. The Chinese herbal formulas for sprains have proven effective through their long history of use for treating injuries incurred in the performance of Chinese martial arts.

Chin Koo Tieh Shang Wan (Muscle and Bone Traumatic Injury Pill); also known as Jin Gu Die Shang Wan

Description: This patent formula is used for relief of bruising and swelling due to traumatic injuries such as strains, sprains, and fractures.

Caution: This formula is prohibited for use during pregnancy.

Dosage: It comes in bottles of 120 pills, with complete instructions on dosage.

Hsiung Tan Tieh Ta Wan (Bear Gallbladder Traumatic Injury Pill); also known as Xiong Dan Die Dan Wan

Description: This patent formula relieves swelling due to sprains, trauma, and bruises. It promotes healing and repairs injured blood vessels. This formula is popular in China for injuries due to sports or martial arts training.

Caution: This formula is prohibited for use during pregnancy.

Dosage: This patent medicine comes in boxes of ten pills, with complete instructions on dosage.

Zheng Gu Shui (Rectify Bone Liquid)

Description: This patent formula is useful for sprains, fractures, ligament strains and tears, and bruising.

Dosage: It comes in bottles of 30cc or 100cc, with complete instructions on dosage.

Hu Gu Gao (Tiger Balm)

Description: This patent formula is used for sprains, strains, contusions, bruises, and fractures. It reduces pain and improves circulation, and it relaxes muscles and tendons.

Dosage: It comes in a jar containing eighteen grams, with complete instructions on dosage.

Stomatitis (see also Fever Blister; Herpes [Oral]; Ulcer)

Although stomach heat and hyperacidity can cause this condition, clinically speaking, stomatitis is any kind of inflammation or ulcer in the mouth. Examples of stomatitis are mouth ulcers, canker sores, cold sores, candidiasis (thrush), and Vincent's angina.

Traditional Chinese medicine treats oral inflammations with the following formulas:

Niu Huang Shang Qing Wan (Cow Gallstone Upper Clear Pill); also known as Niu Huang Shang Ching Wan

Description: This patent formula clears heat from the upper body; it is useful for treating inflammation or infection in the mouth—with or without fever—such as oral herpes, canker sores, and fever blisters.

Caution: This formula is prohibited for use during pregnancy.

Dosage: It comes in bottles of fifty pills, with complete instructions on dosage.

Liu Shen Wan (Six Spirit Pills); also known as Lu Shen Wan

Description: This patent formula resolves infection, decreases inflammation, stops pain, and is useful for treating stomatitis, tonsillitis, and Vincent's angina.

Caution: This formula is prohibited for use during pregnancy.

Dosage: It comes in bottles of thirty or one hundred pills, with complete instructions on dosage.

Xi Gua Shuang (Watermelon Frost); also known as Xi Gua Shuang Run Ho Pian, or Xi Gua Shuang Pen Ji

Description: This patent formula is used for treating diseases in the mouth, including sores, ulcers, stomatitis, and Vincent's angina.

Dosage: It comes in three different forms: powder, spray, and lozenges. The powder (Xi Gua Shuang) comes in vials containing two grams of powder. The powder form, the spray form (Xi Gua Shuang Pen Ji), and the lozenge form (Xi Gua Shuang Run Ho Pian) all come with instructions on dosage.

Strep Throat—see Sore Throat

Stress

The long list of diseases known to be stress related—such as hypertension, gastrointestinal disorders, migraine headaches, and the number one cause of death in the United States, heart disease—clearly point out the profound effect stress bears on overall physical health.

When we consider the constant pressure of modern society, managing one's emotions is easier said than done. But we must overcome the inability to cope and develop a wholesome mental attitude if good health and long life are going to be realistic expectations. Many factors can interfere with a person's mental well-being. They range from mundane daily activities to significant life events such as the death of a loved one, divorce, childbirth, or ill health. Developing techniques for managing the minor stress that is a part of daily affairs is fairly easy. More challenging is acquiring the ability to manage major emotional trauma resulting from deeply emotional life experiences. Doing so usually requires drawing upon spiritual resources. When these stressful situations are left unresolved, they become progressively worse, injuring physical health and developing into more serious mental disorders such as anxiety, depression, or post-traumatic stress syndrome.

Of course, the first order of business in managing stress is to identify the source or underlying cause. Once this is done, certain relaxation techniques can be applied whenever the causative circumstances occur. These techniques, designed to bring about a state of physical and mental calm, focus on regulating breathing, relaxing muscle tension, and subjugating mental activity. Even though the techniques employ the same principles used in meditation, the user need not be religious to experience the physical benefits provided by practicing them. To be sure, however, utilizing the spiritual component of meditation is also highly recommended. Chinese medicine believes that the practice of meditation for nurturing the spirit as well as reducing stress levels is a key factor in maintaining the mental and physical well-being required to live a long life. Chinese medicine's theory concerning the relationship between stress and disease is demonstrated by the fact that stress levels are always considered as part of any diagnosis when determining the root cause of physical disease, and more often than not meditation is part of the curative recommendation.

Realizing that there are differences in physical capability, Chinese medicine offers a variety of meditative postures that can be useful regardless of one's current state of health. For the most debilitated, reclining meditation is an option, followed by sitting, kneeling, standing, walking, and moving meditation, more popularly known as Tai Chi Chuan.

Two excellent reference sources on meditation are *Tao of Meditation,* by Stephen Chang (Tao Publishing, San Francisco, CA), and *Transcendental Meditation,* by Robert Roth (Donald I. Fine, Inc., New York, NY).

Along with choosing a form of meditation, the use of herbs for enhancing the process might also be considered. Herbal formulas that have a long history of use for relaxing the body and calming the mind are known to have a sedative effect and can be used several different ways: more generally, for reducing agitation, abating restlessness, and diminishing mental hyperactivity or simply as an adjunct to intensify meditation. Several herbal formulas follow that should prove useful in managing and reducing stress levels. It has been said, "You are what you eat." To that I might add: you are what you think, and what you think has a profound effect upon your state of health.

An Shen Jing Nao Fang (Calm the Spirit and Tranquilize the Mind Decoction)

Source: *Shaolin Secret Formulas for the Treatment of External Injury*
Ingredients:

Quantity (Grams)	Chinese Herbs	English Translation
9	Fu Shen	Tuckahoe Spirit Fungus
9	Yi Zhi Ren	Alpinia Fruit
.3	Zhen Zhu	Pearl
.3	Peng Sha	Borax
.6	Hu Po	Amber
.6	Zhu Sha	Cinnabar
1.5	Mu Xiang	Costus Root

Description: The qualities of certain formulas appeal to us for personal reasons. This is not to say that one is better than another. Our preference is sometimes based on taste or simply on the way a particular formula makes us feel. This formula, whose indications are similar to that of the next formula, is useful for enhancing meditation.

Analysis: The herbs Fu Shen, Yi Zhi Ren, Zhen Zhu, and Hu Po all sedate, pacify the spirit, and tranquilize the mind. Zhu Sha also has a mild sedative effect. Mu Xiang promotes the flow of vital energy (Chi), and Peng Sha clears heat.

Dosage and Method of Preparation: The herbs in this formula should be ground into a fine powder and kept in a bottle for later use. This can be done by grinding the herbs in a blender, or they can be purchased ground from the herb supplier. Mix .06 grams of powder with two ounces of sweet rice wine and two ounces of tepid water. Drink three times daily. Because this formula calms the spirit and abates restlessness, it can be used to achieve deeper levels of meditation.

Er Miao An Shen Tang (Two-Herb Formula for Calming the Spirit)

Ingredients:

Quantity (Grams)	Chinese Herbs	English Translation
15	Long Gu	Dragon Bones
9	Suan Zao Ren	Sour Jujube Seeds

Description: This herbal formula is used to tranquilize the mind; it calms the spirit and abates restlessness. While the use of this formula will not cause drowsiness or cause the user to become stupefied, its effects are noticeable, and its use during meditation is recommended.

Analysis: Long Gu settles and calms the spirit and is used to abate restlessness and subdue agitation. Suan Zao Ren calms the spirit and cures irritability.

Dosage and Method of Preparation: Prepare a decoction. Drink four ounces of Er Miao An Shen Tang tea, as needed.

An Mien Pien (Peaceful Sleep Tablets); also known as An Mian Pian

Description: This patent formula is used to calm the spirit and tranquilize the mind.

Dosage: It comes in bottles of sixty tablets, with complete instructions on dosage.

Suan Zao Ren Tang Pien (Ziziyphus Seed Soup Tablet); also known as Tabellae Suanzaoren Tang

Description: This patent formula is a classical prescription for insomnia, restlessness, palpitations, and mental agitation. It is commonly used for stress relief.

Dosage: It comes in bottles of forty-eight tablets, with complete instructions on dosage.

Bu Nao Wan (Supplement Brain Pills); also known as Cerebral Tonic Pills

Description: This patent formula is used for stress; it improves poor concentration and memory and calms restlessness, mental agitation, manic episodes, and insomnia.

Dosage: It comes in bottles of three hundred pills, with complete instructions on dosage.

Deng Xin Wan (Stabilize Heart Pills); also known as Ding Xin Wan

Description: This patent formula is used for stress relief; it calms restlessness, anxiety, palpitations, and insomnia, and improves poor memory.

Dosage: It comes in bottles of one hundred pills, with complete instructions on dosage.

Jian Nao Wan (Healthy Brain Pill)

Description: This patent formula is useful for stress; it calms agitation, mental exhaustion, palpitations, and insomnia.

Dosage: It comes in bottles of three hundred pills, with complete instructions on dosage.

Stroke

A stroke results from damage to part of the brain caused by interruption of its blood supply. There are three principal causes: cerebral thrombosis, blockage by a clot that has built up on the wall of an artery; cerebral embolism, blockage by a clot that has swept into an artery from another site in the body; and cerebral hemorrhage, rupture of a blood vessel, causing bleeding within the brain. One of the leading causes of death in developed countries, strokes are more easily prevented than cured. Certain factors increase the risk of suffering a stroke, such as hypertension, which does so by weakening the arteries, making them more susceptible to rupture (cerebral hemorrhage); and arteriosclerosis, which narrows the arteries, impeding blood flow and making blockage (cerebral embolism) more likely. Other factors that increase risk are arterial fibrillation (irregular heartbeat), a damaged heart value, and a recent heart attack. Each of these conditions can create blood clots in the heart that could potentially break off and travel to the brain, causing a stroke.

Symptoms of a stroke include headache, dizziness, confusion, visual disturbance, slurred speech or loss of speech, and difficulty swallowing. **Note:** If these symptoms are exhibited, emergency medical attention should be sought.

Risk factors include aging, high blood pressure, arteriosclerosis, heart disease, diabetes mellitus, smoking, polycythemia (excess red blood cells), hyperlipidemia (high levels of fatty substances in the blood), and the use of estrogen supplements.

Traditional Chinese medicine emphasizes preventive measures (wholesome diet, adequate amounts of exercise, all things in moderation, and avoidance of stress), along with the recommended herbal formulas, which can be useful in prestroke conditions or following its occurrence.

Bu Yang Huan Wu Tang (Tonify the Yang to Restore Five [Tenths] Decoction)

Original Source: *Yi Lin Gai Cuo* (according to *Chinese Herbal Medicine Formulas and Strategies*)

Ingredients:

Quantity (Grams)	Chinese Herbs	English Translation
120	Huang Qi	Milk-Vetch Root
6	Dang Gui	Tangkuei

3	Chuan Xiong	Szechuan Lovage Root
4.5	Chi Shao	Red Peony Root
3	Tao Ren	Peach Kernel
3	Hong Hua	Safflower Flowers
3	Di Long	Earthworm

Description: This herbal formula is used for treating stroke with hemiplegia and atrophy of the lower limbs, facial paralysis, and slurred speech. Because this formula is an anticoagulant (breaks up clotting), it should not be used when the cause of stroke is cerebral hemorrhage. Until the etiology is established and cerebral hemorrhage is ruled out, do not use this formula. It can be safely used when the patient is fully conscious, body temperature has normalized, and when there is no presence of hemorrhage.

Caution: This formula is prohibited for use during pregnancy.

Analysis: The chief herb, Huang Qi, powerfully tonifies the vital energy (Chi). Dang Gui, Chuan Xiong, and Chi Shao together nourish and circulate the blood. Tao Ren and Hong Hua assist in blood circulation by unblocking the channels. Di Long unblocks the meridians, allowing efficient circulation of both blood and Chi to the lower extremities.

Dosage and Method of Preparation: Prepare a decoction. Drink four ounces of Bu Yang Huan Wu Tang tea three times daily, as needed.

Mao Dong Ching (Ilex Root); also known as Mao Dang Qing

Description: This patent formula is a single-herb remedy used for numbness in the limbs and poor circulation. It is useful as a treatment and preventive measure in strokes, embolism, heart disease, and arteriosclerosis. Studies indicate the most effective treatment plan for stroke victims is to use this formula for a course of seven days, taking three capsules three times daily, followed by a rest period for three days. If the symptoms persist, repeat the procedure.

Dosage: It comes in a bottle of thirty capsules, with complete instructions on dosage.

中草藥

Ren Shen Zai Zao Wan (Ginseng Restorative Pills); also known as Tsai Tsao Wan

Description: This patent formula is primarily used to address symptoms related to stroke, including hemiplegia, speech disturbances, and contractive or flaccid muscle tone in the extremities.

Caution: This formula is prohibited for use during pregnancy.

Dosage: It comes in boxes containing ten wax, egg-shaped capsules encasing the herbs, with complete instructions on dosage.

Yan Shen Jai Jao Wan (Ginseng Restorative Pills); also known as Ren Shen Zai Zao Wan

Description: This patent formula has the same name as the previously mentioned patent formula, yet a significantly different prescription. It is used for stroke symptoms such as hemiplegia, spastic paralysis, facial distortion, and difficulty speaking. It is excellent for stroke symptoms if administered immediately following the stroke but is less effective after the onset of flaccid paralysis.

Caution: This formula is prohibited for use during pregnancy.

Dosage: This patent medicine comes in boxes containing ten wax, egg-shaped capsules encasing the herbs, with complete instructions on dosage.

Sunburn

Sunburn is inflammation of the skin caused by overexposure to the sun. Although it is more common in fair-skinned people, whose skin produces lower amounts of the protective pigment melanin, anyone can suffer from it. In mild cases, the affected skin becomes reddened or inflamed and may become blistered. In severe cases, symptoms such as those associated with sunstroke may also be experienced, including dehydration, fever, and exhaustion. After several days, the dead skin cells are shed by peeling. A word of warning: repeated overexposure to sunlight can prematurely age the skin and increase the risk of skin cancer.

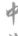

According to both Western and traditional Chinese medicine, prevention is the best course of action against sunburn through the use of sunscreen lotions with the appropriate protection factor. If, however, sunburn occurs, several herbal formulas are useful for treating it.

Jing Wan Hong (Capitol City [Beijing] Many Red Colors); also known as Ching Wan Hung

Description: This patent formula is useful for treating any kind of burn (first, second, or third degree), including sunburn, burns caused by steam, hot water, flame, hot oil, chemical burns, radiation burns (including burns from radiation therapy), and electrical burns. Pain stops immediately upon applying this ointment.

Dosage: It comes in tubes of thirty or five hundred grams, with complete instructions on dosage.

Xi Gua Shuang (Watermelon Frost); also known as Xi Gua Shuang Pen Ji

Description: This patent formula is useful for treating skin burns of various types.

Dosage: It comes in powder or spray. In powdered form (Xi Gua Shuang), the package instructions recommend mixing the powder with mineral or corn oil and applying the mixture directly to the burn. The spray form (Xi Gua Shuang Pen Jie) is sprayed directly onto the affected area. Both are available with instructions on dosage.

Sunstroke

Sunstroke is heatstroke caused by direct exposure to the sun. It typically exhibits symptoms such as high body temperature, a cessation of sweating (brought on by dehydration), dizziness, dry mouth, and exhaustion. Treatment is directed at reestablishing the body's fluid balance and clearing the senses. The following Chinese herbal formulas can be helpful:

Sheng Mai Tang (Generate the Pulse Decoction)

Original Source: *Nei Wai Shang Bian Huo Lun* (according to *Chinese Herbal Medicine Formulas and Strategies*)

Ingredients:

Quantity (Grams)	Chinese Herbs	English Translation
15	Ren Shen	Ginseng
12	Mei Men Dong	Lush Winter Wheat Tuber
6	Wu Wei Zi	Schizandra Fruit

Description: This herbal formula is used to treat symptoms of sunstroke such as spontaneous sweating, dry mouth, and fatigue.

Analysis: The chief herb, Ren Shen, strengthens the vital energy (Chi) and nourishes the fluids. Wu Wei Zi and Mei Men Dong assist the chief herb with their ability to moisten, which is necessary because of the dryness associated with heated conditions.

Dosage and Method of Preparation: Prepare a decoction. Drink four ounces of Sheng Mai Tang tea three times daily, as needed.

Ji Zhong Shui (Benefit Many Problems Liquid); also known as Liu Shen Shui or Chi Chung Shui

Description: This patent formula is useful in an emergency for treating symptoms of sunstroke such as dizziness, dehydration, and exhaustion.

Caution: This formula is prohibited for use during pregnancy.

Dosage: It comes in box of twelve vials, 2cc per vial, with complete instructions for dosage.

Zi Jin Ding (Purple Gold Ding); also known as Yu Zhu Dan

Description: This patent formula is useful for treating heatstroke with dizziness, semiconsciousness, overheatedness, and exhaustion.

Caution: This formula is prohibited for use during pregnancy.

Dosage: It comes in vials of three grams each, with complete instructions on dosage.

Tendonitis

Inflammation of a tendon, known as tendonitis, most often occurs during athletic activities. It can also be a residual condition associated with chronic arthritis. Symptoms include pain, tenderness, and occasionally restricted movement of the muscle attached to the affected tendon. Traditional Chinese medicine treats this condition with acupuncture, massage, and herbal therapy. The following formulas are useful for internal and external treatment of tendonitis:

Tu Zhung Feng Shi Wan (Eucommia Bark Wind Damp Pills); also known as Du Zhong Feng Shi Wan

Description: This patent formula is used to strengthen the bones and tendons; it improves circulation, stops pain, and reduces inflammation.

Caution: This formula is prohibited for use during pregnancy.

Dosage: It comes in bottles of 60 or 120 pills, with complete instructions on dosage.

Zheng Gu Shui (Rectify Bone Liquid)

Description: This patent formula is used for tendonitis, sprains, aching muscles, and inflammation of ligaments. Zheng Gu Shui promotes circulation, decreases swelling, and stops pain.

Note: For external use only.

Dosage: It comes in bottles of 3.4 fluid ounces, with complete instructions on dosage.

Hu Gu Gao (Tiger Balm)

Description: This patent formula is used for tendonitis, sprains, strains, and contusions; to improve circulation; soothe muscles and tendons; relieve inflammation; and decrease swelling.

Dosage: It comes in jars containing .63 ounces, with complete instructions on dosage.

Thrush—see Candidiasis

Thyroid, Disorders of—see Goiter

Tinnitus (see also Ear, Disorders of; Otitis Media)

Unlike normal sound, which is transmitted by the acoustic nerve from external stimuli, tinnitus is a ringing or buzzing noise heard in the ear that originates inside the head or within the ear itself. Tinnitus can be a symptom of ear disorders such as labyrinthitis (inflammation), Ménière's disease, otitis media (ear infection), otosclerosis (chronic progressive deafness), or simply blockage of the outer ear canal caused by a buildup of ear wax. In rare cases, it is symptomatic of an aneurysm or tumor pressing on a blood vessel in the head. Although it is usually continuous, the ringing may change in nature or intensity. Some people learn to accept the condition without distress, while others find it almost intolerable. When it is caused by any of the above disorders, treating the underlying condition can often bring relief. Some find a "tinnitus masker," earphones that play white noise, particularly effective. Another source of relief is the use of the following Chinese herbal formulas:

Er Ming Zuo Ci Wan (Ear Ringing, Left Loving Pills); also known as Tso-Tzu Otic Pills

Description: This patent formula is used for treating ear ringing, headache, eye pressure, and insomnia.

Dosage: It comes in bottles of two hundred pills, with complete instructions on dosage.

Sheng Jing Shuai Rou Wan (Nerve Neurasthenia Weakness Pills); also known as Shen Ching Shuai Jao Wan

Description: This patent formula relieves tinnitus, insomnia, restlessness, and vertigo.

Dosage: It comes in bottles of two hundred pills, with complete instructions on dosage.

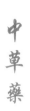

Tonsillitis

Tonsillitis is inflammation of the tonsils caused by infection. Mainly occurring in children under age nine, tonsillitis only occasionally occurs in adolescents and young adults. The main symptoms are a sore throat with difficulty swallowing, fever, headache, earache, unpleasant-smelling breath, and enlarged glands in the neck. In most cases tonsillitis can be treated without resorting to surgery. Quinsy, a complication of tonsillitis resulting in abscessed tissue near the tonsil, exhibits similar but more severe symptoms. Antibiotic herbs are often effective for resolving quinsy; however, in some cases surgical removal of the tonsils is required.

Traditional Chinese medicine's standard treatment involves taking herbal formulas to eliminate infection, reduce fever, and stop pain, as well as gargling with a saline solution (water and salt). If the patient experiences persistent pain (beyond twenty-four to forty-eight hours) and pus is visible on the tonsils, he or she should be examined by a physician.

Chuan Xin Lian-Antiphlogistic Pills (Penetrate Heart, Repeatedly Fighting Heat Pills); also known as Chuan Xin Lian Kang Yan Pian

Description: This patent formula clears infection with fever, resolves inflammation with swollen glands, and is beneficial in viral infections. When fighting the symptoms of tonsillitis, the best results are seen when use of this formula is combined with the formula that follows (Liu Shen Wan).

Dosage: It comes in bottles of sixty pills, with complete instructions on dosage.

Liu Shen Wan (Six Spirit Pills); also known as Lu Shen Wan

Description: This patent formula is useful for a variety of problems characterized by a sore throat (e.g., tonsillitis, mumps, etc.). It reduces fever, clears infection, and stops pain. When treating tonsillitis, the best results are seen when this formula is taken in combination with the preceding formula (Chuan Xin Lian-Antiphlogistic Pills).

Caution: This formula is prohibited for use during pregnancy.

Dosage: It comes in bottles of ten, thirty, or one hundred pills, with complete instructions on dosage

Tooth Abscess

A dental abscess develops when a pus-filled sac forms in the tissue at the root of a tooth. There are several possible causes: bacteria invading an injured tooth (possibly through a fracture), tooth decay infecting the root, or the accumulation of bacteria in deep pockets that form between the teeth and gums. This causes the affected tooth to throb and ache, making biting or chewing painful. If left untreated, infection will usually spread through surrounding tissue and bone, causing the glands in the neck and face to become swollen. In most cases the swelling is accompanied by common symptoms associated with infection, such as headache and low-grade fever.

The following Chinese herbal formulas can be useful for clearing infection and reducing pain. If unsuccessful, the recurrence of pain and swelling usually means root canal treatment is needed.

Qing Wei Tang (Clear Stomach Decoction)

Original Source: *Yi Zong Jin Jian* (according to *Chinese Herbal Medicine Formulas and Strategies*)

Ingredients:

Quantity (Grams)	Chinese Herbs	English Translation
6	Huang Lian	Golden Thread Root
6	Sheng Ma	Black Cohosh Rhizome
9	Mu Dan Pi	Tree Peony Root, Bark of
12	Sheng Di Huang	Chinese Foxglove Root, Raw
12	Dang Gui	Tangkuei

Description: This herbal formula relieves toothache, facial swelling, pain, bad breath, mouth sores, and abscess on the gums.

Analysis: Huang Lian reduces stomach heat. Sheng Ma assists and also relieves toxicity. Mu Dan Pi and Sheng Di Huang cool the blood. Dang Gui reduces swelling and alleviates pain.

Dosage and Method of Preparation: Make a decoction. Drink four ounces of Qing Wei Tang three times daily, as needed.

Note: If the abscess is aggravated by heat, drink this decoction cool.

Niu Huang Jie Du Pian (Ox Gallstone Dispel Toxin); also known as Niu Huang Chieh Tu Pien, or Bezoar Antipyretic Pills

Description: This patent formula is useful for eliminating abscess and infection, inflammation of the gums, oral ulcers, and toothache.

Caution: This formula is prohibited for use during pregnancy.

Dosage: It comes in bottles of eight or twenty tablets, with complete instructions on dosage.

Trichinosis—see Roundworms

Trichomoniasis (see also Candidiasis; Leukorrhea; Vaginal Discharge)

Trichomonas vaginalis is a single-celled microorganism that causes a vaginal infection called trichomoniasis. In the majority of cases it is sexually transmitted, although it is occasionally contracted from a secondary source such as an infected washcloth or towel. The infectious organism can inhabit the vagina for years without causing symptoms. Symptoms, when they do occur, include inflammation and itching of the vagina and vulva, and a profuse, yellow, odorous discharge. Because of the inflammation, sexual intercourse is usually painful. Normally, male sexual partners experience no symptoms; however, exceptions occasionally occur in men who have engaged in intercourse with an infected partner, such as urethral discomfort and/or inflammation of the head of the penis.

Traditional Chinese medicine suggests that both sex partners be treated at the same time to prevent re-infection or the spreading of infection (if multiple sex partners are involved). The following recommended herbal formulas are used internally as well as topically. Additional suggestions include the avoidance of casual sex and of dusting powders, deodorants, perfumed tampons, and other "scented" substances until the infection has been resolved.

She Chuang Zi Tang (Cnidium Decoction)

Original Source: *Zhong Yi Fang Ji Ling Chuang Shou Ce* (according to *Chinese Herbal Medicine Formulas and Strategies*)

Ingredients:

Quantity (Grams)	Chinese Herbs	English Translation
15	She Chuang Zi	Cnidium Fruit Seed
15	Chuan Jiao	Szechuan Pepper Fruit
15	Ku Shen	Bitter Root
15	Bai Bu	Stemona Root
15	Ming Fan★	Alum, Mineral

★See special instructions for preparation below.

Description: This herbal formula is used to dry dampness and to stop itching; it will clear infection and is useful for trichomoniasis vaginitis.

Note: This formula for external use only; do not drink it.

Analysis: She Chuang Zi benefits the kidneys, is antiparasitic (kills germs), and eliminates infection. Chuan Jiao assists the chief herb by reinforcing its actions. Ku Shen also eliminates infection and is specific for use in cases of trichomoniasis. Bai Bu is antibacterial, antiparasitic, and antifungal. Ming Fan, in addition to eliminating infection, is effective for resolving itching.

Dosage and Method of Preparation: Make a decoction. Ming Fan should not be cooked with the other herbs, but added after the normal cooking procedure, then allowed to steep with the decoction for thirty minutes before straining. This formula is used as a douche (for women) or topical application (for both men and women) for bathing external genitalia. Douche with eight ounces of She Chuan Zi Tang tea two to three times daily for five days, then douche with eight ounces of tea mixed with eight ounces of warm water once daily, as needed. For external application to genitalia, apply eight ounces of room-temperature decoction two to three times daily, as needed.

Chien Chin Chih Tai Wan (Thousand Pieces of Gold Stop Leukorrhea Pills); also known as Qian Jin Zhi Dai Wan

Description: This patent formula clears infection, astringes discharge, stops pain, and is useful for treating vaginal infections, including trichomoniasis.

Dosage: It comes in bottles of 120 pills, with complete instructions on dosage.

Tuberculosis

More commonly called TB—or, in days of yore, consumption—tuberculosis is an infectious disease caused by the tubercle bacillus. There are two types of TB. The more familiar form, pulmonary tuberculosis, primarily affects the lungs and is spread from person to person by coughing and/or sneezing. The lesser-known variety, called bovine tuberculosis, involves the intestines, bones, and other organs and is transmitted through contaminated cow's milk. The incidence of TB is higher in certain racial or social groups, including Hispanics, Haitians, and Southeast Asians. The disease is also more common in the elderly, people with immunodeficiency disorders, diabetics, and alcoholics. Because the more common form of TB usually affects the lungs, the main symptoms include coughing (sometimes bringing up blood), chest pain, shortness of breath, fever, night sweats, poor appetite, and loss of weight. Possible complications of tuberculosis of the lungs are pleural effusion (fluid between the lungs and chest wall) and pneumothorax (air between the lungs and chest wall).

Traditional Chinese medicine uses the following herbal formulas to treat tuberculosis:

Ke Xue Fang Tang (Coughing of Blood Decoction)

Original Source: *Dan Xi Xin Fa* (according to *Chinese Herbal Medicine Formulas and Strategies*)

Ingredients:

Quantity (Grams)	Chinese Herbs	English Translation
9	Qing Dai	Indigo Powder

9	Zhi Zi	Gardenia Fruit
9	Gua Lou Ren	Trichosanthes Seed
9	Fu Hai Shi	Pumice
9	He Zi	Myrobalan Fruit

Description: This herbal formula is used to reduce fever, fortify and strengthen the lungs, and stop coughing and bleeding; it is useful for pulmonary tuberculosis.

Analysis: The chief ingredients, Qing Dai and Zhi Zi, benefit the liver and stop bleeding by clearing heat and cooling the blood. Gua Lou Ren and Fu Hai Shi transform phlegm and reduce heat (fever). He Zi transforms phlegm and alleviates coughing.

Dosage and Method of Preparation: Prepare a decoction. Drink four ounces of Ke Xue Fang Tang tea three times daily, as needed.

Chuang Xin Lian-Antiphlogistic Pills (Penetrate Heart, Repeatedly Fighting Heat Pills); also known as Chuang Xin Lian Kang Yan Pian

Description: This patent formula is used to treat pulmonary abscess, tuberculosis, pneumonia, and other infections associated with lung heat (infection).

Dosage: It comes in bottles of thirty-six pills, with complete instructions on dosage.

Da Bu Yin Wan (Super Supplement Yin Pill)

Description: This patent formula is used for tuberculosis and will relieve night sweats, dizziness, fever, and coughing or vomiting with blood; it is used for kidney, bone, or lung TB.

Dosage: It comes in bottles of two hundred pills, with complete instructions on dosage.

Li Fei Tang Yi Pian (Benefit Lungs-Sugar-Coated Pills); also known as Pulmonary Tonic Pills-Sugar-Coated Pills

Description: This patent formula is used for TB with fever, coughing with blood, night sweats, and pain as seen in tuberculosis.

Dosage: It comes in bottles of sixty tablets, with complete instructions on dosage.

Zhi Sou Ding Chuan Wan (Stop Cough, Stop Asthma Pills)

Description: This patent formula is useful for treating TB with shortness of breath, fever, pain, cough with blood, sweating, and is also useful for treating pneumonia.

Dosage: This patent medicine comes in bottles of 150 pills, with complete instructions on dosage.

Ulcer

An ulcer is an open sore on the skin or mucus membrane. Although skin ulcers are fairly common, usually when we think of ulcers, we think of those affecting the digestive system, namely oral ulcers, which occur in the mouth and are commonly called canker sores (see also Fever Blister; Herpes [Oral]; Stomatitis); peptic ulcers, which affect the stomach, esophagus, or duodenum; or intestinal ulcers, which affect the small and large intestines, colon, and rectum in a condition known as ulcerative colitis. Somewhat less common are ulcers affecting the genitals, which are usually transmitted through sexual intercourse, and corneal ulcers, which develop on the front of the eyeball. In a majority of cases, skin ulcers occur on the leg and are usually caused by inadequate blood supply. Although rare, skin ulcers can also develop in basal cell carcinomas, a form of skin cancer.

In addition to the oral ulcers that can develop on the inside of the cheek, lips, and tongue, mouth ulcers caused by the herpes simplex virus are also fairly common. While most are not serious, caution is advised, because ulcers can be the first indication of oral cancer. Rare types of mouth ulcers include those that occur in tuberculosis, syphilis, leukemia, Bechet's syndrome, and Vincent's disease. The commonly occurring peptic ulcer can develop in the esophagus, stomach, or duodenum (between the stomach and the small intestine); the principal cause is erosion of the mucus membrane from stomach acid (hydrochloric acid). Gastric ulcers are peptic ulcers that develop in the stomach, and duodenal ulcers, as their name implies, develop in the duodenum.

A possible complication of ulcers is bleeding, which if considerable, can cause the vomiting of blood and passing of blood in the feces. The loss of a large amount of blood can be serious and should be attended to by a physician.

Traditional Chinese medicine attributes peptic ulcers to stagnation of stomach and liver Chi, and in addition to recommending herbal therapy, also makes strong dietary recommendations that include the avoidance of alcohol, smoking, caffeine, and spicy foods.

Bai Tou Weng Tang (Pulsatilla Decoction)

Original Source: *Shang Han Lun* (according to *Chinese Herbal Medicine Formulas and Strategies*)

Ingredients:

Quantity (Grams)	Chinese Herbs	English Translation
9	Huang Lian	Golden Thread Root
18	Bai Tou Weng	Chinese Anemone Root (Pulsatilla)
9	Huang Bai	Amur Cork Tree Bark
9	Qin Pi	Korean Ash Branches, Bark of

Description: This herbal formula is used for ulcerative colitis or dysentery, with symptoms of lower abdominal pain, burning sensation around the anus, and diarrhea containing blood and/or pus.

Analysis: Bai Tou Weng, the chief herb, is very effective and well known for its ability to eliminate infection and relieve fire toxins (fever and pus). Huang Lian clears infection, especially from the stomach and intestines, and it is assisted by Huang Bai and Qin Pi, which restrain diarrhea and enhance the actions of the other herbs in the formula.

Dosage and Method of Preparation: Prepare a decoction. Drink four ounces of Bai Tou Weng Tang tea three times daily, as needed.

Fu Zi Li Zhong Wan (Aconite Regulate the Center Pills); also known as Carmichaeli Tea Pills, or Fu Tzu Li Chung Wan

中
草
藥

Description: This patent formula is useful for gastric and duodenal ulcers, colitis, and gastroenteritis.

Dosage: It comes in bottles of one hundred pills or boxes of ten honey pills, with complete instructions on dosage.

Chen Xiang Hua Qi Wan (Aquilariae Move Chi Pills)

Description: This patent formula is useful for treating gastritis, stomach ulcers, and duodenal ulcers with poor appetite, belching, and sour regurgitation.

Dosage: It comes in bottles of one hundred pills, with complete instructions on dosage.

Xiang Sha Liu Jun Wan (Saussurea Amomum Six Gentlemen Pills); also known as Aplotaxis-Amomum Pills, or Six Gentlemen Tea Pills

Description: This patent formula is used for treating gastric or duodenal ulcers with the following symptoms: poor digestion, vomiting, nausea, burping, acid regurgitation, and stomachache.

Dosage: It comes in bottles of one hundred pills, with complete instructions on dosage.

Sai Mei An (The Race Between Rot and Peaceful Health)

Description: This patent formula is used to treat gastric and duodenal ulcers, neutralize excessive stomach acid, stop pain, and relieve nausea.

Dosage: It comes in bottles of fifty capsules, with complete instructions on dosage.

Wei Yao (Gastropathy Capsules); also known as 707 Gastropathy Capsules

Description: This patent formula is used to reduce excess stomach acid, stop bleeding, stop pain, and treat gastric and duodenal ulcers.

Dosage: It comes in boxes of forty-two capsules, with complete instructions on dosage.

Urethritis

Urethritis, or inflammation of the urethra, often results from infection by the bacteria that cause gonorrhea. The condition known as nonspecific urethritis can be caused by any number of different microorganisms, including bacteria, yeast, and chlamydial infection, or bacteria from the rectum that is spread (often during sex) and infects the urethra. Other possible causes include trauma resulting from an accident or from surgically introduced instruments (catheter or cystoscope) and irritating chemicals such as antiseptics and spermicidal preparations.

Urethritis causes a burning sensation and pain when passing urine. The pain can be severe and blood-stained, with accompanying pus-filled discharge, particularly when gonorrhea is the cause. The following Chinese herbal formulas can be useful for treating it:

Lung Tan Xie Gan Wan (Gentiana Purge Liver Pills); also known as Long Dan Xie Gan Wan

Description: This patent formula eliminates infection and inflammation of the urethra. It stops pain and is useful for urethritis, pelvic inflammatory disease, vulvitis, and prostatitis.

Dosage: It comes in bottles of one hundred pills, with complete instructions on dosage.

Shi Lin Tong Pian (Stone Dysuria Open Tablets); also known as Te Xiao Pai Shi Wan

Description: This patent formula is used to clear up infection of the urethra. It stops pain and is useful for urinary tract infection and for urethritis with inflammation and pain.

Dosage: It comes in bottles of one hundred tablets, with complete instructions on dosage.

Urinary Tract Infection

Infection can occur anywhere in the urinary tract and affect any of the organs in the urogenital system. Structures in the urinary tract include the urethra, urinary bladder, and kidneys. (See also Cystitis;

Kidney, Disorders of; Pyelonephritis; and Urethritis for herbal formulas to treat inflammation or infection involving these organs.)

Generally, urinary tract infections can be caused by a calculus (stone) in one of the organs of the urinary tract (bladder or kidneys), a bladder tumor, or a congenital abnormality such as a double kidney on one side of the body. Other possible causes include failure of the bladder to empty completely as a result of spina bifida or a spinal-cord injury. Although rare, infections can also be blood borne. By far the most common cause of urinary tract infection is the spread of organisms from the rectum via the urethra to the bladder or kidneys.

Traditional Chinese medicine offers herbal antibiotics that are very effective for treating urinary tract infection.

Wu Wei Xiao Du Yin (Decoction to Eliminate Toxin)

Original Source: *Yi Zong Jin Jian* (according to *Chinese Herbal Medicine Formula and Strategies*)

Ingredients:

Quantity (Grams)	Chinese Herbs	English Translation
9	Jin Yin Hua	Honeysuckle Flowers
3.6	Pu Gong Ying	Dandelion Herb
3.6	Zi Hua Di Ding	Yedeon's Violet Plant
3.6	Ye Ju Hua	Wild Chrysanthemum Flower
3.6	Zi Bei Tian Kuei	Begonia

Description: This herbal formula is used for urinary tract infections; it reduces fever, clears infection, cools the blood, eliminates inflammation, and stops pain.

Analysis: The chief herb, Jin Yin Hua, clears heat and infection and reduces swelling. Pu Gong Ying, Zi Hua Di Ding, Ye Ju Hua, and Zi Bei Tian Kuei all clear heat and cool the blood and are useful for treating poisonous lesions.

Dosage and Method of Preparation: Make a decoction. Drink four ounces of Wu Wei Xiao Du Yin three times daily, as needed.

Lung Tan Xie Gan Wan (Gentiana Purge Liver Pill); also known as Long Dan Xie Gan Wan

Description: This patent formula is used for urinary tract infections; it reduces fever and clears up infection.

Dosage: It comes in bottles of one hundred pills, with complete instructions on dosage.

Shi Lin Tong Pian (Stone Dysuria Open Tablets); also known as Te Xiao Pai Shi Wan

Description: This patent formula is used to treat urinary tract infection, urinary tract stones, and kidney stones. It clears up infection and reduces fever.

Dosage: It comes in bottles of one hundred pills, with complete instructions on dosage.

Urination, Excessive or Frequent

A number of possible causes exist for excessive or frequent urination. Although both terms imply "too much" urination, they by definition slightly differ. Excessive urination, which refers to a volume of more than 2.5 liters per day, is clinically known as polyuria. Frequent urination, which is simply called "frequency," refers to passing urine more than four to six times a day. Both usually signify illness.

Illnesses that cause excessive urination can be physical or psychosomatic. One example of excessive urination with a psychosomatic cause is a condition known as polydipsia, seen in certain psychiatric illnesses. Polydipsia can cause a person to drink (nonalcoholic fluids) compulsively, which inevitably leads to a high output of urine. On the physical side, both forms of diabetes (insipidus and mellitus) can cause excessive urination, as can certain kidney diseases.

Frequent urination, on the other hand, in some cases is the inevitable result of excessive production of urine, while in other cases the total volume produced is not high—the person simply urinates frequently but in small amounts. Other causes for urinary frequency include cystitis (bladder infection), bladder stones, enlarged prostate in men, renal failure, and in rare cases bladder tumors. (See also entries for specific causes, e.g., Cystitis; Diabetes; Kidney, Disorders of; Prostate, Disorders of.)

Whether urination is excessive or frequent, it is always the underlying cause that is treated in an attempt to resolve the condition.

Sang Piao Xiao Tang (Mantis Egg Case Decoction)

Original Source: *Ben Cao Yan Yi* (according to *Chinese Herbal Medicine Formulas and Strategies*)

Ingredients:

Quantity (Grams)	Chinese Herbs	English Translation
12	Sang Piao Xiao	Praying Mantis Egg Case
30	Long Gu	Dragon Bones
12	Ren Shen	Ginseng
12	Fu Shen	Tuckahoe Spirit Fungus
6	Yuan Zhi	Root of Chinese Senega
9	Chang Pu	Sweet Flag Rhizome
15	Zhi Gui Ban	Honey-Fried Land Tortoise Shell
9	Dang Gui	Tangkuei

Description: This herbal formula is used for frequent urination with backache and insomnia.

Analysis: Sang Piao Xiao benefits the kidneys and stops "dribble" or leakage. The other chief ingredient, Long Gu, assists the chief herb in these actions in addition to calming and steadying the will. Ren Shen, Fu Shen, Yuan Zhi, and Chang Pu combine to increase the vital energy (Chi) and benefit the heart and kidneys. Dang Gui and Zhi Gui Ban together strengthen both Chi and blood.

Dosage and Method of Preparation: Make a decoction. Drink four ounces of Sang Piao Xiao Tang tea three times daily, as needed.

Ba Wei Di Huang Wan (Eight Flavor Rehmannia Pill)

Description: This patent formula is used for profuse urination with poor circulation, back pain, and kidney deficiency.

Dosage: It comes in bottles of 240 pills, with complete instructions on dosage.

Du Zhong Bu Tian Su (Eucommia Benefit Heaven Basic Pill)

Description: This patent formula is used for frequent urination with backache and fatigue and insomnia.

Dosage: It comes in boxes of twelve vials, eight tablets per vial, with complete instructions on dosage.

Jie Jie Wan (Dispel [Prostate] Swelling Pills); also known as Kai Kit Pill

Description: This patent formula provides relief from painful urination. It resolves pain and reduces enlarged prostate with accompanying symptoms.

Dosage: This patent medicine comes in bottles of fifty-four pills, with complete instructions on dosage.

Urine Retention

The inability to empty the bladder can take two forms. In one case urinary retention is complete, and urine cannot voluntarily be passed at all (even though there may be some leakage). In the other case retention is incomplete, in which case some urine may be passed, but the bladder fails to empty completely.

Although this condition can affect both sexes, most often it affects men. Possible causes include phimosis (tight foreskin), urethral stricture, bladder stones, prostatitis (inflammation of the prostate), enlargement of the prostate, or a tumor of the prostate gland. In women, urinary retention may be caused by pressure on the urethra from uterine fibroids. In either sex, it can be due to defective nerve functioning, diseases, injury to the spinal cord, or a bladder tumor. (See also entries for specific causes, e.g., Bladder Cancer; Prostate, Disorders of.)

The main symptom is discomfort and pain in the lower abdomen, which can be severe. There is a risk that urinary retention will lead to kidney damage (as a result of back-pressure in the urinary tract) and that incomplete emptying will lead to an increased incidence of urinary tract infection. The underlying cause for complete and incomplete urinary retention must be determined through diagnosis by a physician. Traditional Chinese medicine recommends the following herbal formulas that can be helpful for treating some of the associated problems:

Ming Mu Shang Ching Pien (Bright Eyes Upper Clearing Tablet); also known as Ming Mu Shang Qing Pian

Description: This patent formula is used for urine retention. It reduces fever and clears up symptoms that include concentrated urine and constipation.

Caution: This formula is prohibited for use during pregnancy.

Dosage: It comes in boxes of twelve vials, eight tablets per vial, with complete instructions on dosage.

Niu Huang Shang Qing Wan (Cow Gallstone Upper Clear Pills); also known as Niu Huang Shang Ching Wan

Description: This patent formula is used for complete and incomplete urine retention. It resolves infection, reduces fever, and is useful for concentrated urine and constipation.

Caution: This formula is prohibited for use during pregnancy.

Dosage: It comes in bottles of fifty pills, with complete instructions on dosage.

Uterus, Disorders of: Infection, Inflammation, Tumors, Prolapsed, Cancer (see also Endometriosis; Fibroid Tumors)

A major gynecological concern is the list of disorders affecting the uterus, which includes infection and inflammation, benign polyps and tumors, hormonal and congenital disorders, and malignancy. Many of these disorders are either directly responsible for or are contributing factors in infertility. One of the more common and frequently seen problems is infection and inflammation of the lining of the uterus, known as endometriosis. This infection can originate in the uterus, or it can spread from elsewhere in the reproductive tract. Another possible cause of endometriosis is infection that can develop as a result of placental fragments remaining in the uterus after child-birth or miscarriage.

Benign tumors of the uterus, which include polyps and fibroids, are also fairly common. They can arise from the cervix or endometrium and cause excessive menstrual bleeding, infertility, and painful intercourse. Hormonal disorders include excessive production of prostaglandin (a fatty-acid derivative that performs hormonelike actions), causing painful or heavy menstrual periods. Occasionally, the uterus may move from its normal position; this condition is called prolapse and can cause menstrual irregularities and pain during sex. Injury to the uterus, which is rare, is only likely to occur following surgery, particularly after an abortion.

Also fairly uncommon is the incidence of uterine cancer. Worldwide, it affects approximately one hundred thousand women annually and is known to occur more frequently in women who have an excess of the hormone estrogen in their systems. Risk factors that increase estrogen levels include obesity, a history of failure to ovulate, and long-term use of estrogen hormones. Unlike cervical cancer, uterine cancer can occur in women who have never had sexual intercourse and is more common in women who have had few or no children. Symptoms of uterine or endometrial cancer after menopause usually include blood-stained vaginal discharge and a vague feeling of abdominal discomfort. In younger women, the first symptom may be heavy periods, bleeding between periods, or bleeding after sexual intercourse. Needless to say, any abnormal bleeding should be immediately investigated by a gyne-cologist.

Traditional Chinese medicine is well recognized for its ability to successfully treat many gynecological problems. The following herbal formulas have proven useful for uterine disorders:

Qing Re Zhi Beng Tang (Clear Heat and Stop Excessive Uterine Bleeding Decoction)

Original Source: *Zhong Yi Fu Ke Zhi Liao Xue* (according to *Chinese Herbal Medicine Formulas and Strategies*)

Ingredients:

Quantity (Grams)	Chinese Herbs	English Translation
9	Zhi Zi	Gardenia Fruit
15	Chao Huang Qin	Stir-fried Baical Skullcap Root
9	Huang Bai	Amur Cork Tree Bark
24	Sheng Di Huang	Chinese Foxglove Root, Raw
9	Mu Dan Pi	Tree Peony Root, Bark of
24	Di Yu	Burnet-Bloodwort Root
30	Ce Bai Ye Tan	Leafy Twig of Arborvitae
30	Chun Gen Bai Pi	Ailanthus Bark
15	Duan Gui Ban	Land Tortoise Shell, Calcined
30	Bai Shao	White Peony Root

Description: This herbal formula is useful for abnormal uterine bleeding characterized by large quantities of bright-red blood.

Analysis: The first group of herbs in this formula, Zhi Zi, Chao Huang Qin, and Huang Bai, combine energies to clear heat from the liver. Sheng Di Huang and Mu Dan Pi assist in cooling the liver and blood. Di Yu, Ce Bai Ye Tan, and Chun Gen Bai Pi all address the root cause by eliminating heat from the lower body and stopping bleeding. Duan Gui Ban and Bai Shao nourish the blood and assist in a less primary way to stop bleeding.

Dosage and Method of Preparation: Prepare a decoction. Drink four ounces of Qing Re Zhi Beng Tang tea three times daily, as needed.

Gui Zhi Fu Ling Tang (Cinnamon Twig and Poria Tea)

Original Source: *Jin Gui Yao Lue* (according to *Chinese Herbal Medicine Formulas and Strategies*)

Ingredients:

Quantity (Grams)	Chinese Herbs	English Translation
12	Gui Zhi	Saigon Cinnamon Twig
12	Fu Ling	Tuckahoe Root

中草藥

15	Chi Shao Yao	Red Peony Root
12	Mu Dan Pi	Tree Peony Root, Bark of
12	Tao Ren	Peach Kernel

Description: This herbal formula relieves persistent uterine bleeding, fibroid tumors, painful menstrual periods, endometriosis, amenorrhea with abdominal distention and pain, and mild uterine bleeding of purple or dark blood during pregnancy.

Note: To gain the best results, the user should take this formula for six months or longer.

Analysis: The combined energies of the two chief herbs, Gui Zhi and Fu Ling, unblock blood vessels and reduce blood stasis (poor circulation), in addition to promoting urination. Chi Shao Yao promotes circulation of blood. Mu Dan Pi and Tao Ren assist, while cooling the blood and reducing fixed lower-abdominal masses.

Dosage and Method of Preparation: Make a decoction. Drink four ounces of Gui Zhi Fu Ling Tang tea at room temperature three times daily, as needed.

Uterine Cancer Formula

An excellent book on Chinese medicines used to fight cancer is *Anticancer Medicinal Herbs,* by Chang Minyi. According to the author, the following formula has been used to treat uterine cancer in the primary stage:

Ingredients:

Quantity (Grams)	Chinese Herbs	English Translation
2	Da Huang	Rhubarb Root
3	Mang Xiao	Mirabilite
4	Mu Dan Pi	Peony Tree Root, Bark of
4	Tao Ren	Peach Kernel
4	Dong Gua Zi	Wintermelon Seed's Pulp
4	Cang Zhu	Atractylodes Cangzhu
8	Yi Yi Ren	Seeds of Job's Tears
1	Gan Cao	Licorice Root

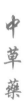

Description: For treatment of uterine cancer in the primary stage.

Analysis: Da Huang and Mang Xiao drain heat from the intestines, relieve abdominal distention and pain, and promote bowel movement. Mu Dan Pi and Tao Ren cool the blood, improve circulation, and reduce firm masses (lumps and tumors). Dong Gua Zi treats infection and eliminates intestinal abscesses. Cang Zhu strengthens the spleen. Yi Yi Ren reinforces the previous actions while assisting in eliminating abscesses and infection. Gan Cao harmonizes the actions of the other herbs and improves the taste of the formula.

Dosage and Method of Preparation: Make a decoction. Drink eight ounces of the formula daily, as needed.

Fu Ke Zhong Zi Wan (Gynecology Pregnancy Pills); also known as De Sheng Dan, or Zhong Zi Wan

Description: This patent formula is used for irregular menstruation with blood clots and abdominal pain; it is useful for treating stagnation of Chi and blood in the abdomen that has caused uterine tumors or endometriosis.

Caution: This formula is prohibited for use during pregnancy.

Dosage: It comes in bottles of one hundred pills, complete with instruction on dosage.

Bu Zhong Yi Qi Wan (Tonify Center to Invigorate Qi Pills); also known as Central Qi Pills, or Bu Zhong Yi Chi Wan

Description: This patent formula is used for treating organ prolapse such as uterine prolapse, anal prolapse, or gastroptosis. It aids with the symptoms of fatigue, irregular menstrual periods, pain, and heavy bleeding.

Dosage: It comes in bottles of one hundred pills, with complete instructions on dosage.

Ci Wu Jia Pian (Acanthopanax Senticosus)

Description: This patent formula is useful for patients undergoing radiation therapy. It strengthens the immune system and protects the body from damage due to radiation. In China, this herbal formula is used for uterine cancer and is considered preferable to Ginseng.

Dosage: It comes in bottles of one hundred tablets, with complete instructions on dosage.

Ji Xue Teng Qin Gao Pian (Millettia Reticulata Liquid Extract Tablets); also known as Caulis Millentiae

Description: This is another patent formula used to aid those undergoing radiation therapy. It is said to increase the white blood cell count in such patients.

Dosage: It comes in bottles of one hundred pills, with complete instructions on dosage.

Yung Sheng He Ah Chiao (Externally Vigorous Combination Donkey Skin Glue); also known as Yong Sheng He A Jiao

Description: This patent formula nourishes blood and stops internal bleeding. It is useful in excessive-bleeding disorders, including uterine and menstrual.

Note: Do not use this formula for bleeding from gastrointestinal disorders.

Dosage: This patent medicine comes in solid blocks of thirty grams. Dissolve fifteen grams in twelve ounces of boiling water or hot rice wine; drink four ounces twice daily, as needed.

Yu Dai Wan (Heal Leukorrhea Pill); also known as Yudai Wan

Description: This patent formula strengthens the blood, astringes discharge, and clears infection in the uterus and the kidneys, with symptoms of backache, fatigue, and lower abdominal pain.

Dosage: It comes in bottles of one hundred pills, with complete instructions on dosage.

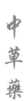

Vagina, Disorders of—see entry for specific condition, e.g., Candidiasis; Pelvic Inflammatory Disease; Trichomoniasis; Vaginal Itching; etc.

Vaginal Bleeding (see also Menorrhagia)

Vaginal bleeding normally has three possible sources: the uterus, the cervix, or the vagina itself.

Of the three, the most likely source is the uterus, and the most likely reason for bleeding is irregular menstruation. Possible causes for uterine bleeding unrelated to menstruation include endometriosis (infection of the lining of the uterus), endometrial or uterine cancer, or the use of hormones such as birth control pills (spotting from oral contraceptives can be remedied by an adjustment in dosage). Bleeding from the uterus during the early months of pregnancy may be a sign of threatened miscarriage. Later in pregnancy it may indicate serious fetal or maternal problems.

Bleeding from the cervix is usually attributable to cervical erosion; bleeding from this cause typically occurs following sexual intercourse. Infection of the cervix and the presence of polyps can also cause bleeding. Another possibility is cervical cancer.

Blood originating from the wall of the vagina is the least common source. The probable cause would be injury during intercourse, especially after menopause, when the vaginal walls become thinner and more fragile. Occasionally, vaginitis can be the cause, and in rare cases vaginal bleeding is caused by vaginal cancer.

Any abnormal vaginal bleeding (i.e., not caused by menstruation) should be investigated and the cause determined before making a decision concerning treatment. The following Chinese herbal formulas have proven effective for treating vaginal bleeding and cause no known side effects:

Wen Jing Tang (Warm the Menses Decoction)

Original Source: *Jin Gui Yao Lue* (according to *Chinese Herbal Medicine Formulas and Strategies*)

Ingredients:

Quantity (Grams)	Chinese Herbs	English Translation
9	Wu Zhu Yu	Evodia Fruit
6	Gui Zhi	Saigon Cinnamon Twig
9	Dang Gui	Tangkuei
6	Chuan Xiong	Szechuan Lovage Root
6	Shao Yao	Peony Root
9	Mai Men Dong	Lush Winter Wheat Tuber
6	Mu Dan Pi	Tree Peony Root, Bark of
6	Ren Shen	Ginseng
6	Gan Cao	Licorice Root
6	Sheng Jiang	Fresh Ginger Root
6	Ban Xia	Half Summer
6	E Jiao★	Donkey Skin Glue

★See special instructions for preparation below.

Description: This formula is used for mild persistent uterine bleeding, irregular menstruation, bleeding between periods, painful menstruation, as well as for infertility due to polycystic ovaries, chronic pelvic inflammatory disease, and dysmenorrhea.

Analysis: Wu Zhu Yu and Gui Zhi, the chief ingredients, unblock the blood vessels and improve blood circulation. Dang Gui, Chuan Xiong, and Shao Yao nourish the blood and counteract anemia while assisting in promoting circulation. Mai Men Dong reduces feverishness by increasing body fluids. Mu Dan Pi assists the chief herbs. Ren Shen, Sheng Jiang, Ban Xia, and Gan Cao strengthen the Chi and benefit the spleen and stomach. E Jiao powerfully addresses the chief complaint by effectively stopping bleeding.

Dosage and Method of Preparation: Make a decoction. E Jiao should not be cooked with the other ingredients; it should be added after the formula has been completely cooked and strained. Stir E Jiao into the decoction and allow the herb to dissolve. Allow the decoction to sit for thirty minutes. It will not be necessary to re-strain the decoction. Drink four ounces of Wen Jing Tang tea three times daily, as needed.

Bu Xue Tiao Jing Pian (Nourish Blood Adjust Period Tablets); also known as Bu Tiao Tablets

Description: This patent formula is used for vaginal bleeding; it nourishes the blood, inhibits bleeding, and is used for irregular periods and excessive cramping.

Dosage: It comes in bottles of one hundred pills, with complete instructions on dosage.

Kwei Be Wan (Restore Spleen Pills); also known as Gui Pi Wan, or Angelicae Longana Tea

Description: This patent formula is useful for treating chronic bleeding associated with functional uterine bleeding, aplastic anemia, and irregular menstruation.

Dosage: It comes in bottles of two hundred pills, with complete instructions on dosage.

Vaginal Discharge (see also specific causes, e.g., Candidiasis; Leukorrhea; Pelvic Inflammatory Disease; Trichomoniasis)

What is considered a normal amount of vaginal discharge varies considerably among women. The amount and nature of the discharge can be influenced by different times in the menstrual cycle, sexual stimulation, pregnancy, or taking birth control pills. Discharge is considered abnormal when it is excessive, smells "off," is yellow or green in color, or causes itching. Most often, vaginal discharge fitting this description is associated with vaginitis, candidiasis, or trichomoniasis.

In a majority of cases, treatment for abnormal vaginal discharge would involve the use of antibiotics and antifungal Chinese herbal formulas to treat the most probable cause: infection. The following formula can be used as a douche for treating most nonspecific vaginal infections with discharge:

Vaginal Douche Formula

Ingredients:

Quantity (Grams)	Chinese Herbs	English Translation
9	Chuan Lian Zi	Fruit of Szechuan Pagoda Tree
12	Gou Qi Gen	Matrimony Vine Root
9	Huang Bai	Amur Cork Tree Bark
12	Ku Shen	Bitter Root
9	She Chuang Zi	Cnidium Fruit
9	Ku Fan★	Alum, Mineral Salt

★See special instructions for preparation below.

Description: This vaginal douche is for all vaginal infections with discharge, foul odor, itching, irritation, lower abdominal discomfort, and discomfort when urinating.

Caution: This formula is for external use only, as a douche; do not drink this formula.

Analysis: Chuan Lian Zi circulates the vital energy (Chi) and relieves pain. Gou Qi Gen and Huang Bai eliminate heat, detoxify poisons, and clear infection. Ku Shen also effectively clears infection. She Chuang Zi is antiparasitic and also benefits the kidneys. Ku Fan dries dampness and eliminates itching.

Dosage and Method of Preparation: Make a decoction. Ku Fan should not be cooked with the other ingredients but added after the normal cooking procedure, then allowed to steep with the decoction for thirty minutes before straining. Douche with eight ounces of this decocted tea at room temperature twice daily, as needed.

Vaginal or Vulval Itching

What most women refer to as "vaginal itching" in fact usually affects the external genitalia, or vulva, rather than the interior canal, or vagina. Technically called pruritus vulvae, the condition results from infection or from an allergic reaction to chemicals in soaps, deodorants, spermicides, creams, and douches. Itching after menopause (due to low estrogen levels) is also fairly common. Traditional Chinese medicine recommends the following formulas for relief of vulval or vaginal itching:

Yu Dai Wan (Heal Leukorrhea Pills); also known as Yudai Wan

Description: This patent formula relieves vaginal itching and clears up infection, pain, and vaginal odor.

Dosage: It comes in bottles of one hundred pills, with complete instructions on dosage.

San She Jie Yang Wan (Three Snake Dispel Itching Pills); also known as Tri-Snake Itch Removing Pills

Description: This patent formula is useful for all types of skin itching, including pruritus vulvae, pruritus, dermatitis, eczema, acne, fungal infections, and vaginal infections.

Caution: This formula is prohibited for use during pregnancy.

Dosage: It comes in bottles of thirty pills, with complete instructions on dosage.

Vaginal Douche Formula

Simple vaginal itching that is not a result of serious infection can usually be cured with a few applications of a topical herbal bath made from the following formula:

Ingredients:

Quantity (Grams)	Chinese Herbs	English Translation
9	Chuan Lian Zi	Fruit of Szechuan Pagoda Tree
12	Gou Qi Gen	Matrimony Vine Root
9	Huang Bai	Amur Cork Tree Bark
12	Ku Shen	Bitter Root
9	She Chuang Zi	Cnidium Fruit
9	Ku Fan★	Alum, Mineral Salt

★See special instructions for preparation below.

Description: This vaginal douche offers relief from all types of vaginal itching with discharge, foul odor, irritation, lower abdominal discomfort, and discomfort when urinating.

Caution: This formula is for external use only, as a douche; do not drink this formula.

Analysis: Chuan Lian Zi circulates the vital energy (Chi) and relieves pain. Gou Qi Gen and Huang Bai eliminate heat, detoxify poisons, and clear infection. Ku Shen also effectively clears infection. She Chuang Zi is antiparasitic and also benefits the kidneys. Ku Fan dries dampness and eliminates itching.

Dosage and Method of Preparation: Make a decoction. Ku Fan should not be cooked with the other herbs but added after the normal cooking procedure, then allowed to steep with the decoction for thirty minutes before straining. Douche with eight ounces of this decocted tea at room temperature twice daily, as needed.

Vaginitis—see Candidiasis; Leukorrhea; Trichomoniasis; Vaginal Discharge

Varicose Veins

Varicose veins occur when valves in the veins become defective, causing blood to pool in the superficial veins just beneath the skin. Most often occurring in the legs, they can also develop in the anus (in which case they are called hemorrhoids), the esophagus, and the scrotum. There are several factors that may contribute to the development of varicose veins, namely obesity, hormonal changes during pregnancy or menopause, and standing for long periods of time.

In traditional Chinese medicine, poor circulation of the blood and Chi deficiency are regarded as the primary causes of varicose veins; weight loss and exercise are encouraged along with the use of herbs that invigorate (circulate) the blood. Some sufferers of varicose veins experience no symptoms, while others experience a severe aching in the affected area that is aggravated by prolonged standing. Swelling of the ankles and feet and persistent itching are also fairly common.

Relief from the pain and discomfort can often be provided by sitting with the legs raised. If severe bleeding occurs after a varicose vein is bumped or struck, bleeding can be stopped by keeping the affected leg elevated and applying direct pressure, after which a physician should be consulted.

Normally the following formula can be used for treating varicose veins:

Bu Zhong Yi Qi Wan (Tonify Center to Invigorate Qi Pills); also known as Central Qi Pills, or Bu Zhong Yi Chi Wan

Description: This patent formula is used to stop pain and bleeding, invigorate the blood, and provide relief from varicose veins, hemorrhoids, and prolapsed uterus and colon.

Dosage: It comes in bottles of one hundred pills, with complete instructions on dosage.

Vertigo

Vertigo is the sensation that one's head or one's surroundings are spinning. A fairly common complaint, the term is sometimes used erroneously to describe dizziness or feeling lightheaded (compare Dizziness). Severe vertigo with accompanying symptoms may indicate a disease such as labyrinthitis (inflammation of the semi-circular ear canals), influenza, hypertension, anemia, ear infection, or the more serious Ménière's disease. Elderly people suffering from arteriosclerosis often suffer from vertigo. Less commonly, vertigo can be caused by a brain tumor or multiple sclerosis.

Traditional Chinese medicine regards vertigo as a symptom of an underlying disorder. An example of a disorder with which it is commonly associated is hypertension. With the exception of brain tumors and multiple sclerosis, all of the other possible causes can be treated with Chinese herbs. For more information on herbal formulas useful for treating vertigo, see entries on underlying causes, e.g., Anemia; Colds and Flu; Ear, Disorders of; Hypertension; Tinnitus.

Vomiting

Traditional Chinese medicine unequivocally considers vomiting a symptom, not an illness. In the case of food poisoning or alcohol hangover, for example, once the stomach contents have been expelled, acute symptoms and vomiting should end. If vomiting recurs over several days or longer, professional help should definitely be sought.

Once diagnosed, many of the following underlying causes can be treated with Chinese herbs. See the specific entry in this chapter.

- overindulgence in food or alcohol, indigestion
- an adverse reaction to certain drugs
- a reaction to general anesthesia
- morning sickness (associated with pregnancy)
- disorders of the stomach and intestines (peptic ulcers, gastroenteritis, appendicitis, etc.)
- intestinal obstruction (due to narrowing of the intestinal tract or tumor)
- inflammation of organs associated with digestion, e.g. the liver (hepatitis), pancreas (pancreatitis), gallbladder (cholecystitis), etc.
- increased brain pressure resulting from encephalitis, hydrocephalus, brain tumor, or trauma
- Ménière's disease
- migraine headache
- motion sickness
- influenza
- internal bleeding from the esophagus, stomach, or duodenum
- psychological or emotional disorders

Whooping Cough—see Pertussis

Resources and Indexes

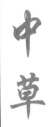

To further assist the reader, a general index (of medical symptoms and disorders) has been provided, as well as indexes of raw herb and patent formulas and a cross reference for the Chinese (in Pinyin, which is a system for transliterating the Chinese into the Latin alphabet), English, and Latin names of the ingredients found in the raw herb formulas.

Sources for
Herbal and Patent Formulas

To purchase herbs in bulk, patent formulas, or any of the raw herbal formulas already prepared, contact the following company. They specialize in mail-order sales of Chinese herbal formulas and will supply you with a catalog on request. This is the only firm we located that supplies all of the formulas described in this book.

Treasures from the Sea of Chi
360 Grand St., Suite 124
Oakland CA 94610
(510) 451-7470
(510) 452-3550, fax
TJSeaofChi@aol.com
http://hometownaol.com/tjseaofchi/myhomepage/ index.html

The following company sells herbs in bulk and patent formulas:

Mayway Trading Company
1338 Cypress St.
Oakland CA 94607
(510) 208-3123

Chinese patent medicines may be purchased from the following Chinese herb stores from throughout the United States. All of these companies speak English.

BAC-A1 Pharmacy
216B Canal St.
New York NY 10013
(212) 513-1344

North South China Herb Company
1556 Stockton St.
San Francisco CA 94134
(415) 421-4907

Wing Gung Tai Ginseng Company
833 N. Broadway
Los Angeles CA 90012
(213) 617-0699

Essential Chinese Herb Store
646 N. Spring St.
Los Angeles CA 90012
(213) 680-1374

Golden Import
46 Beach St.
Boston MA 02111
(617) 350-7001

Cheng Kwong Market
73-79 Essex St.
Boston MA 02111
(617) 482-3221

The following mail-order herb companies sell a variety of Western and Chinese herbs. Call for one of their catalogs, or place an order over the phone. All speak English.

Kwok Shing Import Export, Inc.
1818 Harrison St.
San Francisco CA 94103
(415) 861-1668

Nuherbs
3820 Penniman Ave.
Oakland CA 94510
(510) 534-HERB (534-4372)

Penn Herb Company
10601 Decatur Rd. #2
Philadelphia PA 19154
(800) 523-9971

Reference Books

AIDS and Chinese Medicine, by Qing Cai Zhang and Hong Yen Hsu (Ohai Press, 1990).

AIDS and Its Treatment by Traditional Chinese Medicine, by Huang Bing-Shan (Blue Poppy Press, 1991).

The American Medical Association Encyclopedia of Medicine, by Charles Clayman (Random House, 1989).

Anti-Cancer Medicinal Herbs, by Chang Minyi (Hunan Science and Technology Publishing House, 1992).

Chinese Herbal Medicine Formulas and Strategies, by Dan Bensky and Randall Barolet (Eastland Press, 1990).

Chinese Herbal Medicine: Materia Medica, by Dan Bensky (Eastland Press, 1985).

Chinese Herbal Patent Formulas, by Jake Fratkin (Institute of Traditional Medicine, 1986).

Chinese System of Food Cures, Prevention, and Remedies, by Henry C. Lu (Sterling Publishing Company, 1986).

Gynecology According to Traditional Chinese Medicine, by Susan Chen (Vantage Press, 1993).

Handbook of Chinese Herbs and Formulas, vols. I and II, by Him-Che Yeung (Institute of Chinese Medicine, 1985).

The Merck Manual, 14th ed., by Robert Berkow (Merck Sharp and Dohme Research Labs, 1982).

Outline Guide to Chinese Herbal Patent Medicine in Pill Form, by Margaret Naeser (Boston Chinese Medicine, 1990).

Shaolin Secret Formulas for the Treatment of External Injury, by Patriarch De Chan (Blue Poppy Press, 1995).

Taber's Cyclopedic Medical Dictionary, by Clayton Thomas (F. A. Davis Company, 1981).

Treating Cancer with Chinese Herbs, by Hong Yen Hsu (Oriental Healing Arts Institute, 1982).

Glossary of Chinese Medical Terms

Abate restlessness—to stop agitation

Benefit the stomach—to clear up nausea, gas, stomachache

Blood cleanser—formula to purify the blood

Blood tonic—formula to enrich and strengthen the blood

Calm restlessness—to stop agitation

Calm the spirit—to tranquilize the spirit

Calm stomach heat—to balance the temperature of the stomach

Central Chi deficiency—general weakness of the body's digestive organs (spleen, stomach, etc.)

Chi—vital energy of the body

Chi tonic—formula to strengthen the body's vital energy

Chi deficiency—lack of energy

Chi Kung—breathing exercises

Clear heat—to reduce fever

Clear liver heat—to reduce fever in the liver

Clear lung heat—to reduce fever in the lungs

Clear the surface—to resolve skin infections and rashes

Cool heat—to reduce the internal body temperature

Cool blood—to reduce the temperature of the blood

Cool the intestines—to reduce the temperature in the intestines

Damp heat—bacterial and viral infection

Dampness—edema

Deer, the—reflexology exercise

Deficiency of the kidneys—insufficient kidney function

Deficiency of the liver and kidney Chi—lack of liver and kidney energy and function of the organs

Emperor of the body—the heart

Fire organ—the heart

Harmonize the center—to settle the stomach

Heat and poison in the lungs—infection and inflammation in the lungs

Heat and stagnation of fluids in the lungs—phlegm and fever

Heat in the blood, stomach, and lungs—viral infection

Heavens grade—top grade of Ginseng

Imbalance between kidneys and liver—menopause

Liver stagnation—hepatitis

Lung heat—fever in the lungs

Moving the stagnation—invigorating or speeding up the function of a part of the body that has become sluggish

Moxabustion—heat therapy

Negative emotions—fear, grief, and anger, for example

Nourish the liver, blood, Chi, fetus, lungs, fluids, etc.—to provide beneficial nutrients

Nurture the yin—to replenish body fluids

On the surface—just beneath skin level

Pacify the spirit—to develop the higher nature of the spirit

Perverse energies—illness that has invaded the body from an external source

Purge heat—to eliminate fever

Rebellious Chi—acid reflux; rising energy

Sacral pump—exercise for the anal sphincter muscle

Shiwara—breaking technique

Source of 10,001 diseases—the intestine/bowels

Stagnation of blood and Chi, or stomach and liver Chi—when energy is not moving normally (too slowly)

Stomach heat—stomach fever

Strengthen the organs of the stomach, digestive system, kidneys, blood, and Chi—to strengthen the stomach, spleen, the kidneys, or nourish the blood and increase the vital energy (Chi)

Support the kidneys—to contribute to the efficient functioning of the kidneys

Tai Chi Chuan—combined physical therapy and meditation

Tonify the Chi—to improve, increase, or strengthen the vital energy (Chi)

Tonify the bones or deficient organs—to strengthen the bones or any of the five viscera (heart, liver, lungs, spleen, kidneys)

Tonifying effects—effects of the strengthening formulas

To the surface—to the skin level

Toxic heat—fever or poison

Tranquilize the mind—to reduce mental agitation

Tui Na—Chinese massage

Vaginal damp heat—vaginal infection

Warm the intestines or the uterus—to invigorate the circulation of blood and Chi

Wei Chi—immune system

Wind—the cooling wind from outside; an external element

Wind damp—wind and atmospheric moisture; external elements

Wind invasion—the external element "wind" entering the body

Cross-Reference Table of Herbs by Chinese, Latin, and English Names

Mandarin Chinese	Latin Botanical	English Translation
Ah Wei	Resina Ferulae	Asafoetida Gum Resin
Ai Ye	Folium Artemisiae	Mugwort Leaf
An Xi Xiang	Benzoinum	Benzoin Resin
Bai Bian Dou	Semen Dolichoris Lablab	Hyacinth Bean
Bai Bu	Radix Stemonae	Stemona Root
Bai Dou Kou	Fructus Amoni Cardamomi	White Cardamon Fruit
Bai Fu Zi	Rhizoma Typhonii Gigantei	White Appendage Rhizome
Bai Hua She She Cao	Herba Oldenlandine Diffusae	White Patterned Snake's Tongue
Bai Ji	Bletilla Striata (Thumb) Reich	Bletilla Rhizome
Bai Jiang Cao	Patrina Scabiosaefolia	Herba Baijiangcao
Bai Qian	Rhizoma Cynanchi Stauntonii	White Before Rhizome
Bai Shao	Radix Paconiae Laciflorae	White Peony Root
Bai Shao Yao	Radix Paconiae Laciflorae	White Peony Root
Bai Tou Weng	Radix Pulsatillae Chinensis	Chinese Anemone Root
Bai Zhi	Radix Angelicae	Angelica Dahuricae Root
Bai Zhu	Rhizoma Atractylodis Macrocephalae	Atractylodes Rhizome
Bai Zi Ren	Semen Biotae Orientalis	Arborvitae Seeds
Ba Ji Tian	Radix Morindae Officinalis	Morinda Root
Ban Lan Gen	Radix Isatidis Seu Baphicacanthi	Woad Root

Mandarin Chinese	Latin Botanical	English Translation
Ban Mao	Mylabris	Cantharides
Ban Xia	Rhizoma Pinelliae Ternatae	Half Summer
Ban Zhi Lian	Herba Scutellariae Barbatae	Scutellaria Barbatae
Bei Xie	Rhizoma Discoreae	Fish-Poison Yam Rhizome
Bian Xu	Herba Polygoni Avicularis	Knotweed Plant
Bing Lang	Areca Catechu	Betel Nut
Bing Pian	Bornelol	Resin of Borneol Camphor
Bi Yu San	Jasper	Jasper Powder
Bo He	Herba Menthae	Peppermint
Bu Gu Zhi	Fructus Psoraleae Corylifoliae	Scuffy Pea Fruit
Cang Er Zi	Fructus Xanthii	Xanthium Fruit
Cang Zhu	Rhizoma Atractylodis	Atractylodes Cangzhu
Cao Guo	Fructus Amomi Tsao-Ko	Grass Fruit
Cao Wu	Radix Aconiti Kusnezoffii	Aconite Beiwutou
Ce Bai Ye Tan	Cacumen Biotae Orientalis	Leafy Twig of Arborvitae
Chai Hu	Radix Bupleuri	Bupleurum Hare's Ear Root
Chang Pu	Rhizoma Acori Graminei	Sweet Flag Rhizome
Chan Tui	Periostracum Cicadae	Cicada Molting
Chao Bai Zhu	Rhizoma Atractylodis Macrocephalae	Dry-Fried Atractylodes Rhizome
Chao Huang Qin	Radix Scutellariae Baicalensis	Stir-Fried Baical Skullcap Root
Chao Pu Huang	Typha Pollen	Dry-Fried Cattail Pollen
Chen Pi	Pericarpium Citri Reticulatae	Ripe Tangerine Peel
Chen Xiang	Lignum Aquilariae	Aloeswood

中草藥

Mandarin Chinese	Latin Botanical	English Translation
Che Qian Cao	Herba Plantaginis	Plantago Plant
Che Qian Zi	Semen Plantaginis	Plantago Seed
Chi Fu Ling	Sclerotium Poriae Cocos Rubrae	Red Tuckahoe Root
Chi Shao	Radix Paeoniae Rubrae	Red Peony Root
Chi Shao Yao	Radix Paeoniae Rubrae	Red Peony Root
Chi Xiao Dou	Semen Phaseoli Calcarati	Aduki Beans
Chuan Bei Mu	Bulbus Fritillariae Cirrhosae	Fritillaria Bulb
Chuan Jiao	Pericarpium Zanthoxyli Bungeani	Szechuan Pepper Fruit
Chuan Lian Zi	Frutus Meliae Toosendan	Fruit of Szechuan Pagoda Tree
Chuan Shan Jia	Squama Manitis Pentadactylae	Pangolin Scales
Chuan Wu Tou	Radix Aconiti/processed	Aconitum Appendage
Chuan Xiong	Radix Ligustici Wallichii	Szechuan Lovage Root
Chun Gen Bai Pi	Cortex Ailanthi Altissimae	Ailanthus Bark
Ci Wei Pi	Corium Erinacei	Hedgehog Skin
Cong Bai	Herba Allii Fistulosi	Scallion
Da Fu Pi	Pericarpium Arecae Catechu	Betel Husk
Da Huang	Radix Et Rhizoma Rhei	Rhubarb Root
Dai Mao	Carapax Ertmochelydis Imbricatae	Hawksbill Turtle Shell
Dai Zhe Shi	Haematitum	Red Stone from Dai County
Dan Dou Chi	Semen Sojae Praeparatum	Prepared Blackbean
Dang Gui	Radix Angelicae Sinensis	Tangkuei
Dang Gui Wei	Radix Angelicae Sinensis Root	Tangkuei Root
Dang Shen	Radix Codonopsis Pilosulae	Relative Root

Mandarin Chinese	Latin Botanical	English Translation
Dan Shen	Radix Salviai Miltiorrhizae	Salvia Root
Dan Zhu Ye	Herba Lophatheri Gracilis	Bland Bamboo Leaves
Da Zao	Fructus Ziziphi Jujubae	Jujube Fruit
Deng Xin Cao	Medulla Junci Effusi	Rush Pith
Di Gu	Lycii Chinensis Radicis	Wolfberry Root
Di Gu Pi	Cortex Lycii Chinensis Radicis	Wolfberry Root Bark
Di Long	Lumbricus	Earthworm
Ding Xiang	Flos Caryophylli	Clove Flowerbud
Di Yu	Radix Sanguisorbae Officinalis	Burnet-Bloodwort Root
Dong Chong Xiao Cao	Cordyceps Sinesis	Cordyceps
Dong Gua Pi	Cortex Fructus Benincasae Hispidae	Wintermelon Seed's Husk
Dong Gua Ren	Semen Benincasae Hispidae	Wintermelon Seed
Dong Gua Zi	Semen Benincasse	Wintermelon Seed's Pulp
Duan Gui Ban	Calcined Plastrum Testudinis	Land Tortoise Shell, Calcined
Du Huo	Radix Dunhuo	Self-Reliant Existence Root
Du Zhong	Cortex Eucommiae Ulmoidis	Eucommia Bark
E Jiao	Gelatinum Asini	Donkey-Skin Glue
E Zhu	Rhizoma Zedoariae Curcumae	Zedoary Rhizome
Fang Feng	Radix Ledebouriellae Sesloidis	Guard Against the Wind Root
Feng Wang Jiang	Queen Bee Royal Essence	Royal Jelly
Feng Wei Cao	Pteris Multifida	Phoenix Tail Fern
Fu Hai Shi	Lapis Pumicis	Pumice
Fu Ling	Poriae Cocos Sclerotium	Tuckahoe Root

中
草
藥

中草藥

Mandarin Chinese	Latin Botanical	English Translation
Fu Ling Pi	Cortex Poriae Cocos	Tuckahoe Root Skin
Fu Shen	Sclerotium Poriae Cocos Pararadicis	Tuckahoe Spirit Fungus
Fu Xiao Mai	Fructus Levis Tritici	Wheat Grain
Fu Zi	Lateralis Aconiti Carmichaeli Praeparata	Accessory Root Szechuan Aconite
Gan Cao	Radix Glycyrrhizae Uralensis	Licorice Root
Gan Jiang	Rhizoma Zingiberis Officinalis	Dried Ginger Root
Gan Qi	Lacca Sinica Exsiccatae	Dried Lacca Sinica
Ge Gen	Radix Puerariae	Kudzu Root
Ge Jie	Gecko	Gecko Lizard
Geng Mi	Nonglutinous Rice	Raw Rice
Gou Ji	Rhizoma Cibotii	Lamb of Tatary Rhizome
Gou Qi Gen	Lycii Chinensis Radix	Matrimony Vine Root
Gou Qi Zi	Fructus Lycii Chinensis	Matrimony Vine Fruit
Gou Ten	Ramulus Cum Uncis Uncariae	Stem and Thorns Gambir Vine
Gua Di	Pedicellus Cucumeris	Melon Pedicle
Gua Lou Pi	Trichosanthis Pericarpium	Trichosanthes Fruit Seed's Husk
Gua Lou Ren	Fructus Trichosanthis	Trichosanthes Seed
Guan Gui	Cortex Cinnamomi Cassiae	Inner Bark of Saigon Cinnamon
Gui Ban	Plastrum Testudinis	Land–Tortoise Shell
Gui Zhi	Ramulus Cinnamomi Cassiae	Saigon Cinnamon Twig
Hai Dai	Herba Laminariae Japonicae	Laminaria Plant
Hai Feng Teng	Caulis Piperis Futokadsurae	Sea Wind Vine Stem
Hai Gou Shen	Otoriae Testes et Penis	Seal, Male Sexual Organ (Penis)

Mandarin Chinese	Latin Botanical	English Translation
Hai Long	Hailong	Pipe Fish
Hai Ma	Hippocampus	Seahorse
Hai Zao	Sargassuii Herba	Seaweed Plant
Han Lian Cao	Herba Ecliptae Prostratae	Eclipta Plant
Hei Zhi Ma	Semen Sesami Indici	Black Sesame Seeds
He Shou Wu	Radix Polygoni Multiflori	Polygonum Shouwu Root
He Zi	Fructus Terminaliae Chebulae	Myrobalan Fruit
Hong Hua	Flos Carthami Tinctorii	Safflower Flower
Hong Teng	Caulis Sargentodoxae	Sargentodoxa Stem
Huai Hua	Sophorae Japonicae Immaturis Flos	Sophorae Flower of Pagoda Tree
Huai Jiao	Fructus Sophorae Japonicae	Fruit of Pagoda Tree
Huai Niu Xi	Radix Achyranthis Bidentatae	Ox Knee Root
Huang Bai	Cortex Phillodendri	Amur Cork Tree Bark
Huang Lian	Rhizoma Coptidis	Golden Thread Root
Huang Qi	Radix Astragali Membranacai	Milk-Vetch Root
Huang Qin	Radix Scutellariae Baicalensis	Baical Skullcap Root
Huang Yao Zi	Radix Dioscorae Bulbiferae	Dioscorae Tuber
Hua Shi	Talcum	Talcum, Mineral
Hu Ma Ren	Semen Sesami Indici	Black Sesame Seeds
Huo Ma Ren	Semen Cannabis Sativae	Cannabis Seed
Huo Po	Cortex Magnoliae Officinalis	Magnolia Bark
Huo Xiang	Herba Agastaches Seu Pagostemi	Patchouli
Hu Po	Succinum	Amber

中草藥

Mandarin Chinese	Latin Botanical	English Translation
Jiang Can	Bombyx Batryticatus	Dead Body of Sick Silkworm
Jie Geng	Radix Platycodi Grandiflori	Balloon Flower Root
Ji Nei Jin	Endothelium Corneum Gigeriae Galli	Chicken Gizzard Lining
Jing Da Zi	Semen Euphorbiae Lathyridis	Peking Spurge Seed
Jing Jie	Herba Schizonepetae Tenuifoliae	Schizonepeta Stem/Bud
Jing Jie Sui	Schizonepetae Tenuifoliae	Schizonepeta Spike
Jin Qian Cao	Herba Lysimachiae	Lysimachia Plant
Jin Sha Teng	Lygodii Japonici	Climbing Japanese Fern
Jin Yin Hua	Flos Lonicerae Japonicae	Honeysuckle Flower
Jiu Chao Huang Lian	Rhizoma Coptidis	Wine-Fried Coptis (Golden Thread) Root
Jiu Chao Huang Qin	Radix Scutellariae Baicalensis	Wine-Fried Baical Skullcap Root
Jiu Da Huang	Radix Et Rhizoma Rhei	Wine-Treated Rhubarb Rhizome
Jiu Zi	Semen Allii Tuberosi	Chinese Leek Seed
Ji Xue Teng	Radix Et Caulis Jixueteng	Millettia Root and Vine
Ji Zi Huang	Gallus Ovum	Chicken Egg Yolk
Ju Hua	Flos Chrysanthemi Morifolii	Chrysanthemum Flower
Kuan Dong Hua	Flos Tussilaginis Farfarae	Tussilago Flower
Ku Fan	Alum, Calcined	Alum, Mineral Salt
Kun Bu	Algae Thallus	Kelp Thallus
Ku Shen	Flos Sophorae Flavescentus	Bitter Root
Lai Fu Zi	Semen Raphani Sativi	Radish Seed
Lao Guan Cao	Herba Geranii Et Erodii	Erodium Plant
Lian Qiao	Fructus Forsythiae Suspensae	Forsythia Fruit

Mandarin Chinese	Latin Botanical	English Translation
Lian Zi	Semen Nelumbinis Nuciferae	Lotus Seeds
Ling Yang Jiao	Cornu Antelopis	Antelope Horn
Li Pi	Fructus Pyrus	Pear Peel
Long Dan Cao	Gentianne Scabrae Radix	Chinese Getiana Root
Long Gu	Os Draconis	Dragon Bones
Lu Gen	Rhizoma Phragmitis Communis	Reed Rhizome Root
Luo Shi Teng	Caulis Trachelospermi Jasminoidis	Star Jasmine Stem
Lu Rong	Cervi Parvum Cornu	Young Deer Horn Velvet
Ma Bo	Fructificatio Lasiosphaerae Seu Calatiae	Puffball Fruit
Ma Huang	Herba Ephedrae	Yellow Hemp Root
Mai Men Dong	Tuber Ophopogonis Japonici	Lush Winter Wheat Tuber
Mai Ya	Fructus Hordei Vulgaris Germinantus	Barley Sprout
Mang Xiao	Mirabilitum	Mirabilite
Meng Chong	Tabanus	Horse Flies
Ming Fan	Alum	Alum, Mineral
Ming Tian Ma	Rhizoma Gastrodiae Elatae	Gastrodia–Heavenly Hemp Root
Mi Tuo Seng	Lithargyrum	Galena
Mo Yao	Myrrha	Resin of Myrrh
Mu Dan Pi	Moutan Radicis, Cortex	Tree Peony Root, Bark of
Mu Li	Concha Ostreae	Oyster Shell
Mu Tong	Caulis Mutong	Wood with Holes
Mu Xiang	Radix Saussureae Seu Vladimiriae	Costus Root
Mu Yao	Lindera Strychnifolia	Strychnifolia Root

中草藥

Mandarin Chinese	Latin Botanical	English Translation
Nan Xing	Rhizoma Arisaematis	Jack in the Pulpit Rhizome
Niu Bang Zi	Fructus Arctii Lappae	Great Burdock Fruit
Niu Huang	Calculus Bovis	Cow/Water Buffalo Gallbladder Calculae
Niu Xi	Radix Achyranthis Bidentatae	Ox Knee Root
Nu Zhen Zi	Ligustri Lucidi, Frutus	Privet Fruit
Ou Jie	Nodus Nelumbinis Nuciferae Rhizomatis	Lotus Rhizome, Node
Pai Ying	Herba Solani Lyrati	White Nightshade
Peng Sha	Borax	Borax, Mineral Salt
Pu Gong Ying	Herba Taraxaci Mongolici Cum Radice	Dandelion Herb
Qiang Huo	Radix et Rhizoma Notopterygii	Notopterygium Rhizome
Qian Shi	Semen Euryales Ferox	Euralye Seed
Qi Cao	Holotrichia	Dried Larva of Scarab
Qing Dai	Indigo Pulverata Levis	Indigo Powder
Qing Hao	Herba Arthemisiae Apiaceae	Wormwood
Qing Pi	Pericarpium Citri Reticulatae Viride	Green Tangerine Peel
Qin Jiao	Radix Gentianae Macrophyllae	Gentiana Qinjiao Root
Qin Pi	Cortex Fraxini	Korean Ash Branches, Bark of
Quan Xie	Buthus Martensi	Scorpion, Entire Animal
Qu Mai	Diathus Herba	Fringed Pink Flower Plant
Ren Shen	Radix Panax Ginseng	Ginseng Root
Rou Cong Rong	Herba Cistanches	Fleshy Stem of Broomrape
Rou Dou Kou	Semen Myristicae Fragrantis	Nutmeg Seeds
Rou Gui	Cortex Cinnamomi Cassiae	Saigon Cinnamon Inner Bark

Mandarin Chinese	Latin Botanical	English Translation
Ru Xiang	Gummi Olibanum	Frankincense Resin
Sang Bai Pi	Cortex Mori Albae Radicis	Bark Mulberry Root
Sang Ji Sheng	Loranthi Seu Visci, Ramus	Mulberry Parasite Stem
Sang Piao Xiao	Ootheca Mantidis	Praying Mantis Egg Case
Sang Shen Jiu	Mori Albae	Mulberry Wine
Sang Ye	Folium Mori Albae	White Mulberry Leaf
Sang Zhi	Ramulus Mori Albae	Mulberry Twigs
San Leng	Rhizoma Sparganii	Bur Reed Rhizome
San Qi	Radix Pseudo Ginseng	Pseudo Ginseng Root
Shan Dou Gen	Radix Sophorae Subprosteatae	Mountain Bean Root
Shan Yao	Radix Dioscoreae Oppositae	Chinese Yam Root
Shan Zha	Fructus Crataegi	Hawthorne Fruit
Shan Zhu Yu	Fructus Corni Officinalis	Fruit Asiatic Cornelian Cherry
Shao Yao	Radix Paeoniae Lactiflorae	Peony Root
Sha Ren	Fructus Seu Semen Amomi	Grains of Paradise Seeds/Fruit
Sha Shen	Glehniae Littoralis Radix	Root of Silvertop Beech Tree
She Chuang Zi	Cnidii Monnieri Semen	Cnidium Fruit Seed
She Gan	Rhizoma Belameandae Chinensis	Arrow Shaft Rhizome
Sheng Di Huang	Radix Rehmanniae Glutinosae	Chinese Foxglove Root, Raw
Sheng Jiang	Rhizoma Zingiberis Officinalis Recens	Fresh Ginger Root
Sheng Jiang Pi	Cortex Zingiberis Officinalis Recens	Fresh Ginger Root, Skin
Sheng Ma	Rhizoma Cimicifugae	Black Cohosh Rhizome
Shen Qu	Massa Fermentata	Medicated Leaven

中草藥

中
草
藥

Mandarin Chinese	Latin Botanical	English Translation
She Xiang	Secretio Moschus	Musk Deer Gland Secretions
She Zong Guan	Herba Isodi	Isodon Glaucocalyx Plant
Shi Chang Pu	Rhizoma Acori Graminei	Sweet Flag Rhizome
Shi Gao	Fibrosum Gypsum	Gypsum, Mineral
Shi Jue Ming	Concha Haliotidis	Abalone Shell
Shu Di Huang	Rehmanniae Glutinosae Conquitare	Chinese Foxglove Root, Wine-Cooked
Shui Zhi	Hirudo Seu Whitmaniae	Leech
Suan Zao Ren	Ziziphus Jujuba	Sour Jujube Seeds
Su Zi	Fructus Perillae Frutescentis	Purple Perilla Fruit
Tao Ren	Semen Persicae	Peach Kernel
Tian Hua Fen	Radix Trichosanthis Kirilowii	Heavenly Flower Root
Tian Ma	Rhizoma Gastrodiae Elatae	Gastrodia Rhizome
Tian Men Dong	Tuber Asparagi Cochinchinensis	Tuber of Chinese Asparagus
Tian Nan Xing	Rhizoma Arisaematis	Jack in the Pulpit Rhizome
Tong Cao	Medulla Tetrapanacis	Rice Paper Pith
Tu Bie Chong	Eupolyphaga Seu Optisthoplatia	Wingless Cockroach
Tu Su Zi	Semen Cuscutae Chinensis	Dodder Seeds
Wang Bu Liu Xing	Vaccaria Segetailis Semen	Vacarria Seed
Wei Ling Xian	Radix Clematidis Chinensis	Chinese Clematis Root
Wei Rou Dou Kou	Semen Myristicae Fragrantis	Dry-Fried Nutmeg Seeds
Wu Gong	Scolopendra Subspinipes	Centipede
Wu Jia Pi	Cortex Acanthopanacis Radicis	Five Bark Root, Bark
Wu Mei	Fructus Pruni Mume	Dark Plum Fruit

Mandarin Chinese	Latin Botanical	English Translation
Wu Shao She	Zaocys Dhumnades	Black Striped Snake
Wu Wei Zi	Fructus Schisandrae Chinensis	Schizandra Fruit
Wu Yao	Radix Linderae Strychnifoliae	Lindera Root
Wu Zhu Yu	Fructus Evondiae Rutaecarpae	Evodia Fruit
Xia Ku Cao	Spica Prunellae Vulgaris	Self-Heal Spike Prunella
Xiang Fu	Rhizoma Cyperi Rotundi	Nut Grass Rhizome
Xiang Ru	Herba Elsholtziae Splendentis	Aromatic Madder Plant
Xian Lu Gen	Rhizoma Phragmitis Communis Recens	Reed Root
Xian Mao	Rhizoma Curculiginia Orchioidis	Golden Eye-Grass Rhizome
Xiao Hui Xiang	Fructus Foeniculi Vulgaris	Fennel Fruit
Xiao Ji	Herba Cephalanoplos Segeti	Small Thistle Plant
Xi Jiao	Rhinoceri Cornu	Rhinoceros Horn
Xing Ren	Semen Pruni Armeniacae	Almond Kernel
Xin Yi Hua	Flos Magnoliae Liliflorae	Magnolia Flower
Xiong Dan	Fel Ursi	Bear Gallbladder
Xiong Huang	Realgar	Realgar
Xi Xin	Herba Cum Radice Asari	Chinese Wild Ginger Plant
Xuan Shen	Radix Scrophulariae	Ningpo Figwort Root
Xu Dan	Radix Dipsaci	Teasel Root
Xu Jie	Sanguis Draconis	Dragon's Blood Resin
Yan Hu Sou	Rhizoma Corydalis Yanhusuo	Corydalis Rhizome
Ye Ju Hua	Flos Chrysanthemi Indici	Wild Chrysanthemum Flower
Ye Ming Sha	Excrementum Vespertilionis	Bat Feces

中草藥

Mandarin Chinese	Latin Botanical	English Translation
Yi Mu Cao	Herba Leonuri	Chinese Motherwort Plant
Yin Chen Hao	Artemesiae Capillaris Herba	Capillaris Herb
Yin Yang Huo	Herba Epimedii	Licentious Goat Wort Leaf
Yin Xing	Semen Ginkgo Bilobae	Ginkgo Nut Seed
Yi Tang	Saccharum Granorum	Barley Malt Sugar
Yi Yi Ren	Coicis Lachryma-jobi Semen	Seeds of Job's Tears
Yi Zhi Ren	Fructus Alpiniae Oxyphyllae	Alpinia Fruit
Yuan Zhi	Radix Polygalae Tenuifoliae	Root of Chinese Senega
Yu Zhu	Rhizoma Polygonati Odorati	Rhizome of Solomon's Seal
Zao Jiao Ci	Spina Gleditsiae Sinensis	Spine Chinese Honeylocust Fruit
Ze Lan	Herba Lycopi	Marsh Orchid Aerial
Ze Xie	Rhizoma Alismatis Orientalis	Water Plantain Rhizome
Zha Sha	Cinnabaris	Cinnabar
Zhe Bei Mu	Bulbus Fritillariae Thunbergii	Fritillaria Zhebei Bulb
Zhen Zhu	Magarita	Pearl
Zhi Da Huang	Treated Radix Et Rhizoma Rhei	Treated Rhubarb Root
Zhi Gan Cao	Honey-Fried Radix Glycyrrhizae Uralensis	Honey-Cooked Licorice Root
Zhi Gui Ban	Plastrum Testudinis	Honey-Fried Land–Tortoise Shell
Zhi Hua Di Ding	Violae Cum Radice Herba	Yedeon's Violet Root
Zhi Ke	Frutus Citri Seu Ponciri	Bitter Orange Fruit, Ripe
Zhi Mu	Radix Anemarrhenae Asphodeloidis	Anemarrhena Root
Zhi Ran Tong	Pyritum	Pyrite
Zhi Shi	Fructus Immaturus Citri Aurantii	Green Bitter Orange Fruit

Mandarin Chinese	Latin Botanical	English Translation
Zhi Ying Su Ke	Pericarpium Papaveris Somniferi	Honey-Fried Opium Poppy Husk
Zhi Zi	Fructus Gardeniae Jasminoidis	Gardenia Fruit
Zhu Ling	Polypori Unbellatus	Polyporous Fungus
Zhu Ru	Caulis Bambusae in Taeniis	Bamboo Shavings
Zhu Sha	Cinnabaris	Cinnabar
Zi Bei Tian Kuei	Herba Begoniae Fimbristipulatae	Begonia
Zi Cao	Radix Arnebiae Seu Lithospermi	Groomwell Root
Zi Hua Di Ding	Violae Cum Radice, Herba	Yedeon's Violet Plant
Zi Su Ye	Perillae Frutescentis Folium	Perilla Leaf
★	Nasturtium Officinale	Watercress Plant
★	Thymus	Thyme, Herb

★No Chinese name available for this herb.

General Index (Including Medical Terms, Disorders, and Symptoms)

中草藥

Alphabetical Index of Raw Herb Formulas (in Chinese)

Alphabetical Index of Raw Herb Formulas (in English)

Alphabetical Index of Patent Formulas (in Chinese)

中
草
藥

Alphabetical Index of Patent Formulas (in English)